GETTING WELL NATURALLY FROM THE SOIL TO THE STOMACH

GETTING WELL NATURALLY FROM THE SOIL TO THE STOMACH

UNDERSTANDING THE CONNECTION BETWEEN
YOUR HEALTH AND THE EARTH

Penny Kelly, N.D.

Originally published as *From The Soil to The Stomach* © 2001,
Second edition *From The Soil to The Stomach* © 2005
Third edition *Getting Well Again, Naturally* © 2010
Fourth edition *Getting Well Naturally from The Soil to The Stomach* © 2021

Lily Hill Publishing
ISBN 978-0-9857480-9-8

Cover design by Penny Kelly

We are deeply grateful to the Weston A. Price Foundation
for permission to reprint the excerpt on hydrogenation from
Sally Fallon's book *Nourishing Tradition* on pp. 137-138.

The information, procedures, suggestions, and ideas contained in this book are not meant to take the place of your physician. All use of this information is at your own discretion. Neither the author nor the publisher will be held liable for any injury, damage, or loss as a result of the information contained in this book. You should consult with your physician before beginning any program of healing.

Nutrition/Health/Natural Healing/Holistic & Alternative Medicine/Organics

Dedication

This book is dedicated to my parents,

Hugh and Shirley Kelly,

who brought me up

with my hands, feet,

head, and eventually

my heart,

in the garden…

which led to a deep

and intimate connection

with Mother Earth.

Other Books by Penny Kelly:

The Evolving Human
The Elves of Lily Hill Farm
Robes: A Book of Coming Changes
Consciousness and Energy, Vol. 1
Consciousness and Energy, Vol. 2
Consciousness and Energy, Vol. 3
Consciousness and Energy, Vol. 4

Poetry:
Child of the Brown Earth

Table of Contents

*Part 1*_____

The Basics

1
Healing is a Way of Life

THE BEGINNINGS WERE SO SUBTLE. First, there was a fatigue that rose early in the afternoons and would not go away. I was frequently aware that I was pushing myself to keep up with the people around me and with the daily schedule I had always maintained so easily. I stopped exercising because I was too tired to care about what it might be doing for me. The bathroom scales crept persistently upward, and I was 30 pounds heavier than I had been only ten years earlier. One day, in a fit of frustration, I went shopping and bought $800-worth of size 12 clothing because I was tired of not being able to reach, bend, or breathe in the shirts, jeans, and skirts that choked my freedom of movement.

My dark, curly hair, once a source of pride, was lifeless. I would look at it in the mirror and tell myself it was just my imagination that it was getting thin. I stopped plucking my eyebrows because they quit growing, and even my eyelashes were becoming sparse.

One spring day, my eyes burned and itched until I peeled the contact lenses off my dry eyeballs and put on the glasses I hated. The lenses were old, and soon it was obvious I needed an eye exam and an updated prescription. New glasses helped for a while, but over the next year my vision worsened slowly and steadily. I went back, got another exam and stronger glasses.

One day, while working in one of our small vineyards, I noticed that my ring finger hurt. Upon examination, I saw that it was bright red, rather swollen, and throbbed slowly unless I tried to bend it...then it protested with violent, excruciating pain. A few days later, I decided it must be a little arthritis, and when it went away on its own, I dismissed the whole experience...for a short time.

The following week the pain in my finger was replaced by an itch in the skin of my hands, wrists, and forearms. This was no ordinary itch. It was a deep, driving itch that caused me to scratch and dig at my skin even when I consciously tried not to. It would itch so badly that I would sometimes shake all over in an effort to discipline myself and resist scratching. Oddly, the places where the itching seemed worst showed no signs of rash or injury. I could not imagine why I had this maddening itch. When summer ended, so did the itch, and again I forgot about it. A year went by.

The next May, I went out to trim vines in the back vineyard. At the end of the first day, the elbow of my right arm was sore and painful. I tried to work the next day, but my arm hurt too much. I had overworked the muscles the first day and realized I needed to give them a couple of days to rest and heal.

A couple of days later, however, my arm was so sore I couldn't move it or my fingers. A month went by and now my right shoulder was as stiff and sore as my elbow and fingers. My back was also getting stiff to the point I could not bend or lean over at all.

I went to see my doctor who told me point blank, "You have rheumatoid arthritis and there is nothing we can do for it except make you comfortable." It sounded like a death sentence.

She gave me a prescription for naproxen, a painkiller also known as a non-steroidal, anti-inflammatory drug, or "NSAID"[1] for short. I didn't start taking it immediately, but when the arthritis suddenly spread to my other elbow and shoulder, my knees, ankles, and the fingers of my left hand, I got the prescription filled and started taking it. Not until then did I understand the term "side effects."

"Dry mouth" was listed as a minor side effect, and this was quite an understatement. Imagine trying to run across a freshly tarred parking lot

---

1 Pronounced *"EN-sed"*.

wearing a pair of rubber boots in the hot sun. That image is similar to the effort needed just to speak while under the influence of an NSAID. Speech was not only slowed, it was often slightly slurred just from the necessity of having to take time to peel my tongue off the roof of my mouth or disengage the inside of my cheek from the teeth it was clinging to. Ditto for the eyelids, which required constant doses of my contact lens wetting solution just to allow the eyelid to slide over the eyeball while wearing my glasses, since contact lenses were now absolutely out of the question.

Before the arthritis, I did not like to bother with either cooking or eating, so meals were quick, often whatever I could find. Under the influence of the naproxen, I had no appetite at all. When I did eat, I felt slightly nauseous for a while. Pain played constantly in the background, fatigue was center stage, and I was now a non-performing act, too tired to do things as simple as walk across the room to get something I needed or wanted. I began to wait until someone came in the room and then ask them to please get whatever it was I needed, a trick of servitude I had always resented when others did it to me. If no one arrived to rescue me, I calculated long and hard about how much I really needed that item across the room. Often I was so drowsy that I simply sat, as if in a stupor. Other effects were heart palpitations when I did get up and move, constipation, a worsening of my eyesight, and sometimes even the feeling that it took great effort just to breathe.

In spite of the fatigue and drowsiness, at night I slept poorly. Every roll or shift of position triggered waves of pain that woke me up. In the morning, I would not feel rested, restored, or energized. Movement was slow and tentative; I needed help with everything, from carrying water to my chickens, to handling milk cartons, to opening the catsup bottle.

By midsummer, my right arm was in a sling, and I often used a walking stick to get around. The walking stick was a graceful thing with a bunch of grapes carved into the top, a gift from my uncle, meant to be decorative. Now it was an essential tool in any kind of movement.

At times, I caught a glimpse of myself in the mirror and was shocked at how old I looked. One day, while moving slowly back and forth in the garden, I noticed my bent shadow. That couldn't be me, could it? Other times I found myself in a moment of self-perception in which I seemed ancient and used up, withdrawn from the world and wishing it would go away. This was a drastic change from the way I usually saw myself, but I didn't – or couldn't – care. Pain was becoming the lens through which I kept seeing my life and myself within that life. Fatigue was undoing everything I had once been.

One July evening after heat and humidity had steam-baked the family all day, my husband, Jim, asked if I wanted to go shopping with him in Kalamazoo. Although I seriously disliked any kind of shopping, the thought of being in an air-conditioned store changed my usual mind about such excursions.

In the store, I followed him about like a quiet puppy, content to be cool, saving my energy. He was looking at something near the book section, and I was leaning against the end of a display shelf when I noticed a thick book lying open almost in front of me. Casually scanning the page, my eyes fell on the words, "One side effect of aspirin and other NSAIDs that is often not mentioned is their inhibition of cartilage repair … and acceleration of cartilage destruction in experimental studies. Since osteoarthritis is caused by a degeneration of cartilage, it appears that, while NSAIDs are fairly effective in suppressing the symptoms, they possibly worsen the condition by inhibiting the cartilage formation and accelerating cartilage destruction." [2]

I was stunned. What was my doctor thinking in giving me something that would only make the whole arthritis problem worse? How stupid!

I bought the book, took it home, and read both chapters on arthritis. Then I got out the bottle of naproxen, opened it up, and dumped the medication into the toilet. "There! That's what I think of your medicine!" I said to the absent doctor as I flushed the pills away. Over the next few days, I alternated between fury at our medical system and the pure entrapment I felt in having to rely on its methods of healing. These methods were not really designed to heal; they were designed to cover up the symptoms. As the doctor had said, they would make me comfortable – while I continued to degenerate.

---

2 Michael Murray ND and Joseph Pizzorno ND, *Encyclopedia of Natural Medicine* (Rocklin, CA: Prima Publishing, 1991) p. 449.

Still, I was uncertain about what to do next. I had an aunt who had severe arthritis and was in a wheelchair. Her hands grew backwards along her forearms toward her elbows, a condition known as *ulnar drift*. She could not brush her hair or pick up a spoon. I loved her, but I didn't want to end up like her. She was in her late 70s and had seemed fine to me until just recently. Then, it seemed like her condition worsened dramatically. Thus, the first decision I made was simple…I was not going to end up like my aunt.

❖

That was the summer of 1994. At that point in my life, I had spent more than 15 years studying the mind, writing, exploring consciousness, experimenting with perception, teaching people to develop and use high levels of intuition, and working with researchers to understand subtle energies and the connections between science and the mind.

About ten years into this work I had become increasingly discouraged. Yes, I *was* able to teach people to awaken their intuition and to become extremely good with it. Often, they would astound me, as well as themselves, with what they could do after only a short period of learning and practice. But something always happened to get in the way of their continued development. They would *begin*, but they wouldn't *maintain* high levels of spiritual awareness and evolved practices. Since the expanded awareness and advanced practices were meant to improve everyday life, it seemed tragic that they couldn't implement what they knew.

"I'm wasting my time," I said to my husband one day. "They come out here, they awaken, and then they stumble…or forget…or get sick… or get caught up in some drama and fail to use what they have learned! At the critical moment, they stop believing in themselves. What's wrong? It's almost as if they don't have enough strength to maintain their own minds. If they can't maintain high levels of awareness and consciousness, how are they ever going to keep progressing? If they can't change their views of how and why things are happening, how can they ever *respond* differently to change their lives?"

For nearly five years, I had asked myself these same questions. But there were no answers, and I was coping with a growing sense of futility in my work. Maybe spiritual awakening, the development of intuitive abilities, a satisfying life of extraordinary creativity, and deep inner peace was not possible for the masses of humanity. I had just decided to do something else with my life, something that had more lasting effects, when arthritis appeared and took center stage.

One day, I was eating lunch alone at the kitchen table, staring blankly at the pile of mail I had intended to read while eating. Unexpectedly, the words on the top piece of mail stood out, "Nutrition as it is today does not supply the strength necessary for manifesting the spirit in physical life. A bridge can no longer be built from thinking to will and action. Food plants no longer contain the forces people need for this." [3]

My reaction was one of disbelief. "Nutrition?" I thought, "What does that have to do with anything?" The idea that nutrition could affect the mind or one's will power seemed absurd, yet I couldn't forget those words.

Now, years later, in coming to understand the grip of rheumatoid arthritis and the dozens of other degenerative diseases plaguing us, I have come to realize *exactly* what nutrition has to do with things. After years of concentrating on the mind and consciousness, arthritis forced me to focus on the body and begin to understand it at a deeper level. In doing so, I began to understand that *body, mind, and Earth are an integrated system of life*. Each part depends on the rest of the system for its health and successful function. Disturb any part of this system, and the whole thing suffers. I have come to understand that people cannot maintain high levels of awareness or deep inner peace because they just don't have the energy to do so. They don't feel good. They aren't healthy. Very few realize that perception, emotion, attitude, and intuition are directly produced by biochemical conditions in the body. Even fewer know that those biochemical conditions are produced by the ever-changing, dynamic fields of mineral-based plasma that make up the entire body. Every human is a collection of plasmas, something we will talk about later in the book.

My own illness thus served as a conduit that led me to rediscover what has always been true...that the body affects the mind and the mind

---

3 The words were on the back of a newsletter from the Josephine Porter Institute in Woolwine, VA. It was a quote from Rudolf Steiner's *Agriculture*, a series of lectures on farming.

affects the body for good or ill. They are equal partners in the body/mind system, and the body/mind is embedded in the feedback system of life that has developed here on Earth over uncountable years.

Since those days, I have made a commitment to learn what I really need to know to get well and stay well. This decision led me to discover much of what is presented in this book. As I have gone through this process of learning, nothing has surprised me as much as the fact that so few of us know the information presented here when it is so vital, so basic, *and so interesting*. For me and my bones, for my husband and his lungs, and for others in our family with failing hearts, kidneys, or reproductive systems, this information has been the difference between healthy lives and lives spent coping with pain or disability.

Somewhere along the way, we realized that the commitment to good health might mean we had to change our way of life. Of course, many changes did become necessary, and the changes were much more extensive than we imagined. Therefore, I tell people right up front that a true commitment to health often requires that you let go of old ideas and beliefs about food and health. You must greatly expand the base of information you are operating from, and this ends up changing everything about your life. You start changing what you eat, what you wear, your daily routine, the way your kitchen is arranged, your bathroom setup, your bedroom, your sleep or rest routines, the work you are willing to do, your relationships, how you think and feel about money, your perception of real medicine, your yard, your neighborhood, and maybe more. In spite of the changes required, people get excited as they heal. They develop a new awareness of food and the other energies that we use to sustain us, and this can only be good for us and our planet.

For these reasons, I have attempted to present this information in such a way that you will come to understand the whole, integrated system – the body, the mind, your relationships with food, water, air, plants, animals, the Earth, and all of Nature. A little friend of mine often encourages me to "explore the nature of balance rather than attempt to restore the balance of Nature," and I will encourage you to do the same. This requires you to drop preconceived notions. Doing so allows you to make the right decisions in the process of healing yourself. It is like the old saying about Caesar and God, but with a couple of modifications, "Give unto Bodies the things that are physical, and unto Minds the things of the spirit."

Although some people, especially New Age people, want to change the condition and health of their bodies using only their minds and attitudes, it seems quite obvious to me that most of us have not evolved far enough to simply "think our bodies well and *voilà!* It is done!!" Although it certainly helps to think like that, for most people, nothing happens. Why? Because we are 3-dimensional, physical beings living in a 3-dimensional, physical world. Because physical stuff is heavy and stable, we must take physical action to change it, and that action must be appropriate. If you're talking about healing, that action has to be what the body needs, and it must not contradict or destroy the integrated system the body is embedded in.

Your body is your unique home. If you are going to become well, you must learn to honor your body and its unique needs, not necessarily the way you were raised or following the latest food fad. It is my hope that this book will help you understand why too many of us are getting sick, falling apart, dying early, or holding ourselves together with a regimen of drugs that lead to further dependence on heavier chemicals later on. Too often, the illness and the chemicals we take for relief from symptoms produce fatigue and fuzzy thinking, which lead to an inability to see your whole situation clearly. This lack of clarity results in poor decision-making around the subject of health and healing.

It has been my experience that miracles do happen, and it is my wish that, if you need one for your own health, you will come to understand how to make this miracle happen for you whether it appears as a quick change or takes a few years to create. Your body knows how to heal. All you have to do is support that effort. Once you do, you will discover you are the best doctor you will ever have! ❖

2
The Basics of Healing

IT HAS ALWAYS ASTOUNDED ME that we are not taught much about how to care for the physical body. Since each of us has one, this would seem to be quite an oversight, if not outright negligence. Most of the people I know have learned what they know about health care from television and magazine ads selling pills, potions, lotions, exercise programs, diets, cold and flu remedies, fast foods, and drugs. The message always implies, and sometimes states quite boldly, that the product being advertised will do something wonderful for a sense of health and well-being, a claim that is often pure marketing baloney.

Of course, these products would not be for sale if they did any immediate or overt damage, yet they have serious side effects that often create the need for additional products. They also distract us from what we really need to know and do to remain healthy. Thus, ongoing damage occurs while we neglect what our bodies require, and we continue thinking we are taking care of ourselves.

A great many healing techniques have been lost over the last 100 years, partly because so many of our old people have been cast into nursing homes along with their wisdom and knowledge, and partly because of our complete reliance on the medical profession and its emphasis on drugs and surgery. Drugs and surgery are very important, but they should be the final step in the process of healing, after the natural – and much cheaper, more body-friendly – methods have been employed.

When drugs and surgery are the first or only choice, the result, for millions of people is a sense of helplessness when it comes to healing themselves. They can't afford the excessive fees that doctors and hospitals charge, and they have no idea of what to do to heal themselves...I mean *really* heal, not just cover up symptoms. If you only want to cover up symptoms, that's your choice, but the choice you are making will be expensive, the results will be limited and short-term, and you will find yourself enjoying life less and less. Eventually, you will be unable to participate at all. When people can no longer enjoy and contribute to life in a meaningful way, they usually shrivel up and die. Don't be one of them!

When I was studying to become a naturopath, it was drilled into me again and again that, except for a dozen or so states in the U.S.,[4] naturopaths were not allowed to *diagnose, treat,* or *cure* people. We were not allowed to use the word *Doctor* or *Dr.* with our name, nor could we *examine, prescribe, administer, advise,* or *dispense* because these words have been copyrighted by the American Medical Association. For anyone other than a licensed medical doctor, these words were illegal to use in states that did not accept naturopathic medicine.

At first, this seemed to be a great disadvantage. How could we possibly work as healers if we couldn't diagnose and treat? However, as it turned out, there was no reason to know the technical name of every disease or every single, minute detail of the body's biochemical processes. Being able to give a technically impressive name to a disease does not mean you can heal it or make it go away. A precise biochemical diagnosis is only necessary if the intent is to prescribe a specific chemical that will suppress the exact symptoms and signals the body is displaying. Since we aren't dispensing drugs, it is unnecessary to pinpoint specific chemical sequences that characterize the processes of various organs.

Instead, naturopaths learn the basic systems of the body, how they cooperate and contribute to one another's functions, and what their basic

---

4   Happily, the number of states that recognize Naturopathic medicine have increased over the years. These now include: Alaska, Arizona, California, Colorado, Connecticut, Florida, Hawaii, Idaho, Kansas, Maine, Maryland, Massachusetts, Minnesota, Montana, New Hampshire, New Mexico, North Dakota, Ohio, Oregon, Pennsylvania, Rhode Island, Utah, Vermont, Washington, District of Columbia, Puerto Rico, and the Virgin Islands.

distress signals are. We think in terms of the whole body/mind system and the lifestyle of the individual.

Before the American Medical Association took over medicine, the only kind of medical practice that existed was naturopathy. Gradually, as naturopathy was outlawed, those who studied naturopathic medicine were not allowed to practice medicine at all unless they lived in one of the few states that recognized it. However, with or without state recognition, the legal system allowed naturopaths to *teach* people how to go about healing themselves.

Back when I was studying naturopathy, there were almost no accredited schools. I think there might have been one, maybe two. It was a chicken-and-egg situation. With hardly any states recognizing naturopathy, there was little demand for accredited schools. As more states began to recognize and license naturopathy, the situation became difficult for those of us who had studied and graduated from schools that did not have accreditation. States that licensed naturopaths required graduation from an accredited school. The result was that the few naturopathic physicians who were in existence were once again being forced out of business, taking their knowledge and experience with them.

Since I am a writer and teacher, I can share what I know. The law says it is okay to say, "If it were me, I would do this (or that or such-and-such). So everything I say in this book is just me sharing what I know and what I would do. Much of it is what I am doing to keep myself and my family healthy.

In teaching, I follow the ancient wisdom, "If you catch a fish for a man, you can help to feed him for a day, but if you teach him how to fish, he can feed himself for the rest of his life." In other words, it is best to teach someone how to heal himself. Then he can do it over and over and even pass on the skills to those he cares about.

Except for accidents and unexpected infections, all illness and disease is the result of a chosen lifestyle. I frequently hear people argue with this saying, "But what about genetics?" Genes and your genetic inheritance do play a role, but genes are turned on and off by frequencies, and these frequencies come from the amount of electricity your body produces as well as the numerous specialized frequencies that come from the amino acids and minerals you are supposed to be taking in regularly. Although the general public does not quite understand this yet, research is moving forward with investigations into how to use and apply frequencies to turn genes on and off. At the moment they mostly use chemicals to do so, but the time is not far off when we will be able to apply frequencies directly.

In the meantime, lifestyle is the biggest determinant of health and includes, among other things, what you eat and how you prepare it; how much exercise you get; the water you drink; the way you handle your relationships with family and others; the amount of physical, mental, and emotional stress in your life; the kind of work you do for a living; how much sleep you get; whether or not you smoke, drink, or take drugs – both prescription and over-the-counter; your creative endeavors; your level of debt; your involvement in personal growth and spiritual awakening; where you live; the conditions in your local environment; and many other factors that make up your daily routines, along with the traditions of your culture.

As naturopaths, we are taught to think in terms of correcting the source of the problem, and we are shown again and again that the body will heal itself if we remove the irritating factors or supply the missing nutrients. The *body* is the great healer, not the naturopath or the allopath (*allopath* is the name for today's medical doctor).

If you go to see a naturopath, you will often be asked to sign a paper acknowledging that *you* – not the doctor – will remain fully responsible for your own healing processes. When you go to see an allopath, you are asked to sign papers giving the doctor full responsibility for your healing processes. This is not really fair to the medical doctor simply because he or she cannot force you to make the changes that will make you well again. If the entire burden of healing you is on the doctor, he or she is then open to being sued if the prescribed ideas and procedures do not work for you. It also means that you do not have to do anything different and that you're expecting drugs or surgery to remove the indications that you are living in a way that does not support and sustain life.

Although most people willingly sign over all responsibility for their healing to someone else, this non-participation adds to subtle levels of anxiety about whether or not the desired healing will take place. It is as if something deep inside of us knows that we need to take responsibility for our life if we want to heal. If the drugs and surgery don't do the whole job, and you were not allowed to be part and parcel of the decision-making process, the results are anger, accusations, and lawsuits, all fueled by the subtle anxieties that were generated by being left out in the first place.

Medical doctors are doing the best they can. Several of my close friends are MD's, and I have never met a medical doctor who is not acutely conscious of wanting to help others feel better and who isn't cautious in the attempt to avoid hurting or causing further damage. When something goes wrong, they agonize just like you or I would.

Allopathic medicine is wonderful for a crisis, emergency, acute trauma, or other situation where "rescue medicine" can save your life long enough for the body's own healing mechanisms to take over. If it were not for the intervention of allopathic medicine, I would probably have only two children living instead of the four I gave birth to. One daughter would have been lost giving birth to my grandson. Another daughter would have been lost when infections got out of control. Thanks to the rescue medicine of allopathic doctors, I still have both of them.

Medical doctors seldom know much about nutrition, and yet a huge majority of the chronic illnesses and degenerative diseases they are struggling with are the direct results of poor and missing nutrition. To heal these, a different set of healing skills is necessary.

You can easily learn these skills. To do so, you must be fully involved with the healing process. To be fully involved means that you must be willing to do the work and to follow the techniques that support the body, not just take a quick pill and keep on running through life. You must also know that your medicine is sustainable. For your medicine to be sustainable, you must be confidant that what you do to heal yourself in one part of the body doesn't undo another part of the body.

When my doctor told me I had arthritis, she also announced that nothing could be done about it except to take painkillers. This is an example of very bad mental and emotional programming. It is also a perfect example of medicine that is not sustainable over the long haul because it neither addresses the source of the problem nor brings true healing.

Although not everything that goes wrong in your body may be fixed to perfection, beware of accepting the idea that "nothing can be done about the problem" except to cover up the pain by altering your brain with chemicals so you can't feel the warning signs your body is giving you. The body sends these signals out for a reason! They are to notify you that you must do something different with your life if you wish to continue living. Covering up symptoms may make you feel better for a short time, but it is not true healing.

Understanding the connection between the soil and your stomach... learning a few detoxification techniques...coming to grips with the nutritional requirements of your body...filling in areas where your nutrition is lacking by using supplements...learning to trust the gentle, patient, healing ways of foods and herbs...doing a bit of exercise in order to increase the electrical energy that drives nutritional transactions...delivery of those nutrients to all areas of the body...practicing a peaceful mind... these are the things that lead to balance, healing, and the return of youthful energy and looks. *This* is true healing. As Dr. Richard Schulz often says, "There are no incurable diseases, there are only incurable people."

To heal yourself completely you need to be able to create a complete and workable healing program for yourself. You have to know how, when, and why to incorporate the six basic aspects of a good healing program. These basic six are:

> **Food, Water & Air** – organic, high-nutrition, whole foods consisting of meats, dairy, fruits, vegetables, and grains, as well as access to living water and fresh air.
>
> **Supplements** – Amino acids, minerals, vitamins, enzymes, glandulars, herbs, essential oils, flower essences.
>
> **Detoxification** – The Liver Flush, Colon Sweep, Purge, Castor Oil/Olive Oil Sweat Bath, fasting, castor oil pack, clay poultices, a variety of soaks and enemas.
>
> **Exercise** – Regular stretching, walking, yoga, and some physical labor or weight-lifting that will generate the electricity your body needs.

Psychological/Spiritual Support – a person, family, group, or belief system that will encourage you to start healing and keep it up, even if things get worse before they get better, which is often the case.

Home and Work – assessing your environment; collecting the tools and equipment needed for healing; rearranging your life, your space, and your schedule to eliminate various stressors; and carry out the various healing routines that support good health.

A few comments I hear frequently from people who are desperately ill include: "Oh, I tried herbs already…" or "I take vitamins, and they really haven't done anything as far as I can tell…" or "I can't afford organic food…"

These comments usually come from people who try one thing for a few days or weeks, then jump to another thing for a few months, then skip to something else for a while, all the while hoping that they have found the magic bullet that destroys their problem. They want healing that will take little effort.

Let me say something right up front. *There is no magic bullet.* The only magic is your willingness to be flexible enough to do what your body needs. The old saying that, "You cannot serve two masters," is applicable here. You cannot serve what the world would have you believe, and honor what your body will teach you. If you do what everyone else is doing, you will go down with the crowd and health will be lost.

Consider the rule we have at our house that says, "First you take care of yourself, then you can think about taking care of others." This is not selfish, it is common sense. If you don't take care of yourself, you will end up becoming a burden to others and you'll feel bad when you discover no one else really wants to take care of you.

Now let me add a few other things. First, if you have a catastrophic illness, taking a few commercial herbs is not likely to do anything by itself. It might help, but it's seldom enough. Ditto for taking vitamins, especially since most people do not know how to take supplements properly in the first place. A huge number of people do not realize the importance of high-quality nutrition, thus they fail to make the necessary changes in their diet.

Do not force your body to process foods that do not have a payoff in terms of good quality aminos, minerals, and vitamins!

Almost no one knows or understands that the body is an electrical and electromagnetic structure that generates light, heat, and must be in motion to maintain and regenerate itself. In fact, many people make an endless effort to avoid work. They act like physical labor is beneath them. Keep up this attitude and you will be six feet beneath the soil. Exercise is critical in healing yourself and restoring energy.

Lots of people feel helpless to do anything about their water supply, even though this is one of the easier problems to correct. Hardly anyone understands the devastating physiological effects of stress – whether physical, emotional, mental, or external – and thus they tend to discount the necessity of eliminating stressors, especially if the stress involves a wife, a child, a change of house, or a different kind of work. And almost everyone blanches when they hear the word "enema!"

If you have a catastrophic illness and you really want to heal, *you have to do everything at once*. You have to make the changes in your food and water, get the right assortment of supplements that will work synergistically, detoxify your body continuously, exercise lightly every day – not strenuously, just regularly. If you love strenuous exercise you can do this three or four times a week for 15 to 30 minutes, but more is not required.

As you make the various changes that are needed, hold a picture in your mind of yourself in a beautifully healthy condition. Believe in what you're doing as well as your body's innate healing abilities, and organize your home and work to support the food, water, detox, and exercise routines that will gradually become a way of life. ❖

3

An Early Pioneer

IN 1931, A SMALL, ENERGETIC MAN with perceptive blue eyes was making preparations for a trip to Switzerland. Weston Price was a dentist in Cleveland, Ohio, and, over the previous decade, he had noticed a dramatic rise in tooth decay. Large numbers of people were suffering from cavities and many of them had lost 80% of their teeth by the time they were 20 years old. This was unprecedented! In the past, people had enjoyed excellent teeth that were perfectly formed and beautifully maintained with almost no cavities.

Like many health professionals of his day, Price was focused on trying to find the invading organism as suggested by Pasteur's discovery of bacteria. He was convinced that human teeth were under attack by some strange and, so far, unknown variety of bacteria.

Dentists were not the only ones dealing with an increase in health problems. Professionals from medical science, psychology, social science, anthropology, law, and other disciplines were noticing a steady increase in health abnormalities. Since 1907, heart disease had gone up 60%. Cancer had gone up 90% over the same time period, and the tuberculosis that terrified everyone was still spreading. People displayed an increasingly poor immune response, delinquency was rising, and there was a strange disappearance of creativity, motivation, and inventiveness in school-age children. Birth defects such as clubfoot, cleft palate, and mental retardation were up, as was infant mortality. Most disturbing were subtle personality changes and depressive character traits in people across the spectrum.

Working in his private clinic and research laboratory, Price, like his peers, methodically examined every possible theory and supposed cause of rotting teeth he could come up with. He searched diligently through his microscope for signs of unidentified and possibly injurious bacteria, but the result was the same every time – a dead end.

Meanwhile, at Harvard University, Earnest Hoonton had established the Institute of Clinical Anthropology in order to find out "what man is like biologically when he does not need a doctor, in order to ascertain what he should be like after the doctor has finished with him." [5] After thinking about this, it occurred to Price that maybe the problem was due to the *absence* of something rather than the *presence* of a mysterious pathogen. He began to suspect that the sudden, serious degeneration of modern people had something to do with what they were eating or perhaps not eating. Influenced by Hoonton's work, Price decided it might prove fruitful to examine the teeth of indigenous peoples who had not been introduced to the modern Western diet, which was based on white flour, white sugar, canned fruits and vegetables, jams and jellies, coffee, tea, and alcohol.

After writing to many major governments, asking if they knew of any groups of people within their territories who were still eating the traditional diets that had sustained them over thousands of years, he finally found one. The first such group was in the Loetschental (*let*-shen-tull) Valley of Switzerland. Once he found them, he and his wife, Monica Price, a registered nurse, along with a troupe of assistants, clerks, photographers, and other health workers, organized a trip to Switzerland to study them.

When they arrived in the valley, they found a group of about 2,000 Swiss men, women, and children who had been living self-sufficiently for over a dozen centuries and who exhibited some of the most extraordinary health in the world. The Swiss Guards of the Vatican, famed the world over for their amazing physiques and stamina, often came from Loetschental Valley or neighboring valleys with similar indigenous lifestyles.

---

5 Weston A. Price DDS, *Nutrition And Physical Degeneration* (New Canaan, CT: Keats Publishing, 1989) p. 17.

The people were living in small villages at the bottom of the valley, with no cars, trucks, tractors, or even horse-and-wagon transport. People walked everywhere they needed to go, carrying whatever needed to be transported on their backs, and this contributed to both their excellent physiques as well as their strong hearts. Children spent six months of the year learning from books and the other six months helping with the tasks of daily life. Although tuberculosis was rampant all over the developed areas of Switzerland, there was not a single case of it in Loetschental.

In winter, these hardy Swiss stayed in the village tending their herds of cows, sheep, and goats. By early June, the animals began moving up the steep, mountainous hillsides, following the receding snowline in order to feast on the sumptuously green spring grasses that emerged from under the snow. Every June, the milk from these cows turned a rich, creamy yellow color, filled with vitamins, minerals, and butterfat. The villagers harvested this special June milk, making and storing large quantities of cheese and butter that was almost orange, so great was the amount of Vitamin A and beta carotene in it.

In the summer, they added a few greens and vegetables from small gardens to their basic fare, but on the whole, their daily diet consisted of thick slices of whole rye bread spread with butter, large slices of cheese that were as thick as the bread, fresh milk, and a bit of meat in stews or soups about once a week. Today, we would consider such a diet a ticket to the cardiovascular unit of the hospital. Yet Price and his group found it was common for villagers in their 60s and 70s to be spry, willing, and able to carry heavy loads of grain or milk products up and down the hillsides without difficulty or fatigue.

The children of the valley played barefoot and without hats or coats in the cold air of early spring mornings or late fall evenings. They played in the cold water of mountain streams without discomfort and did not contract the colds and flu that were common for children who lived in America on modern foods. These Swiss children had almost no cavities, and Price found that only one out of three had any sign of ever having had a cavity at all.

Young people who had gone to live in nearby cities for a year or two around the age of 18 did show some signs of cavities, and a few had even lost a tooth or two, but as soon as they returned to the village and took up their former diet, the body created a hard, glassy, enamel-like coating over the cavity and the decay processes stopped completely!

Besides the strong hearts, excellent physiques, and absence of dental problems of almost every kind, there were other important differences between the villagers of Loetschental and those people living in more modern settings.

The photographs taken by Price's research assistants showed that they had perfectly developed upper and lower dental arches. These dental arches offered plenty of room for all 32 teeth, which were always perfectly aligned. There was never an overbite in the two maxillary arches (the left and right maxillary bones hold the upper teeth and meet in the center, under the nose) or an underbite in the mandibular arch (the bone holding the lower teeth). The remaining bones of the face were beautifully developed with broad cheekbones, widely set eyes, and wide nasal passages allowing for easy, natural breathing with plenty of oxygen-carbon dioxide exchange.

Just as striking as the physical differences were the differences in emotional, mental, and spiritual character. These were a people who were peaceful; who had consciously decided that the development of individual character was more important than the development of material things. Children seldom cried or fought, they had high integrity, and their reserves of physical energy were astounding.

In sharp contrast to the people of Loetschental Valley were the people of St. Moritz. Oddly, in 1931 St. Moritz was already known as a health resort, and people from all over the world vacationed there year round, feasting on the most sophisticated and modern of foods. Price's shopping list of "modern foods" included anything made with white flour, sugar, jams, jellies, syrups, canned vegetables or fruits, and candy or confections of any sort. Unfortunately, the people of St. Moritz had plenty of access to these goodies.

Traveling to St. Moritz in order to investigate the health and physical condition of its inhabitants and compare this to the residents of Loetschental, Dr. Price found that although it was a beautiful setting, every child in St. Moritz had tooth decay, with children under 15 having cavities in almost 30% of their teeth. In some children, an entire tooth had rotted away to the gum line. Others had abscesses in the jaw or evidence of scars from old abscesses that had eaten right through the cheek or the neck. Many were suffering from tuberculosis.

He was also deeply dismayed to find that the children of St. Moritz had narrowed jawbones and crooked teeth fighting for space. In many, the entire set of facial bones had shrunk, and their pinched nasal passages required them to breathe through the mouth in order to get enough oxygen. There were large numbers of goiters in the adult population, many forms of thyroid trouble, and a dramatic susceptibility to infections and diseases of all kinds at all ages.

After months of travel and study, Price returned to his clinic in Cleveland, armed with a huge amount of data in the form of photographs, measurements, dental records, information on personal diets and lifestyle, and food samples.

The following year, he, his wife, and the entire team returned to Loetschental for further study. This time, he began to suspect that the extraordinary good health of the villagers had something to do with the butter they produced from April through June, and when he left for the second time, he arranged to have samples of the butter produced in Loetschental Valley sent to him at regular, monthly intervals so he could analyze it carefully over the course of a year.

Although he was excited by his discoveries, Price began to worry that the superb physical, mental, emotional, and spiritual conditions exhibited by the Swiss in Loetschental Valley might be a fluke. He began looking for another group of people who had not been introduced to modern foods.

In 1933, he and his troupe of researchers traveled to the Isle of Lewis in the Outer Hebrides off the northwest coast of Scotland. In this barren land of gales and damp, they found a population of about 20,000 Gaelic people living on a basic diet of oatcakes and porridges, fish, lobster, crab, oysters, and clams.

Although the island was cold and covered with peat, residents managed to grow oats in the short growing season available to them. Peat was burned for fuel in homes that often had no chimneys. Instead, the smoke filtered up through a thatched roof, which was replaced every year, and the remains of the old thatch were carefully collected and used to fertilize the soil in their gardens. Houses were so smoky that it was common to see smoke coming out of doors and windows, yet this did not affect their lungs, eyes, or general health in a negative way, and there was *no* evidence of tuberculosis, heart disease, or cancer among them.

As with the Swiss people, they had almost no cavities. Their perfectly developed jawbones were filled with beautifully aligned teeth. They had extraordinary intelligence, along with peacefulness and a gentle, thoughtful character. They also had prodigious amounts of energy, which they used to work long hours, all the while enjoying the work itself.

As unbelievable as it may sound, nearly 5,000 sailors and fishermen would crowd into the port of Stornoway every Saturday night. There, they would sing, dance, and tell stories with never a fight or any kind of violence, and alcoholism did not exist.

I read Price's description of Saturday nights in the port of Stornoway over and over. How was it possible that so many men could be happy and nonviolent in that time and place, whereas we could not even put three sailors on shore leave without drunken excesses, fistfights, brawls, and competitive sexual aggression?

In tragic contrast to conditions on the Isle of Lewis, life on nearby Bardsey Island was much different. Modern processed foods had been introduced there, and people began abandoning their traditional foods and gardening practices. Bread made with white flour and smeared with jelly was common, as was canned fruit, candy, and alcohol. The result was the deterioration and swift death of almost everyone on the island. The cause of death was tuberculosis. When the government sent a second group of about four dozen new families, all young and healthy, to restart the population on the island, they, too, quickly degenerated, all succumbing to TB.

Representatives from the health department went to the island to investigate, hoping to determine why the people should suddenly become susceptible to killer diseases. They decided that it must have been the smoky houses that were causing irritation of the lungs, which then turned into tuberculosis. In spite of the fact that the people on Bardsey Island had lived in smoky houses for centuries, health officials insisted that the people of the island stop their ancient, traditional practice of burning peat and allowing the smoke to filter up through their thatched roofs.

Those who followed the health department recommendations found that, without the smoked thatch from the previous year, their oat crop would not mature in the short, severe growing season that was typical on the island. Without a healthy, mature oat crop, their health soon faltered. A compromise was reached when the villagers finally agreed to move into new houses that the government had built for them, as long as they could continue to maintain the old houses with thatched roofs and burn peat in them all year, a solution that turned out to be both inconvenient and expensive. Yet, those who did so retained their health! And by analyzing the thatch, Price discovered it was loaded with nutrients and ash that gave a boost to the oat crop, bringing it to maturity quickly, a necessity in the short growing season.

With the visit to the Isle of Lewis, Price had found a second example of people following ancient, nourishing traditions and enjoying excellent health. Right next to them on Bardsey Island were the remains of those who had abandoned those traditions, only to suffer miserably and die early.

Each year for another 11 years, Weston Price and his group traveled to a different place in the world, bringing back evidence that everywhere the western European diet of white flour and refined sugar went, a sad trail of degeneration, disease, deformity, disability, and death followed.

Among the groups Price visited and lived with were the Eskimos and natives of Alaska. They lived mainly on salmon, fish eggs, caribou, groundnuts, kelp, a few cranberries, bits of sorrel grass, and seal oil.

He spent time among the Indians of Peru who fished along the Pacific coastline while growing corn, squash, beans, and other plants to combine with the seafood that was a mainstay of their diet. The Indians of the Amazon ate similarly except they also included birds, eggs, animals from the jungle, and yucca root, which is similar to potatoes.

The Melanesians, Micronesians, and New Zealand Maori lived on fish, crab, wild pig, fruits, and a few green plants. Polynesian diets were similar to this, except for a bit of taro root, which they made into poi. All of these groups had little or no tooth decay, extraordinary physiques, high levels of energy and stamina, and no degenerative diseases.

In sharp contrast to the seafood diets of Eskimos and those groups who lived in coastal areas, the tribes of East and Central Africa lived inland mainly on dairy products. Their diet included fresh milk products from cows and goats, some meat, varying amounts of vegetables, a few fruits and insects, and blood from their cows, something they considered to be of the highest value in maintaining good health.

During their trip through Africa, Price, his wife, and their research group had to be constantly on guard against dysentery, malaria, tick-borne fevers, lice, the tsetse fly and its dreaded sleeping sickness, as well as dangerous sunburns. Yet the African tribes who maintained their ancient diets were completely immune to such troubles. Neither were they familiar with arthritis, gallstones, ulcers, cancers, colds, bladder infections, appendicitis, infertility, abscesses, pyorrhea, or tooth decay. Only where the missionaries had succeeded in getting them to abandon their traditional foods had the African people succumbed to the difficulties in their environment or become subject to modern diseases.

After visiting over 30 African tribes on a 6,000-mile journey through their continent, Price wrote, "Their nutrition varied according to their location, but always provided an adequate quantity of body-building and repairing material, even though much effort was required to obtain some of the essential food factors. Many tribes practiced feeding girls special foods for an extended period before marriage (often for at least six months). Spacing of children was provided by a system of plural wives." [6]

Upon visiting the Australian Aborigines, Price felt they were among the most intelligent and skilled of all the groups he had visited. They exhibited the greatest endurance under extreme conditions and lived on fish, kangaroo, wallaby, waterfowl, birds, eggs, insects, and roots. Like the other groups Price had visited, they had minimal levels of tooth decay, no abscesses, no crowded, crooked teeth, and no degenerative diseases.

When he ran out of living people who were still maintaining traditional, pre-modern diets, Price studied the skulls and teeth of the plains Indians of North and South America. He also examined hundreds of ancient Peruvian skulls and skeletons, as well as other collections of bones and teeth wherever he could find them. None showed any evidence of tooth decay or what he referred to as "deformed dental arches" with crooked, crowded teeth.

---

6 Price, p. 138-139.

In the end, the conclusions were unavoidable. Among the living groups he visited, wherever traditional foods had remained in place, people were healthy, happy, peaceful, and beautiful. He confirmed that before the advent of the modern Western diet, people were on intimate terms with food and knew specifically which parts of an animal or plant would provide the nutrients that prevented specific diseases. Again and again, he found that people went to great effort to assure that each generation was superbly nourished.

As for those who did not keep to the traditional foods, Price wrote, "In every instance where individuals…had adopted the foods and food habits of our modern civilization, there was loss of the high immunity (to many diseases)…It rapidly became apparent that a chain of disturbances developed in these people, starting immediately and rapidly increasing in severity with expressions like the characteristic degenerative processes of our modern civilization of America and Europe." And the hundreds of photographs he brought back spoke volumes, certainly more than any words could ever say!

Everywhere he went, he gathered samples of traditional diets and compared their nutritional levels to modern foods. Each trip added to Weston Price's knowledge and understanding of what was happening to people and why degeneration was rampant.

At that time, it was already known that the human digestive system was able to extract and absorb less than one-half of the vitamins and minerals present in any given food. This meant foods had to contain at least twice the amount needed if humans were going to extract the minimums required for good health. When Price calculated the body's need for extra nutrition during periods of growth, pregnancy, lactation, stress, or sickness, he concluded that foods had to supply at least four times the minimum daily requirement in order to safely weather all periods of life without sickness taking over or degeneration setting in.

Price knew that a human being needed an absolute minimum of 680 mg of calcium every single day *just to stay alive*, and more to constantly repair and rebuild the body. He knew we needed 1320 mg of phosphorus, and at least 15 mg of iron. The minimums for magnesium, sodium, potassium, copper, iodine, and other minerals were also known or being studied. Thus, he had a useful yardstick for measuring the differences between traditional diets eaten by indigenous peoples and the modern diets eaten by the average American.

Analysis of foods in the average American diet showed them to be extremely low in vitamins and minerals regardless of where they were produced. People living on foods made from white flour simply could not eat enough to get the minimum amounts of nutrition even if they could afford to buy that much food. An entire day's worth of white-flour food contained barely 500 mg of calcium and sometimes only 300 mg. Phosphorus was present in amounts that reached 600 mg at best, and was often as low as 300 mg. These were far below the minimums needed for survival, and nowhere near the optimum amount needed for good health, high energy, and high levels of immunity to disease and degeneration. It was clear that modern foods were not supplying enough nutrients to build healthy bodies or repair them when they went down.

In sharp contrast to this, the average calcium in traditional indigenous diets was up to 7.5 times the minimum required. Phosphorus levels averaged 8.2 times the minimum daily requirement suggested by American nutritionists. Magnesium ranged up to 28.5 times the minimum. Iron was 58.2 times the basic need. Levels of iodine were 49 times the necessary requirement. The fat-soluble vitamins of D, E, A, and K were present in at least ten times the amounts found in the modern foods of the 1930's. And in every one of the traditional foods, there were significant increases – usually tenfold and up – in the amount of water-soluble vitamins such as Vitamin C and B-complex.

Because these high levels of available nutrition were missing in the modern American diet of processed food, the result, Price discovered, was an average increase in susceptibility to disease and disability of *thirty-five fold*! Besides illness, cavities, and abscessed teeth, he documented case after case of physical deformity and immediate physical degeneration as soon as a family began eating modern foods. Mothers who changed from traditional diets to modern diets after having one or two children discovered enormous differences in those children born after the diet change. These later children were sickly, weak, and didn't look like the rest of the family. Many had club feet, poor eyesight, suffered from constant colds and flu, lacked strength, energy and motivation, and were relatively less social, seeming to feel and act like outsiders to the family.

The truth is, and always has been, that without enough high-quality nutrition, the body begins to skimp on basic structures. Jawbones shrink, become narrowed, and there is not enough room to accommodate all 32 teeth. The skull and cheekbones get smaller, and the face looks pinched. Often the middle third of the face looks "pushed in" and lacks natural beauty, or there is a jutting jaw with an under bite. Sometimes the lower third of the face is not developed, creating a receding chin and an overbite. Or the upper third of the skull doesn't develop, making the forehead recede, giving the face the overall shape of a ski slope.

In other forms of degeneration, the upper palate in the mouth takes on a high, narrow, tent-like shape, and when an infant sucks or a child chews and swallows, the push-pull stimulation of the tongue against the roof of the mouth does not happen because the tongue can't "reach the ceiling" of the mouth easily. This stimulation is critical for the development of the brain because the structures of the limbic brain, the pituitary, and the pineal gland are just on the other side of the upper palate and require the stimulation of sucking in order to develop fully.

In one amazing reclamation of human life and intelligence, Dr. Price worked with a Mongoloid teen of about 16 years old who was retarded, sexually undeveloped, and unable to function without constant supervision. Price operated on the boy's upper palate, cutting it apart and surgically spreading the two sides to create a wider, more natural shape. Within months there was startling growth. Regarding the young man, Price wrote:

> "With the movement of the maxillary bones laterally, as shown… there was a very great change in his physical development and mentality. He grew three inches in about four months. His mustache started to grow immediately; and in twelve weeks' time, the genitals developed from those of a child to those of a man, and with it, a sense of modesty. His mental change was even more marked. The space between the maxillary bones was widened about one-half inch in about 30 days…The outward movement of the maxillary bones (which form the roof of the mouth and the sides of the nose) by pressure on the temporal bones produced a tension downward on the floor of the anterior part of the brain, thus stimulating the pituitary gland in the base of the brain." (p.368)

This same young man's mental retardation dissolved to the point that he was able to learn to read children's books and newspapers. He then was able to get a job in another city, get himself back and forth to that job, and be a fairly self-sufficient human being in society.

Price also described and detailed other forms of subtle degeneration. A healthy chest and good lungs tend to be broad and shallow, thus breath moves into the bottom of the lungs quickly and is exhaled easily. A narrowing of the shoulders and lengthening of the chest leads to less-efficient breathing, analogous to trying to breathe through a straw. A deep, narrow chest leaves one susceptible to tuberculosis, asthma, and other pulmonary and breathing difficulties.

Similarly, narrowing of the bones in the pelvic cavity leads to great difficulty in giving birth, along with changes in reproductive organs that create numerous increases in miscarriage, stillbirths, premature births, and outright reproductive sterility. While on their trip, Price found extremely healthy women on traditional foods who gave birth in bed in the middle of the night, right next to their husbands, without waking anyone! In contrast, women all over Europe and America were dying in childbirth due to complications of narrowed pelvic bones. When they succeeded in giving birth, their infants were weak and sickly.

Hand-in-hand with deep, narrow lungs, shrunken pelvic bones, and crowded teeth full of cavities went many cases of flat feet, clubbed feet, or instances where one leg was shorter than the other. Price found increasing deficiencies in hearing, huge numbers of children with poor eyesight, children with poor muscle coordination, sometimes cleft palate, or outright absence of the entire upper palate.

As disturbing as the physical deterioration was, the mental deterioration he observed all around him was even more upsetting. A number of his peers were dealing with burgeoning numbers of children exhibiting low intelligence, retardation, regular demonstration of unsocial traits, an inability to learn in school, and a tendency toward delinquency, which often landed them in jail.

Price visited special education classes for slow learners, asylums and institutions for retarded and Mongoloid children, reform schools for the delinquent, and jails for those who had committed serious crimes. He noted that at least 98% of these children had the pinched, undeveloped facial bones and dental deformities that resulted from nutritional deficiency.

When he asked the director of the Ohio State Penitentiary if he had noticed anything special about the mouths of the inmates, the director's reply was that "there was a tendency for the tongue to be too large for the mouth." (p. 357)

In a piece titled *Mental Deficiency*, A. F. Tredgold, as cited in Price's book, wrote:

"The association of abnormalities of the palate with mental deficiency has long been recognized, and there is no doubt that it is one of the commonest malformations occurring in this condition. Many years ago, Langdon Down drew attention to the subject, and more recently Clouston has recorded a large number of observations which show conclusively that, although deformed palates occur in the normal, they are far and away more frequent in neuropaths and the mentally defective. He states that deformed palates are present in 19 percent of the ordinary population, 33 percent of the insane, 55 percent of criminals, but in no less than 61 percent of idiots. Petersen, who has made a most exhaustive study of this question, has compiled an elaborate classification of the various anomalies found in palatal deformities present in no less than 82 percent of aments (mental defectives), in 76 percent of epileptics, and in 80 percent of the insane." (p. 354)

In his travels around the world, Price had been struck by the health, peacefulness, intelligence, and sense of joyful self-responsibility that were so obvious in the groups of indigenous peoples he had visited. They did not have hospitals or jails. They had no need for such institutions and made sure that they continued to have no need for them.

Contrary to popular opinion, Price found that these indigenous people were quite aware of the rest of the world and of how that world lived. They were not naïve, ignorant primitives, wishing to be like us, going through their daily routines because they did not know better and had nothing else to do with their lives. They were wise and aware, and deliberately chose their foods and lifestyles because these ways created healthy, intelligent, peaceful people.

The women and men in native villages went to great lengths and considerable effort to obtain the high-quality foods they needed for themselves and especially for the young couples about to be married. Women went on special diets for a year before allowing themselves to become pregnant. While nursing their children, they continued this careful attention to nutrition. In many of the native groups, special care was taken to avoid another pregnancy until the mother had fully recovered from the previous birth, with a period of at least three years being considered as necessary for the recovery. No one wanted to give birth to a sick, troublesome child, or a child who couldn't or wouldn't do his share of the work.

After years of studying and surveying people who enjoyed superior nutrition, comparing their mental and emotional conditions with those groups who clearly showed signs of nutritional deficiency, Price realized that personality, spirituality, and moral character were far more dependent on the biological condition of human beings than had previously been recognized. He wrote:

> "Thinking is as biologic as is digestion, and brain embryonic defects are as biologic as are club feet. Since both are readily produced by lowered parental reproductive capacity, and since Nature in her large-scale human demonstration reveals that this is chiefly the result of inadequate nutrition of the parents and too frequent or too prolonged child bearing, the way back (to health) is indicated."(p. 7)

Weston Price was aware of modern civilization's growing difficulty in getting good, healthy chicken, beef, pork, and lamb. He was always on the lookout for the possibility of providing high nutrition and maintaining superb health and immunity using vegetarian diets. In the same way that people were degenerating, so were plants and animals. Exhausted soil produced sickly plants with too few minerals in them. As a result, meat, eggs, milk, cheese, and other animal products not only contained fewer nutritional elements, the increasing number of deaths among farm animals due to proliferating diseases made these products harder to get and more expensive. The result was that many groups began experimenting with vegetarian diets. However, after years of research, Price wrote:

"As yet, I have not found a single group (of people) building and maintaining excellent bodies by living entirely on plant foods…In every instance where the groups involved had been long under this teaching, I found evidence of degeneration in the form of dental caries, and in the new generations…abnormal dental arches to an extent very much higher than in the primitive groups who were not under this influence." (p.279)

In the end, Price reluctantly concluded that vegetarianism, as a way of life, was not sustainable because those who practiced this way of eating suffered from the same slow degeneration as those trying to subsist on the modern Western diet.

Recently, while attending a local conference on food, I was seated next to someone who was touting the benefits of vegetarianism as if anyone who ate meat was doing something dirty. I mentioned the work of Dr. Weston Price and the fact that he had traveled around the world for 14 years and not found a single group of indigenous people who thrived and maintained excellent health or lived to advanced ages on a vegetarian diet. I also commented that I had ended up with rheumatoid arthritis after ten years on a vegetarian diet.

The young man immediately protested my statements, insisting that the people of India had survived for years on vegetarian diets. My response to him was, "Have you *seen* the people of India? They may be surviving, but just barely, and they certainly aren't thriving. The poverty and sickness there are devastating, and they don't produce the extraordinary bodies with the health and stamina that were once found among the Swiss people, the Eskimos, the South American Indians, or the Melanesians."

"But they are very spiritual," he argued, as if their vegetarianism was the source of their spirituality.

"Have you been there?" I asked him.

"No," he replied.

"Then what makes you think their poverty or poor health makes them spiritual?" I inquired.

He couldn't answer, and the conversation ended when someone gracefully changed the subject. However, it made me aware that a good many people lack the common sense to recognize groundless logic. India may be highly spiritual, but it is not because her people are hungry or have less food. It *may* be true that vegetarianism decreases aggression over the long haul because you have less energy to fight, but a decrease in aggression is not equivalent to an increase in spirituality. It *is not* true that eating meat increases aggression. The work of Price and others shows that it is *poor nutrition* that increases aggression while decreasing one's sense of social belonging, thus leading to the tendency for destructive behavior and relationships.

I recommend getting Price's book and reading it cover to cover. Even if you don't read it, just look at the photos. They tell a remarkable story all by themselves. What you will see in those photos is that here in America, the epitome of beauty – the tall, gaunt woman with a thin, aquiline nose, long narrow chest, narrow hips, slender face and features, complete with artificially straightened teeth – is actually an icon of physical degeneration. Many of our movie stars and models are a testament to the processes of degeneration and ill health in our country. The pictures in Price's book celebrate another kind of beauty that is just as pleasing to the eye, yet is based on superb health, something we have lost touch with in far too many ways.

Price's research in nutrition is monumental. Of that there is no doubt. For over 60 years it has stood like a beacon for those in the field of health, yet much of what he did has been overshadowed by "modern" science and advertisers who market foods to a public that pays little attention to nutrition. Perhaps Price's work came at a time when too few people were willing to look at the implications of what he presented. Perhaps what he was seeing and saying was too painful. Maybe it didn't seem real to those of his time, or there was nothing anyone could do about the way the world was going at that moment. Maybe they didn't have enough examples of poor nutrition to compare where they had been with where they were at, but if we look back, a clear picture emerges of the forces and factors destroying our health today.

If you are looking for the way back to health, his work illuminates the path, and here at the farm we have discovered that there is no substitute for high-nutrition food. ❖

4

Poor Health Makes The
(Business) World Go 'Round

CITIES HAVE COME AND GONE for thousands of years, and as the Industrial Revolution gained momentum, a slow stream of people began leaving farms for jobs in factories and life in cities. In America, the steady migration of people toward cities continued through the second half of the 19th century.

By the time the 20th century arrived, this slow migration became a flood. People were leaving farms by the thousands. They moved to the cities, took jobs in factories, bought food wherever they could get it, and adopted the white-flour/white-sugar diet because that was what was available.

Generation #1

Between 1900 and 1925, the first generation of Americans to be conceived by parents living mainly on a white-flour/white-sugar diet were being born in large numbers. We will call them Generation #1 because they were one generation away from the soil. As they grew, people like Weston Price and others working in the field of health began noticing problems that had not been prevalent prior to the turn of the century. Besides large numbers of rotting teeth, abscessed jaws, and narrow, degenerated bone structures, this generation was unable to resist even minor infections. Colds, flu, chickenpox, measles, and fevers were springing up everywhere. Although people often survived these milder physical diseases, they were

41

increasingly vulnerable to the more serious diseases of tuberculosis, diphtheria, and pneumonia. Even when they managed to avoid the serious ailments, they were tired all the time and began losing interest in the active and self-sufficient ways of their ancestors. Worse, they began to suffer emotional and mental disturbances, and they could neither relax and rest, nor sleep easily and deeply.

As the health of Generation #1 went down, the number of businesses based on poor health went up. The rise of the dental profession accompanied the sudden rise in cavities. The profession of psychiatry made its first appearance, as did the need for mental institutions to accommodate the increasing number of people with emotional and mental disturbances. Orphanages were organized to take care of street children whose parents had succumbed early to the change in diet. Hospitals, doctors, and nurses began gathering influence and power. Chemists and scientists began to focus on substances that might improve health. And the sudden spread of infection, fatigue, malaise, and disease brought a wave of pills and potions, laying the foundations for the pharmaceutical industry to become the behemoth it is today.

Generation #2

Generation #2, born roughly between 1925 and 1950, was the second generation to be conceived and raised on modern foods. Like the children in Generation #1, these children also suffered from cavities, loss of teeth, and abscessed jaws. However, in addition to cavities and abscesses, they suffered from crowded, crooked teeth that did not fit their mouths. They suffered from constant colds, flu, ear-nose-and-throat infections, and some died from the childhood diseases that had once been considered only nuisance infections.

Over all, they were more susceptible to the diseases that plagued the previous generation, but deeper, more pernicious changes began to be evident. Serious birth defects appeared. Children were born blind, or deaf; they had misshapen legs and feet and serious spinal deformities. Low levels of intelligence began showing up and retardation became more common. As Generation #2 reached adulthood, they suffered from vague depressions and levels of fatigue that left them capable of little more than finding a job and settling for a paycheck, rather than relying on their own skills, creativity, and ingenuity to maintain self-sufficient lives.

Many who escaped being blind or deaf found they needed glasses or hearing aids by the time they were in their 20s and 30s. They argued often, drank too much, and were willing to go to war. Once they passed 50 years of age, they ran into the long-term effects of the white-flour/white-sugar diet as heart disease, osteoporosis, arthritis, diabetes, tumors, and other difficulties began appearing to plague them.

To accommodate this second generation of Americans raised on empty foods, there was an increase in the development of pharmaceutical companies, the appearance of the optometrist and the eyeglasses industry, the hearing specialist and the hearing aid, the podiatrist for foot problems, and surgeons who specialized in removing everything from tonsils to tumors. Associations were formed to help with blindness, alcoholism, or crippled limbs, while nursing homes became the solution for dealing with the early wave of those who were falling apart and no longer able to contribute to society because of poor nutrition.

The easy availability of modern processed foods and "imitation" foods made new increases in population possible, and the dangers hidden in this kind of this population explosion were ignored under the banner of economic growth for our nation. As the population grew, so did the cities, and as the cities grew, so did a variety of transportation, communication, and manufacturing businesses. As these businesses grew, still more people left the land to take jobs in these industries. With fewer and fewer people farming, it became harder for individual farmers to do the amount of work required to renew the soil each year. Crops began faltering and the result was the early appearance of chemical companies producing NPK (nitrogen-phosphorus-potassium) fertilizers, herbicides, pesticides, and fungicides. Deliberately overlooking the fact that they were highly toxic, these chemical solutions were designed to push the soil to produce enough food for the burgeoning population.

Generation #3

Generation #3, the third generation of Americans to be conceived and birthed from parents living on foods without enough nutrition, was born between 1950 and 1975. All of the same difficulties that plagued Generations #1 and #2 also plagued Generation #3, plus a few new ones. Physical degeneration was now accelerating as the toxic chemicals introduced into agriculture began compounding the problems of poor nutrition. In addition to the cavities, loss of teeth, birth defects, poor bone structure, low immune response and its resulting string of infections, there now came a wave of allergies, asthmatics, and ADHD children. There were large numbers of slow, remedial schoolchildren who had difficulty concentrating on anything. To make matters worse, eyesight problems made glasses necessary for thousands of 10- and 12-year-olds.

As the potent pesticides and plant sprays worked their way into the human metabolism, immune system function dropped to new lows and a subtle derangement of the glands that make up the endocrine system began to show up in people and animals. The endocrine system, responsible for producing the neurotransmitters, enzymes, and hormones that stabilize physical, mental, and emotional conditions within the body, began showing signs of serious disruption. Skin was suddenly full of pimples and blackheads. Thyroids became dysfunctional. Pituitary and pancreatic glands collapsed, adrenal glands exhausted themselves trying to cope with rising stress levels, digestion suffered, weight went up, and sexual and menstrual difficulties mushroomed. Worse, instead of merely removing tonsils and tumors, surgeons were now replacing heart valves and even hearts, lungs, and kidneys.

To cope with the problems and needs of Generation #3, we added a number of new businesses. The use of chemicals to fluoridate water was an attempt to prevent cavities, with no mention of its deleterious side effects on the brain. The toothpaste, toothbrush, mouthwash, and orthodontic industries became big business, as did the allergists.

The appearance of so many slow, retarded, and remedial children categorized as learning- or emotionally-disabled marked the beginning of the special education classroom, special drugs to "help" them, and specially trained teachers to manage them.

Whole hospitals sprang up just for children. Welfare offices proliferated to assist those who didn't have the health, energy, or motivation to become part of the constantly changing economic landscape. Social services, juvenile detention centers, and jails began appearing in order to cope with the increasing number of youths who were poorly nourished, maladapted, and aggressive. Cancer research and treatment became big business. Cardiac specialists became kings. Psychotherapy – both individual and group – began happening everywhere. We began playing with artificial insemination and test tube babies, cesarean delivery, and neo-natal specialists. And all the while, chemical companies and pharmaceuticals continued to grow.

By this time, Generation #2 was moving into middle age. Sadly, an epidemic of cancers, heart disease, diabetes, high blood pressure, kidney failure, stroke, serious depression, fatigue, and frustrating obesity marked their passage into middle age and beyond.

Meanwhile, the remaining survivors of Generation #1 found themselves unable to focus, think, or act sensibly in response to everyday reality. They were routinely shut out of the economic system and quickly lost any reason for living. When they became unable to walk, too weak to care for their homes, too fragile and confused to live alone or maintain their health, they, too, were shipped off without a second thought to the nursing homes that were now ubiquitous.

Generation #4

The fourth generation of people raised on empty foods was born between 1975 and 2000. Generation #4 suffered from all of the difficulties of Generations 1, 2, and 3. Because the problem of poor nutrition had gone unrecognized, there was a dramatic worsening of conditions in all categories of disease and across all ages and social classes.

Infants were born prematurely, had dangerously low birth weights, could not breathe properly, or were born without an immune system at all. Two-year-olds had cancers, six-year-olds were coming down with arthritis, eight-year-olds had diabetes, and far too many ten-year-olds were bloated and seriously overweight. Children everywhere had killer allergies and asthmas. They suffered from digestive upsets and constant congestion of sinuses due to the body's ongoing efforts to dump waste matter from the system. There were continuous ear-nose-and-throat infections simply because the tubes that drain the ears did not develop fully. These ear tubes were too short and at the wrong angle to allow drainage – all the result of eating food with no nutrition in it, thus hampering the body's ability to build itself out fully and correctly.

Learning disabilities were rampant, making special education and tutoring not just a specialty niche but a major part of the education business. Whole schools began springing up to cater to the learning disabled child.

Other school systems counted on "special needs" children for a major part of their budget money. Mainstream schools complained bitterly about the violence and social problems they were dealing with in their halls and classrooms, yet they continued to feed students fast food lunches that were completely devoid of nutrients.

Formerly, it had been accepted that by age 50 people began falling apart, but suddenly those in their teens and 20s exhibited the same problems and large segments of the population were seriously dependent on drugs, prescription or otherwise, to help them maintain some semblance of everyday life. Young people only 14 years old had heart attacks and died. Others couldn't sleep due to breathing difficulties.

The appearance of whole stores devoted to junk foods that were nothing but sugar and chemicals fueled the spread of poor health, all supported by the demands of an addicted society that was ignorant of anything regarding nutrition. The results were widespread mental and emotional problems that left teens alienated, suicidal, or homicidal. Many of them were simply unable to bond. Jails became a huge segment of the low-wage economy in many states, and some jail populations were as big as whole towns and villages. Teen support groups sprang up for everything from alcoholism, depression, and cancer to stroke, bulimia, and chronic fatigue.

Upon reaching adulthood, many found themselves unable to conceive or carry a child to term. When they did conceive, they needed Cesarean sections to deliver that child, and often the infants were small and sickly.

As they grew older, they found themselves dealing with irritable stomachs, irritable bowels, and irritable moods. Derangement of the endocrine system created dysfunctional ovaries, prostates, adrenal, and thyroid glands. When the glands malfunctioned, people struggled with PMS problems, yeast troubles, urinary infections, weight gain, skin problems, hair loss, depression, and fatigue – all signs that the endocrine system was crashing.

The need for expensive braces and orthodontic bite correction was now something every parent *expected* to pay for. Weight loss centers did a brisk business. And there was a proliferation of equipment – both small and large – to help manage and monitor everything from extra oxygen to blood sugar levels to fetal development.

Those in their 60s and 70s who had spent a lifetime on food with no nutrition in it were needing hip replacements, knee replacements, stents to open up blocked arteries, and adult daycare services because they were unable to participate in normal activities or take care of themselves. Whole industries arose to supply the sick or infirm with everything from special walkers and toilets to mechanical lifts that would lift them in and out of the bathtub or up and down the stairs.

As the number of sick went up, there was a steady increase in the number of doctors and nurses needed, and plenty of financial opportunities for those in the medical field. The explosive rise of medical insurance and managed care industries, along with the now gigantic pharmaceutical companies swept everyone into the medical industry.

Today, thousands of people in Generation #4 are sterile and unable to reproduce. Those who can't conceive pay enormous amounts for the chemicals and drugs that will force their bodies to produce eggs and sperm or hold onto a fetus.

Every year a sizable portion of our financial budget is taken up with the problems created by poor food and its results – physical degeneration.

Generation #5

Today, those who can still reproduce are giving birth to Generation #5. These infants exhibit serious defects in their bone structure, organ structures, brain, and central nervous system. Of the last five infants that I know of born to friends, family, and acquaintances, not a single infant has been healthy and normal. All required extended hospital stays and continued, expensive interventions after being taken home. Statistically, about 15% of newborns are unable to go home with parents and must endure days or weeks in NICU, Neonatal Intensive Care Units. Worse, we have a wave of autism spectrum disorder appearing in our infants that is rapidly getting worse each year. In 2014, it was one child out of every 68 children. Today it is one out of every 40 children.

We are seeing a worsening of conditions in all age groups and an expansion in the kinds of health problems that are appearing. Approximately one out of every two men, and one out of every three women has difficulty or is unable to reproduce. One out of every three people is dealing with some sort of cancer, diabetes is rampant, Parkinson's Disease is spreading, and Alzheimers is ubiquitous.

When my daughter was pregnant with her first child, she was several months along when she went to the hospital for an ultrasound. A month or two later she had another one. When she went back for a third one, I remarked that I thought it odd she should need another one. I had delivered four children without a single ultrasound.

To my surprise, she said she wasn't the only one getting ultrasounds; all her girlfriends who were pregnant had to have a series of them. I couldn't imagine why the doctors would need to peer inside for a look at the fetus again and again, and when I asked her why she needed so many, she didn't know, but promised to ask the doctor the next time she saw him.

His reply to her question was that ultrasounds were necessary these days because too many children were being born with oversized ventricles in the brain (a ventricle is a hollow area or cavity). The enlarged ventricles then filled with fluid, a condition commonly known as "water on the brain," which caused mental retardation and other developmental difficulties. The ultrasounds allowed the doctor to track the size of the ventricles, and if they reached a certain size limit, which was something like 10 mm, delivery was induced. When this happened, the obstetrician invited neonatal specialists to be present in the delivery room in case shunts were needed to relieve the pressure of the fluid in the infant brain, thus preventing serious damage.

I was stunned. The fact that today's infants do not have enough nutritional materials to build enough brain matter to fill the skull without leaving dangerously enlarged ventricles is further evidence of the degenerating condition of the human body.

As things turned out, my tiny grandson's brain ventricles did reach the limits set by today's doctors, and they did have to induce labor, complete with the neonatal specialists present. He turned out to be okay, there was no need for shunts or other intervention procedures and today he is a successful lawyer.

❖

As I write these words, there are over seven billion people on the planet, and most of us are at least one or two generations away from any kind of involvement with the soil. We grew up running to the grocery store for food and believe that someone else will take responsibility for feeding us. We are so comfortable handing over this responsibility that it feels strange, unnatural, to even think about taking on this task for oneself.

Both media and government compound this sense of awkwardness around food, the soil, and Mother Nature by speaking of those who grow their own food as people who live at "subsistence level." They make it sound as if this is something pitiful and as if those who subsist on what they can "wrest" from the soil live miserably. The truth is that Mother Nature is extremely generous, and those who grow their own food enjoy a very full, healthy, and secure way of life. The biggest difference is that this way of life requires a different daily routine with different priorities; however, in addition to high quality food, it returns a sense of capable self-sufficiency to the one who knows how to provide for himself.

A huge segment of our economy is based on ill health. Even the growth in sales of supplements, herbs, and over-the-counter medicines has been nothing short of spectacular and must be counted in this effort to cope with the results of empty food.

Ask yourself, "Could the giant hospital complexes and their related medical businesses, the pharmaceutical industries, the jails, lawyers, and parts of the legal system, the social services industry, the nursing homes, and the biggest industry of all – the chemical (fake) food processing industry – survive if we did not have a large population of sickly people to keep them in business?"

If you look around, you will see a painfully obvious truth: that our entire economic system is based heavily around the premise of sickly, weakened people who are too foggy to see what is happening to them. If we all took a sudden, serious interest in getting healthy, a lot of people would be out of work. This would include those who work in industries focused on food processing; the shipping of food; trucking; packaging; agriculture; over-the-counter drugs; prescription pharmaceuticals; the medical insurance industry; the medical equipment industry, including everything from x-ray machines to hospital gowns; medical personnel of every type including doctors such as heart surgeons, oncologists, orthopedic surgeons, pediatricians, and other specialists; nurses; dentists; orthodontists; lab technicians; optometrists; podiatrists; physical therapists; psychologists; psychiatrists; scientists who do medical research; workers who make prostheses and things like heart valves or other body parts; a good many social workers; a number of police and lawyers; many teachers and tutors; and the tens of thousands of clerical and accounting workers in all of the above offices or trade centers. We all talk about the rise of the service industry, and what we are really referring to is the fact that we all serve the gods of ill health.

As a result of our disconnection from the soil, we have built ourselves an economy that is looking more and more like a house of cards. How can we possibly afford to get well if it puts half of us out of work? Yet how can we maintain ourselves as a peaceful, powerful people if we don't begin to get well and stay well? It is my belief that we can't even begin to approach the creative levels, the insights, and the stamina that will be needed to transition through this dilemma unless we do get well.

Because of our disconnection from the soil, we do not understand how critically important it is to maintain healthy *soil* in order to maintain healthy *people*. When I make this statement about healthy soil to groups of people, the response is almost always the same – blank looks and confusion. The masses of humanity no longer know or understand that we do not have access to food that will sustain human life.

Without a relationship to the soil and Mother Earth, it is easy to be ignorant of the fact that our soils are dead. It is easy to think that putting something in our stomachs is the same thing as nurturing and feeding our bodies. It is easy to believe that factory food is the same thing as real food. It is easy to excuse and overlook the fact that those who are raising our foods are spraying poisonous chemicals on them before they sell it to us.

So what, we think, if there's a little fungicide or a bit of pesticide in our fields and gardens... *so what* if there's no topsoil... *so what* if I eat the modern, white-flour-white-sugar-canned-food-coffee-tea-and-alcohol diet? Everyone else is eating it. I have to make a living and don't have time to grow my own food. I don't even have time to cook any more. Food manufacturers can create something to eat as easily as the local farmer, and all I have to do is open the can or the bag to get a meal. Unfortunately this is not true...and we do not know that we do not know. ❖

5
Connecting Soil and Stomach

MOST OF US THINK OF THE GROUND we walk around on as *dirt*, something unimportant, something to avoid walking through for fear of messing up our shoes or the rug. It's rare that people look at dirt and think of it as *soil*. It's rare that people think of dirt or soil at all. Since the majority of Americans are now several generations removed from any sort of relationship to the soil, news about soil is ignored as meaningless and irrelevant.

Those who have been in love with gardening for years often know "good dirt" from "bad dirt" just by look or feel. They are quite conscientious about adding old leaves and kitchen wastes to the garden plot in the off-season or through composting. Yet even among people who continue to garden, when it is finally time to gather those first peas or pluck that sweet, red tomato, any awareness of the soil and what it has contributed is eclipsed by the excitement of the ripening vegetables. Seldom do you find someone who eats a tomato and remarks on the quality of the soil it was grown in.

If something drastic happened to all the grocery stores tomorrow and we were all left on our own to feed ourselves, would you know how to get from the soil to the stomach and end up with something nutritious to eat? Knowing that food with all the required nutritional elements is the bottom line in staying healthy and alive, could you grow a balanced diet to get what you need? Could you do it year after year? If there was trouble in the garden patch, would you panic and run for chemical fertilizers, weed killers, and insecticides? Or would you know enough to realize that sickly plants, invading insects, and weeds that outgrow your vegetables no matter what you do are the results of sick, faltering soil, and that chemicals only make things worse?

Few of us think of soil as a living thing in its own right, but it is. We don't think of soil as something that needs to be healthy, and we don't worry much when it's sick, but we should. It's hard to find anyone who really knows much about the soil anymore, yet a major part of learning to heal yourself comes when you begin to understand the connection between the soil and the stomach. So let's take a short course on soil that will help you understand the most basic of truths: that healthy soil equals healthy plants, healthy plants equal healthy people, and it is your re-connection to the soil of the earth that will provide the foundation for your healing.

Dead dirt is a combination of particles of sand, silt, clay, minerals, dusts, and miscellaneous forms of carbon-based material such as bits and pieces of leaves and twigs.

Living soil is a combination of all of the above *plus* the bodies of billions of living, highly active fungi, bacteria, and microorganisms with names like actinomycetes, streptococcus, staphylococcus, protozoa, nematodes, flatworms, earthworms, mites, beetles, snails, slugs, and centipedes. Together these elements constitute what is known as healthy, living soil.

Living soil has a structure to it – a crumb structure! This structure is made entirely possible by the presence of those billions of tiny living organisms, bugs, and insects. As these fungi, bacteria, bugs, snails, slugs, and other microorganisms go through the processes of everyday living, they excrete sticky substances as waste matter. They also die, then deteriorate into gooey globs. As we will see, all this sticky, gooey material is very important.

In the first stage of crumb development, the fungi living and growing in the soil put out fine, hair-like arms called *mycelia* that wrap themselves around an assortment of particles of clay, silt, sand, minerals, and decaying matter. This creates individually packaged "crumbs," each containing an assortment of nutritional goodies in them for plants. Once the basic crumb parts have been wrapped in the arms of the fungi, the sticky, gooey waste material from all of the insects and microorganisms acts like a glue that helps bind the crumb of soil together quite firmly. Once bound, the crumb will stay this way until it meets with the root hairs of a plant that then "unlock" its cache of goodies and feast on the minerals and other materials it contains.

SOIL WITH GOOD "CRUMB" STRUCTURE

These crumbs, together with the billions of microorganisms and other tiny critters, form what we call living topsoil. Topsoil should be at least five or six feet deep and have a complex honeycomb of air passages through which the roots of plants move easily in a constant search for nutrients, moisture, and minerals. [7]

A plant growing in good topsoil sends out main roots that descend into the soil at least three or four feet. Vegetables will reach down between three and ten feet, some herbs and weeds will work their way down 20 feet or more. Trees go even farther, as deep as 164 feet. [8]

From these main anchor roots, hundreds of very fine root hairs emerge, and it is the root hairs that do much of the work of feeding the plant. Each root hair extends itself outwardly, moving easily through the air passageways, searching the crumbs of soil for specific nutrients. When the root hair finds something of value in a crumb, it winds itself tightly around that crumb and emits a weak acid called *humic acid*. These plant-emitted acids react with the "glue" and other excretions of the microorganisms living in the soil, creating an additional assortment of mild acids. Some of these acids cause the crumb to break apart, exposing its valuable minerals

7 Deborah L. Martin and Grace Gershuny, Eds, *The Rodale Book of Composting* (Emmaus, PA: Rodale Press, 1992) p. 13-18.

8 Bill Mollison, *Permaculture* (Tyalgum, NSW, Australia: Tagari Press, 1996) p. 223, 252 .

and nutrients. Other acids then react with the exposed minerals, nutrients, and trace elements in the crumb, dissolving them into a solution that can be sucked up by the plant to feed itself and build the structures that will become the vegetable, grain, or fruit the plant was genetically destined to produce. [9]

When growers spray poisonous chemicals on their fields and gardens, *it is the microorganisms that are killed.* In spite of Mother Nature's extraordinary capacity to constantly restore herself, it takes only three years of chemical applications to completely destroy the life in a garden or field. Without the fungi and its mycelial arms, without bacteria, and tiny living organisms to excrete their sticky wastes, the crumbs of soil cannot form. The soil collapses into a compacted mass of packed particles. Without the crumbs, the numerous air passageways do not form, making it extremely difficult for roots to move through soil looking for nutrients. Plants must struggle mightily to work their way through this compacted mass. Their ability to find, dissolve, and uptake the nutrients needed to build themselves into good plant or fruit structures is greatly hampered, and thus, most of their time and energy goes into digging passageways through the soil instead of building healthy plants and an abundant harvest.

Plants raised in poor, dying, or dead soil are not healthy enough to withstand normal cold or heat, droughty periods, rainy periods, or the normal range of pests, fungi, and viruses that live in any healthy soil. These plants suffer from impaired function in themselves, their development is delayed, and the vegetables, fruits, and grains they produce are depleted or even empty of the minerals, carbohydrates, proteins, amino acids, and other nutrient factors that humans *must* have. The result is that *our* development is delayed and we become dysfunctional as well.

When the soil collapses, serious problems appear in other areas of life. Rainwater dropping onto healthy, living soil sinks in immediately and quietly. It does not splash all over the place nor does it create mud. Living soil with good structure does not stick to your shoes and boots. Instead, rain runs through the honeycomb of air passages and goes deeply into the soil. The deepest roots of plants get a drink, and the water not only dilutes

9 Martin and Gershuny, p. 16-23.

the humic acids produced in the soil by roots, it prevents a chemical burn that can be caused by nutrient or fertilizer overdose.

Healthy soil absorbs two to four times its weight in water before the saturation point is reached. [10] An acre of soil is roughly 208 feet by 208 feet, and the actual numbers multiply out to 43,560 square feet. Six inches of living topsoil on that acre will weigh about two million pounds and will hold up to 8 million pounds of water. Twelve inches of topsoil will hold twice that amount, nearly 16 million pounds of water. If the topsoil were five or six feet deep, which is what it should be in a viable soil system, it would hold up to 96 million pounds of water before it started to run off. Imagine, 96 million pounds of water in the space of about four city lots each 75' by 150'. That's 48,000 tons of water. Not only is this powerful protection against flooding, it is quite a reservoir of water.

This also shows why we are suffering from floods and mudslides in so many places, while at the same time running out of good, potable drinking water. We have destroyed our soil, and thus, much of our rainwater runs across the surface of the land and into streams and rivers, carrying precious topsoil with it. From there it goes to the sea where it turns to salt water.

Mother Nature has a water purifying system of her own, but rainwater has to sink deeply into the soil for the system to work. When the rainwater doesn't get down into the deep layers of soil, the aquifers and springs dry up, and we lose clean, clear drinking water.

As of 2001, over 900 million tons of poisonous chemicals were being dumped onto topsoil each year. [11] These chemicals have added exponentially to the problem of collapsed soils around the world. Most fertilizers, pesticides, herbicides, and fungicides are so extremely volatile that heavy metal salts – arsenic, lead, cadmium, nickel, and others – are used to keep them chemically stable long enough to get them out of the bottle or box and onto fields and crops. We all know that poisonous chemicals are very bad for us, but the heavy metal salts are just as bad, if not worse. These metallic salts sink through the few inches of topsoil we

---

10 Dan Skow DVM and Charles Walters Jr, *Mainline Farming for Century 21* (Kansas City, MO: Acres USA Publishing, 1991) p. 35.

11 *Acres USA* newspaper.

have left and settle on top of the subsoil layer. Once there, the salts react with calcium carbonate in the subsoil in a slaking action that produces something very similar to cement.

This cement is called *hardpan*. It forms a thick layer only eight or nine inches below the surface of the ground. This cement-like layer seals off the subsoil quite effectively and contributes to the water run-off mentioned above. Worse, roots cannot work their way past the hardpan into the subsoil, which often has at least some nutrients in it.

Roots end up confined to the top eight or nine inches of soil where they overheat on warm days. At 85° Fahrenheit, plants stop growing and begin to suffer from malaise or failure to thrive. Without plenty of water, things quickly become critical. In shallow soil, they soon use up all available nutrients and end up taking in large amounts of the heavy metals in the subsoil as they try to work their way through it. The heavy metals are then incorporated into the structure of the plant itself as well as the fruit (farmers call everything *fruits*, whether it is a vegetable, grain, or an actual fruit). We eat the fruit and suffer thrice, once from the absence of nutrients, again by the presence of poisonous chemicals, and once more by taking in the heavy metals, something we will come back to in the chapter on chelation.

While this heavy, cement-like layer is forming a few inches under the topsoil, the exact opposite – a fine dust – is forming as the topmost layer of the soil. As bacteria and microorganisms die, the soil making up the top layer becomes a loose, lightweight layer of sand, dust, and silt. Without the sticky glue to create heavy crumbs, this fine, light top layer blows away in the wind, further reducing our ability to produce good food. When we dump toxic chemicals onto the soil, these toxins end up blowing away as well, polluting the air and eventually our lungs.

Over the past 100 years, our topsoil has washed or blown away to the point that its depth has been reduced to less than three inches. In some places there is only an inch left, while other places have none. A desert is essentially a place without topsoil, and this condition is spreading around the globe. Without living topsoil, plants struggle to push their roots through subsoil where they fail to thrive and soon die. Without a good layer of healthy, living topsoil, there will eventually be hunger and famine across the land.

When European settlers first arrived in America, they found virgin topsoil that was three, four, five, even six feet deep. Between 1800 and 1850, New York farmers regularly produced 150 bushels of corn per acre, and yields of 172 bushels per acre were not uncommon. Potato farmers were able to get 800 bushels of potatoes per acre, [12] all without NPK fertilizers, pesticides, fungicides, or herbicides. Today, we can get those yields only with heavy doses of expensive chemical fertilizers and lots of pesticides and fungicides to ward off bugs, molds, and mildews until harvest.

NPK fertilizers will make your plants look big, green, and healthy when they aren't; they're simply bloated and watery – thus tasteless! NPK fertilizers also produce a condition of overgrowth with too many leaves, stems, and shoots that the plant then has difficulty supporting, especially if the soil is dead or has started to collapse. By the time the plant tries to produce fruit, it is nutritionally bankrupt from supporting such a large plant and nothing goes into the fruit. The result is a crop that amounts to garbage, and that is where insects come in.

To understand the role that insects play in food production, it is necessary to revisit the periodic table we all studied in chemistry. Every element of the periodic table is surrounded by a vibrating field of electromagnetic energy. The pattern and color of this energy field is different for every kind of element, each as unique as a fingerprint. Using a device called a spectrometer, we can study this energy field imprint to determine if an element is present in a compound or a living system.

Every kind of matter, every molecule, every plant, animal, and human is also composed of and surrounded by a vibrating field of electromagnetic energy. When a plant has absorbed a particular mineral element, the frequency pattern of the mineral will affect the overall frequency pattern of the plant. The mineral thus becomes a contributor to the total pattern of the plant's electromagnetic field in the same way that a violinist or horn player contributes to the overall sound of a symphony. All of the frequencies of the various minerals and nutrients combine to help drive the plant's operation as a living system, and when complete, this vibrating energy pattern becomes a plant's electromagnetic signature.

---

12 Arden Anderson PhD, DO, *Science in Agriculture* (Kansas City, MO: Acres USA, 1992) p. xv.

Healthy plants that have access to all of the minerals and nutrients necessary to build well-functioning stems, leaves, flowers, and fruits radiate an energetic frequency that has a particular complex of electromagnetic (E-M) signals and tones. These mineral frequencies are the same frequencies that trigger certain genes into action or inaction, and it is critical that our foods be well-mineralized and nutrient-dense. Otherwise, we end up with genetically based diseases, and we spend millions of dollars trying to figure out how or why this gene turned on and that one turned off.

When soil collapses and the plant is unable to find the nutrients it needs to be healthy, it will be short on minerals and nutrients, which mean that certain contributions to the plant's electromagnetic signature will not be made. This causes the plant to radiate an off-color frequency and give off a different E-M signal and tone.

MAN-MADE ANTENNAS

INSECT ANTENNAS

(above drawing) [13]

What you may not have known or realized is that the antennae on insects and bugs are exactly that – an antenna system for picking up electromagnetic wave signals. Not only do they work just like your TV antenna, they are built just like them as well. Insects and pests use their antennae to pick up the altered electromagnetic signals coming from weak, diseased, or dysfunctional plants, then zero in on those plants to destroy them, simply because *that is the purpose of insects*. They are Mother

---

13 This is not my drawing. I found it years ago in a book and never forgot the picture, but I don't know which book it was and couldn't find it after two days of looking. I felt it was too important to leave out, and I will be happy to give credit to the proper source if and when I find it.

Nature's garbage men, as well as her quality control team, disposing of inferior plants and plant or animal wastes in an efficient and timely way.

Many people think that insects and pests will attack any plant and destroy it, but this is not true. When healthy and unhealthy plants in separate pots are placed right next to one another and their stems and leaves intertwined, the insects will ignore the leaves of the healthy plant and go after the leaves of the sickly one. They may take a few bites out of the healthy plant as a means of testing, but they won't destroy it. [14] Why not? Because healthy plants grown in good soil not only give off a different electromagnetic signal, they maintain a very high level of natural sugars in their leaves, stems, and fruit, and this is the magic key to pest control. For farmers and growers, this plant sugar is referred to as *brix*. You might think that insects and pests would be anxious to get to the plants with the highest sugar/brix, but this is not the case. Only humans are foolish enough to eat high amounts of sugar, another topic we will come to later.

Insects munching on plants with high levels of sugar quickly get a paralyzing stomachache and abandon the plant altogether. The high sugar combines with the bugs' internal chemistry to produce an alcohol in their digestive tract. This alcohol quite effectively knocks out the delicately balanced metabolism of insects and pests. Those insects that foolishly continue to eat leaves with high levels of sugar end up falling into the soil in a drunken stupor and become a tasty lunch for the microorganisms, bacteria, and other critters that live in the soil! [15]

In good soil that is fully alive and well-mineralized, a plant builds its structure and begins moving quickly to produce the high levels of sugar that will protect it from attack by insects. Brix can be measured with a pocket refractometer and may range from a low of zero to upwards of 25 to 30%. Once the brix in the leaves reaches about 14%, the plant will not be bothered by insects anymore nor will it succumb to mold, mildew, or rot. In a living soil with healthy plants, each kind of plant achieves this level of brix just about the time that the insects who favor that plant are reaching their maturity, displaying once more the marvels of timing and response we all have to one another in the web of life. Those plants that

---

14 Anderson, p. xi.

15 Skow and Walters, p. 33.

don't make enough brix by the time the first generation of insects reaches maturity will almost certainly feed those insects well enough to allow them to produce a second generation, and then the laggard plants will be completely overwhelmed.

Sometime around 1918, samples of soils from around the world were studied, and it was discovered that these soils were able to produce plants with viable protein levels of only 12%. The minimum level required for human and animal health is 25%. By the 1950s, soils in the United States were down to only 6% viable protein. By the 1970s, U.S. soils had sunk to somewhere between 1.5% and 3.0%. Today, they are certainly no better. [16]

William Albrecht, famed professor of soil science at the University of Missouri for many years, described a plant's struggle as one that strove to synthesize proteins and living tissue to support growth, provide self-protection, and reproduce. [17] The fruit is the plant's way of reproducing. He pointed out that humans and all other warm-blooded bodies were also struggling to get enough proteins and that proteins were synthesized directly from basic elements *only by plants and microbes*. These plants and microbes then feed us. They also feed the animals that feed us.

"Protein contains nitrogen and nitrogen is essential to the construction of a new cell. A deficiency of protein, and thus of nitrogen, will short-circuit new cell construction and this signals the beginning of disease. In humans, this is called degenerative metabolic disease." [18]

The reality of this is now hitting home. There are only a few basic forms of illness. One form is infectious disease, another is degenerative disease, and the rest are accidents. Some have suggested that congenital birth defects are another form of illness, but it turns out that almost all birth defects are due to poor nutrition in the mother, and thus are a form of degenerative disease, which is not rampant in this country. Twelve-year-olds need hip and knee replacements, while thirty-year-olds need

16 Anderson, p. xi.

17 Skow and Walters, p. 169.

18 Skow and Walters, p. 3.

everything from heart transplants to lung and kidney transplants. Each generation is displaying degenerative symptoms at earlier and earlier ages. Almost every family I know has someone seriously sick, seriously overweight, or even terminal. Even those who are health-conscious get sick. Why? Because our soils are, for all practical purposes, dead, and even if we are eating fresh, whole foods that do not come out of boxes and cans, those fresh, whole foods are seriously deficient in nutrition and, unless organic, also laced with heavy metals and poisons.

Over the thousands of years that people have been on Earth, whenever we have overworked our soil or neglected to renew it, famine followed. Dead soils and sickly plants invited attacks by hordes of locusts. When this occurred we simply picked up and moved to new lands. Droughts, or the failure of a group's staple crop such as potatoes or wheat, have been the driving factors in the continuous westward migration of human beings over the past several thousand years. Now we are at the end of the trail. We have migrated all the way around the globe, filling the planet almost beyond capacity with sick and degenerating people, dead soil, and polluted water. There is nowhere left to run, and the dreams of a Green Revolution promised by the chemical factories have proven to be more of a nightmare than a dream.

Fruits, vegetables, and grains that grow in dead soil are almost as dead as the soil they come from. Even when they look beautiful, they have minimal levels of protein, complex carbohydrates, and natural oils; they also lack minerals and vitamins. Worse, they contain chemical residues and other poisons.

We eat this stuff and wonder why we are sick or overweight. It's because the body puts out hunger signals when it is in need of materials for repair and rebuilding. Since cells are always dying and we use up many nutrients in the course of everyday living, the body is in need of a constant supply of top quality building materials – vitamins, minerals, enzymes, proteins, carbohydrates, fats and oils, and other nutrient factors. When you put food in your body, the body goes to work right away, breaking down what you have offered it to find the nutrients contained in the food. When it discovers there is nothing in the food, the body immediately calls for more food. This becomes a vicious circle because you have to eat much more than is healthy to get even a minimum amount of usable nutrition into the body. If you shortchange the body nutritionally for any length of time, you will find you are always hungry, always on edge, always unsatisfied, and driven to eat more. The result is stubborn and intractable weight gain.

People naturally try to figure out why their weight keeps going up. They blame the excess pounds on lack of self-discipline, not enough exercise, their metabolism, lack of time to eat right, laziness, or a bad thyroid. There are cries of despair that sound something like, "I've done everything I know to lose weight..." For most people, dieting becomes an endless circle of hunger, discomfort, denial of the body's call for nutrients, guilt when you can't resist that call, and shame over how you look (overweight) or how weak and undisciplined you are (low self-esteem).

Do not get caught in this circle. Constant dieting when you aren't getting enough nutrition in the first place results in low-level malnutrition, which leads to a lowered thyroid function. The doctor might test you for thyroid activity and tell you you're "low normal," but even a slightly lower thyroid function can result in low levels of the stomach acid that is required for good digestion and absorption of nutrients. Without a good supply of hydrochloric acid in your stomach, your digestive processes will suffer, and you will not be able to extract or absorb useful substances in your food. This leads to a critical shortage of nutrients that the body can use for repair and rebuilding. Because the body very carefully regulates what is in your blood, when the level of various minerals in the blood drops below a certain point, the body robs bones and tissues to get the needed supplies. Let this go on for any length of time and the result is osteoporosis and a host of other degenerative difficulties.

Constant hunger is the body's constant call for *building materials* that it can use to restore itself. When you eat, the body works for hours to extract nutrients, and when it turns out there is nothing useful in the food, your body has used up even more of its precious resources for little or nothing in return. It is like constantly mining for gold without ever hitting pay dirt. There are huge piles of useless waste material everywhere as evidence of how much work was done, but eventually the mining company goes bankrupt. The same thing happens to the body. It has chewed and dug its way through all kinds of food, waste piles up or accumulates in every cell and tissue, interfering with function, and efforts to continue rebuilding eventually go bankrupt because the body never hits the equivalent of pay dirt, which is the nutrition it really needs.

Picture a carpenter about to build a house. He has a life-or-death deadline to get the house built. He also has some of the supplies, but not enough. So he pours cement for the foundations but adds more water than he should to make the cement go farther. He has two-by-fours, but no insulation, a few windows but not enough. The doors that he ordered arrived in the wrong size but there is no time to return them and reorder. Installation of wiring is scant in a few rooms because he ran out of wire. Plumbing producers are on strike so he skimps on plumbing, and there was a shortage of ductwork for the furnace, so a few rooms have no heating or cooling. He does have enough roofing, siding, and paint, and so he proceeds to finish the house and make it look as good as he can.

The owner is pleased with the new house for a while but soon discovers that, although the house looks okay from the outside, it is uncomfortable to live in. Without insulation, he's too hot or too cold. Too few windows require more artificial lighting, but he's short on electricity because there isn't enough wiring. Poorly fitting doors allow drafts and bugs to get inside. The plumbing doesn't work right, some of the rooms cannot be used in certain seasons because they're too hot or too cold, and in a short time the foundation begins to crumble because of soft cement. Slowly the house falls apart.

This is what happens in too many bodies today. The "house" is crumbling. We are degenerating. To make matters worse, the body is not something you build once and then just live in. It has to be rebuilt every single day! When you don't have enough of the right materials to constantly rebuild, the result is a slow, downhill slide into degenerative disease and dysfunction.

When what you eat has been grown in dead, depleted soil, it will be dead, depleted food. Eating this kind of food leads to degeneration at all levels. Degeneration *is*…poor eyesight, loss of hearing, high blood pressure, obesity, heart problems, cancers, diabetes, thyroid problems, arthritis, asthma and breathing difficulties, allergies, eczema, cleft palate, bone deformities, club foot, kidney failure, the need for orthodontic braces, the need for cesarean sections in order to give birth, osteoporosis, aneurysms, dental cavities and orthodontic braces, high levels of cholesterol, psoriasis, and a host of other problems much too numerous to mention. When the soil collapses, we collapse.

It is time to recognize that dead soils produce seriously deficient foods, sometimes with as little as one-quarter to one-eighth the amount of nutrition as we used to grow when our great-grandparents were young. If we try to eat enough of this depleted food to get the minimum recommended requirements in terms of vitamins, minerals, aminos, and other nutrients, we end up eating huge quantities of food that leave us overweight and feeling sluggish, like the snake that swallows a pig. When these deficient foods are also laced with pesticides, herbicides, fungicides, and heavy metals, the degeneration process accelerates and becomes more vicious, more heartbreaking.

The time, money, and effort needed to restore our soils to good condition cannot be any more than the time, money, and effort demanded by the skyrocketing costs and burgeoning complexity of the hospital-medical industry. For those interested in a return to real health and high energy, top quality nutrition is a must. For a serious turnaround of the health problems in this country, we may all have to become gardeners for a while, or at least until those who produce our food understand that neither we nor they can survive on dead and deficient produce and meats laced with even the smallest amounts of poisonous chemicals.

Each time you go to the grocery store, buy at least one organic thing. If the store doesn't have organic food, ask the produce manager where it is, and this will let him know that organic food is important to you. If he says they don't have an organic section, just say thank you and go about your shopping. But keep asking! These requests will eventually filter through to those who make the decisions about what to buy and sell. It also is passed on to those who decide what to plant and how to grow it. If you can't grow your own food, you can at least have a voice in the food that is available to you.

As Weston Price once said, "Life in all its fullness is Mother Nature obeyed." [19] More than anything, before we can begin to heal, we need first to understand our connection to the soil and the food it produces. Once we understand this, we will be able to understand why we are in the condition we're in…and perhaps learn to honor the ancient, sacred path that takes us from the soil to the stomach. ❖

---

19 Price, p. 419.

6

Trees, Earth, Water, & Air

I LIVE IN AN OLD HAYLOFT. A couple of giant linden trees, a silver maple, two red maples, a mulberry, and a Chinese elm extend their lacy boughs onto the third-floor deck that surrounds my loft. Just out of reach are a few river birch, spruce, cedars, pines, a magnolia, and a mountain ash. So close are these leafy neighbors that, at times, it seems I am living in the trees.

Living up here has opened a small window into the tree community, introducing me to the domestic habits of birds, squirrels, butterflies, beetles, cicadas, moths, and several families of tiny organisms that create bumple-sized dwellings on the undersides of leaves.

Over the years, I have become more and more interested in my tree neighbors and their daily lives. Trees are master alchemists who transform the gifts of sun, wind, and water into wood. Wood is a marvelous substance! We use it as fuel to keep us warm, for building boats, homes, garages, picnic tables, telephone poles, and a myriad of other things from rake handles to hairbrushes. Too often we think of trees as useful only after they have been cut down. But the gifts from living trees are far more important and useful than those from dead trees.

Viktor Schauberger, born in 1885, was a brilliant scientist who spent much of his life in the wilderness areas of Austria studying trees, water, air, their relationships, and the motion of the subtle living energies in them. He once calculated that by the time a tree is 100 years old...

...it has processed the carbon dioxide in 18 million cubic meters of air and fixed it as 2,500 kg of pure carbon in the form of wood

...it has *photochemically* converted 9,100 kg of carbon dioxide and 3,700 liters of water

...it has made 6,600 kg of molecular oxygen available for humans and animals

...working against the forces of gravity, it has drawn 2,500 tons of water in through its roots, up the trunk, and through the branches of the tree to its crown where it evaporates into the atmosphere for recycling and, therefore, purifying

... it has supplied one member of society with enough oxygen for 20 years. [20]

Trees are not just part-time producers of oxygen for us on this planet, they are the *major* producers. The question that no one is asking yet is, "Who will dispose of our excess carbon dioxide and supply us with oxygen when all the trees are gone?" The ocean absorbs some carbon dioxide, but would it be enough?

Trees are a key player in the water cycle here on earth and another good question is, "Who will make sure we have enough drinking water when the trees are gone and the water table sinks?" Once again, the ocean is full of water, but it's not drinkable.

If we believe that the government will take care of these problems, or that we can turn our need for oxygen into a manufacturing business and let some commercial supplier sell it in return for money, our existence here will be considerably shorter and more miserable. It would be foolish to set ourselves up to buy and sell oxygen when Mother Nature makes it and gives it to us for free. We have already made the mistake of buying and selling mineral rights, water, and land when they could have been ours for free.

Oxygen is one of the most powerful antibiotics in the entire world, and already the amount of available oxygen in our world has gone down drastically. Ice cores extracted from glaciers at the poles were analyzed to

---

20 Callum Coates, *Living Energies* (Bath, UK: Gateway Books, 1996) p. 216.

see what the make-up of our atmosphere was in the past. To the surprise of the scientists, the amount of available oxygen in the atmosphere used to be almost 50% higher than it is today.[21] [22] Some estimate that oxygen was as high as 38% of the atmosphere. Today, it is around 20%, even lower in some places on the globe, and those who have asthma or lung problems have a much more difficult time getting enough of this critically important element.

When I hear news programs talk about the destruction of the rain forests and its supposed effect on the ozone layer, I wonder why no one ever says anything about the decreasing amount of available oxygen and the increasing numbers of human beings who need that oxygen. The decline in oxygen, combined with the degenerative narrowing of noses and lungs, has led to a steep increase in breathing difficulties. Even more tragic is the increase of infections, cancers, and other problems, many of which heal when exposed to higher levels of oxygen.

Building an environment that will support all plant and animal life, trees patiently create layer upon layer of topsoil, year after year. During the growing season, they send roots deep into the subsoil, and even into the deep rock layer. A good gauge of how deep the roots of a tree go is to look at how high the tree grows. Although some trees are shallower than others and prefer to spread their roots out laterally, there is often as much or more mass below ground as there is above ground.

Tree roots tunneling their way through subsoil and rock create a small mineral-mining operation. As with all plants, tree roots work their way deeply into the earth where they release mild acids from their root hairs. These acids dissolve tiny amounts of minerals from soil and rock and transport them up the tree where they are used to build the trunk, the branches, and thousands of thick, sturdy leaves. Each autumn these leaves fall to the ground, creating a fresh deposit of organically-mined minerals on the surface of the soil.

This layer of dead leaves offers fresh roofing material for an entire community of worms and six-legged "others" who make their homes under anything that provides a sense of shelter. Yet in a quirk of Nature,

---

21 Bio/Tech News, 1998.

22 http://www.npl.washington.edu/av/altvw27.html

the worms and insects end up eating the house! Worms consider leaves to be an extraordinary delicacy and will make their way through a leaf pile with great relish, digesting the carbon-based green matter and leaving behind a trail of mineral-rich worm castings. Insects, micro-organisms, bacteria, fungi, and mycorrhiza breed and die among the fallen leaves, creating the dark, moist, living mass that builds slowly over time into a thick, luxurious, organic topsoil, known as humus. This mineral-rich humus becomes the perfect soil for plants, which then produce delicious, high nutrition food for us.[23]

This same layer of loosely stacked humus also works as a layer of insulation over the surface of the earth, keeping the roots of trees cool and moist, which promotes healthy trees and a good water supply. When the surface of the earth is kept cool and porous, rainwater will easily penetrate and begin to sink into the soil. This is the beginning of the atmosphere-to-earth-to-atmosphere cycle that produces living water.

When I was a girl, I heard an ancient prediction. It went something like, "Long ago, God destroyed the world with water, but then made a pact with Noah not to do that again. The next time God destroys the world it will be with fire."

As we cut trees by the thousands, the soil heats up and dries out, the atmosphere becomes dry and dusty, the water table drops, and the timber turns to tinder. One stray match or lightning strike can turn whole regions into smoke and charcoal.

The world does not need to burn in one great conflagration for the old prediction to be true. All it takes is one drought after the next, followed by repeated fires in one region or another, until one day we look around and say, "Gee, I don't want to live there…it's too hot…not enough rain… nothing will grow there…too dry…there's too much danger of fire…their water is too expensive…they ran out of water…"

While listening to National Public Radio one day, I was astounded to hear a news report of a family in New Jersey preparing for a party, only to discover an hour beforehand that their well had run dry. They ran a hose

---

23 Martin and Gershuny, p. 29-46.

from their neighbor's house to supply water during the party, but their shock at having to face this problem was obvious.

This may be just the tip of the water-shortage iceberg coming toward us. Even if we never have a full-blown water crisis, we certainly have a crisis of ignorance based on the fact that very few people truly understand water or that there is a big difference between *mature*, living water and *immature* water, also known as dead water.

Viktor Schauberger was the first to discover the difference between the two. He came to the conclusion that living water was born, developed to maturity, and sought to change itself into higher forms of energy. After watching the poor results from crops watered with what he called dead, "immature" or "juvenile" water, Schauberger spent years trying to teach people that water matures only when it is allowed to move through its full cycle, called the hydrological cycle.

This cycle begins when water evaporates into the atmosphere. Once aloft, it is carried by the wind until the temperature of the air cools enough to cause the condensation we call rain.

This rain then falls to earth among the trees, sinks through the topsoil, and moves down into the deeper layers of soil and rock. These deep layers of soil are kept cool because of the shade provided by the trees, and the cool temperatures help keep the soil porous. As the rain sinks down through the cool root zone of the trees, the water loses temperature rapidly at first. It continues its descent into the earth until it reaches a level where the pressure coming up from within the earth is equal to the weight of water pressure in the atmosphere. At this point, pressure and heat from deep in the earth begin to warm the water and some of it becomes steam.

The hot steam then binds with carbon in the soil and a chemical reaction takes place: carbon-plus-steam changes to carbon dioxide-plus-hydrogen gas ($C + 2 H_2O \Rightarrow CO_2 + 2 H_2$).

Now the hot hydrogen gas begins to rise upwards again. As it pushes its way upward through the soil, it reacts with the minerals in stones, rocks, and other material in the soil, dissolving a variety of these minerals into itself and carrying these as mineral salts upward toward the surface. As the rising hydrogen gas reaches the cool zone maintained by deep tree roots, these cooler temperatures create an internal motion in the hydrogen molecules that is characterized by a left-hand spin. Known as *centripetal motion*, this motion is very magnetic. The result of this magnetism is that the hydrogen seeks out oxygen and bonds with it, now creating water molecules that have an internal centripetal spin. Water with an internal spin moving in a left-hand direction is known as *mature, living water.*[24]

As this living water continues to move up through the root zone of the trees, some of the mineral salts precipitate out and are deposited in the root regions to become nutrients for the trees and other vegetation. In this way, trees and plants are fed via a slow-growth, mineral-rich system that results in good health for the trees and superior quality wood for building projects.

Only when the water reaches the surface on its own and enters streams, rivers, artesian springs, or pours or drips from other natural sources is it considered ready to be used for drinking and irrigation. When kept cool and moving in rivers and streams, this potent and energetically beneficial water will remain alive and well. Those plants, animals, and people who drink it will maintain strong, stable, energetic, and healthy physical systems. The sick who drink it will be slowly returned to good health.

Schauberger deplored the pumping of "immature" water from deep in the earth to be held in pipes and tanks. He discovered that if water was pumped from the earth before it had risen to the surface on its own, it did not have the internal centripetal motion that was critical to life. Instead, its internal spin was *centrifugal* and was characterized by a right-hand spin, which he described as a "disintegrating, dissipative, destructive, or outwardly exploding force" used by Nature to speed the break-down and dissolution of systems to be recycled. This was just the opposite of the centripetal, magnetic motion used by Nature to attract and hold the particles necessary to build up life-forms and maintain their shape, strength, vitality, and function.[25]

In our present-day world, we do not allow water to come to the surface naturally. Instead, we dig deep wells and pump it forcefully to

---

24 Olof Alexandersson, *Living Water* (Bath, UK; Gateway Books, 1996) p. 55-77.

25 Alexandersson, p. 56 .

the surface. Once there, we hold it quietly in tanks and pipes where it is forced to stop moving and allowed to become warm. Warming has a very poor effect on water because it is another factor causing the water's internal motion to change from centripetal to centrifugal, thus going from magnetic (form-building) to explosive (form-destroying).

As water loses its natural magnetism and becomes dissipative, it begins to throw off its precious load of minerals and trace elements, which is why pipes and plumbing so often become clogged with mineral deposits.

When coupled with the other degenerative pressures of our time, water that is dead, immature, and dissipative contributes to our reduced life span of a mere 70 years. This is a shame when it is fairly well known that human life should be between 120 and 160 years. Scientists are now saying that the cells of the body have no known limits to their ability to continue living and reproducing.

Living water turns out to be water that has matured until it acquires a left-hand spin with natural magnetism. This only happens when it is allowed to pass through the full atmosphere-to-earth-to-atmosphere cycle.

Once it has risen to Earth's surface, it must continue moving in the naturally spiraling ways that are characteristic of living water. Photographs of the inside of a drop of living water reveal extraordinary structure and order in what appear to be whole sets of currents, waterfalls, and oceans of motion inside the molecules, all of which the water uses to maintain itself while carrying the gift of nutrients to plants, animals, and people.

Immature water has not passed through the full hydrological cycle that moves it from atmosphere-to-earth-to-atmosphere. Dead water is that which has been captured in tanks and pipelines where it warms and loses its subtle, life-building, centripetal motion. Whether you call it immature or dead water, its inner motion is sluggish, centrifugal, explosive, and carries few nutrients to the living beings who drink it.

For many of us alive today, water is water. Our education has left us woefully unschooled in Nature's classroom. Said Schauberger, "Water in its natural state shows us how it wishes to flow, so we should follow its wishes." [26]

---

26 Alexandersson, p. 34.

Those twisting, turning, snakelike bends that we see in every natural river course are the water's way of constructing its own path to maintain its high-energy spiral motion. When we straighten out a river, we ruin that motion. When we cut the trees along the banks and eliminate shade, water warms up and becomes lazy. Instead of spiraling along in a manner that literally and continuously excavates its own deep and narrow river courses with a range of temperatures to spur its motion, warm water stops spiraling, gets shallow and spreads out, then slows down and gets muddy.

As pointed out earlier, when we cut too many trees from the land, surface soil heats up, microorganisms die, and the soil collapses. Falling rain cannot sink in deeply. Instead it runs across the surface, carrying topsoil with it. Most of that topsoil ends up in the river, choking the waterways and filling in the channel the river is constantly trying to dig out for itself.

The bottom line is that when water does not sink deeply into the earth, we end up with water that has not passed through the entire water cycle. The water table slowly drops, and there is less fresh water to drink. We end up drinking dead water with centrifugal energies that explode our good health. We water the plants in our garden with dead water and wonder why we're fighting fungus and mildew all season long. The missing minerals and energies that should have been in the water contribute to plants that are structurally weak. In the same way that we use calcium, magnesium, iron, and other minerals to build good, strong bones, plants use the same minerals to build strong, healthy leaves and stems. Without these minerals, they are highly susceptible to the same decays, molds, mildews, and rots that we are.

In the same way that we have been ignorant of the fact that the soil is alive, most of us don't know that water is alive. We didn't know that when we captured water out of the rivers and underground reservoirs, forcing it into pipes, tanks, and drainage ditches, that we were interfering with the internal energies it used to sustain itself and us. We didn't know about water's maturity and powerful abilities to build living forms.

Schauberger predicted the day when a barrel of water would sell for more than a barrel of oil, and he was right. These days a 55-gallon barrel of oil runs between $65 and $100. We pay between $1.50 and $4.00 for a quart of good mineral water. That puts the cost of the water somewhere between $330.00 and $880.00 per barrel!

Schauberger's favorite saying points the path for all of us: "Study Nature and then copy Her." [27]

When I was married, my husband and I had a beautiful chalet in the forests of northern Michigan. When the wind blew with quite a bit of force, you could hear it, and you could see the tops of the tallest trees moving, but on the ground the air was quiet and still.

When it rained, it had to rain long enough and hard enough for water to get to the "through-fall" stage where it actually reached the ground because so much was collected by the trees first. Mud puddles were rare because the soil was so absorbent, and I thought it was my imagination that things rarely got dusty. Later, when I began to study trees, I discovered that 3,000 feet inside the edge of a forest, the trees will have cleaned, sifted, and filtered the air to a sparkling, dust-free state. This, combined with the cool, moist, oxygenated air, made it easier to breathe. My husband's asthma eased greatly, fatigue disappeared, and we were left feeling energized.

When we bought our farm in 1987, there were woefully few trees on the property, which had been farmed for years and sprayed half to death. Each year, we planted at least a dozen more trees in an attempt to restore our little corner of the earth. We celebrated each tree that survived, encouraging it to keep growing with doses of living water.

A full-size tree has been estimated to have as many as 100,000 growing tips on it, and research now suggests that each tip is a unique genetic individual. Cutting a branch off a *deciduous* tree in order to graft it or re-root it elsewhere has occasionally resulted in the growth of an *evergreen* tree. When a mammal produces seed, all the seeds come from within that one body. But when a tree produces seed, each seed comes from a different flower – which may have picked up genes from something in the air, the rain, something carried on a visiting insect, or perhaps it was responding to a unique set of micro-climate conditions on one side of a tree. It is possible that a tree is a collection of compatible genetic individuals, each with a set of persistent characteristics differing from place to place on the tree and responding to changing energies and other stimuli. Cutting

27 Alexandersson, p. 34.

down trees in wholesale fashion destroys 100,000 possibilities for genetic adaptation with every tree that loses to the saw. [28]

If you look back in time just a bit, you will see that for thousands of years, our leafy allies stood quietly on mountainsides, holding on to the soil, keeping it from sliding away and piling itself onto villages below. Trees that didn't mind wet feet stood at the edges of the sea to catch waves that came with great storms. Those trees kept the land from being washed away. Great swamps formed at land's end and whole trees went down in them, becoming huge masses of absorbent carbon to hold water. This created unique neighborhoods for a whole new assortment of flying, crawling, swimming creatures, and an even more varied collection of water-loving plants, flowers, vines, and bushes.

Today, mudslides and floods are a year-round problem. We build dams and dikes costing billions of dollars and tell ourselves we have "created jobs," when a more accurate perception is that we have only ruined Mother Nature and made more work for ourselves. When it comes right down to it, we could not find enough men and money to do the work that trees do, and if we could, the quality of their work would not even come close to the expertise and quality of the work done by trees.

When I drive along certain streets just outside our community, there are huge residential lots with big, expensive houses on them. They have $10,000 worth of landscaping around the foundation and deck of these houses, with a few young trees planted in the yard, some deciduous and some evergreen.

The evergreen trees, which collect and then radiate heat, are often clustered around the air conditioning unit because the wide branches at the base of the tree hide the ugly unit from the street or the neighbors. It would make more sense to shade the compressor unit with a tree that offers shade, rather than one that radiates the heat right back at the compressor, but too often we do things only for looks.

On any hot, summer day the sprinkler system in these yards will be on, watering trees, flowers, and bushes, and it is clear we no longer know or care what young trees need. Trees are extremely sensitive to light and heat. In the forest, young trees that grow to maturity under the shady

---

28 Mollison, p. 139.

protection of the mother trees are healthiest, strongest, straightest. They produce the best wood when grown slowly in cool, diffuse light. Their annual tree rings will be small and close together, which helps the wood maintain its shape when turned into lumber. Their trunks are wide at the bottom and taper nicely to the top, a shape that is essential for the tree's good health. Those with smooth bark prefer dim light and will often be found in the center of the forest. Those with rough or shaggy bark will be okay in the sun at the edge of the tree line.

When shade-loving trees are grown in full sun, their temperature rises, and this is equivalent to being in a "fevered" state. Their internal metabolism is disrupted, and they may be unable to fight invasion by parasites, fungi, or bacteria.

When trees sitting in full sun are watered with dead or immature water, they grow too quickly and their annual rings become widely spaced and corky instead of tight and compact. This results in a weak tree that is not only susceptible to disease, it may suffer violent damage, the loss of limbs, or even uprooting during periods of high wind or ice storms.

When grown in the sun, trunks tend to be straight, round cylinders from bottom to top rather than wide at the bottom and tapering upward. Yet this tapering shape is the key form by which a tree maintains the high-energy metabolism it needs to continue developing, to transport minerals and nutrients all the way up, and to stay healthy throughout its life.

Industry prefers the quick-growing, cylindrical trunks of modern tree farms, but much of the wood is weak, twists out of shape when dried in the kiln, and rots too quickly at the lumberyard. It is ironic that a tree that has stood outside through winter snows, summer rains, spring winds, and numerous temperature changes must now be sheltered from all these once it gets to the lumberyard lest it rot before it is incorporated into a house and sheltered by aluminum or vinyl siding.

My mother worked in a lumberyard when I was a girl, and I remember running and climbing among huge piles of pine and oak that sat outside all year. Nowadays, if you leave piles of wood outside for any length of time, they curl up enough to be suitable only for the bottoms of rocking chairs.

Besides its preference for light and shade, each tree has a personality expressed in its patterns of shape, color, the texture of its bark, and personal rhythms for leafing out, flowering, or closing down as winter approaches. Each has its own sound, expressed by the movement of wind through branches that are plentiful, sparse, tightly compacted, or widely spread.

The trees outside my loft also have a language of sounds by which they send messages to those who are listening. There is the soft hissing sound that is heard at the start of a light summer shower when you can't yet see or feel the first drops of rain. There is the soft soughing sound that pines make when the winds of spring arrive and there will be no more severe winter storms. Once in a while, they have great roaring conversations with a gale wind who comes by to prune dead or weakened limbs. I also overhear shimmery, rustling conversations among them, sometimes strain to hear their whispers, and at times, am in awe of their towering silence. How can anything be so huge and so quiet, like a patient giant standing outside my door?

Once I had a conversation with a tree. I asked if it had anything to add to what I was writing about it.

"Yes," it replied, "the very page from which your words rise is a transformed tree, sacrificed to make paper. Why don't you people learn to communicate and leave us alone?"

Needless to say, my shock was complete. Suddenly, I was aware that every piece of paper, every book, card, or letter expressed the silent voice of the tree from which it had been made. The tree's thoughts, hopes, and presence were woven among the words we placed upon that paper. How many trees had given their lives that we might send letters, invoices, greeting cards, newspapers, and advertisements back and forth and then into the wastebasket?

When I go into the city, I am appalled at the thin, sickly-looking trees growing in small, cement squares along the edges of sidewalks or marooned in an ocean of asphalt laid down to make a parking lot.

"Look at those poor trees," I once said to a friend. "Why did they even bother to plant them in this kind of environment?"

"People like trees," she said, "they like a little greenery."

"But what about the trees?" I asked.

"What about them?" she replied with a small shrug. It was an eloquent testament to the divorce that took place between humans and Nature generations ago, and it also points to the direction we must begin to move. As Schauberger once believed, and I now agree, we will only be able to achieve stability in the world if we immediately return to honoring our soil, water, and forests. What's more, we will not be able to evolve ourselves and our technology wisely in order to join others in the cosmos without aligning ourselves with life and studying Mother Nature, for she holds all the secrets to an advanced understanding of plasma physics and beyond.

Sometimes, I look out across the field and see the ghosts of lost trees, thousands of them. The place I live in – an old barn – was built with a framework of tall, strong tree trunks. The bark is still on some of them. I wonder if the family who built this barn gave any thought to replacing the sixteen trees they cut from the woods and planted among cement and stones to stand for at least a hundred years holding up the small forest of rafters, roof boards, and siding that makes this a barn.

Whether they did or not, it is time for us to begin thinking about such things. Umbrellas in a light rain…specialists in chemical manufacture… modifiers of the wind…end posts on a hammock… monkey bars to a five-year-old…landlord to 10,000 "others"…the tree is a world in itself, a living being that literally makes it possible for us to live, breathe, and share this time and place with it and each other. ❖

7
Somatids, Plasma, and the Electric Body

IN ORDER FOR YOU TO REBUILD AND HEAL yourself at a deep level, it is helpful to expand your knowledge of key aspects of the body. These aspects involve *somatids, plasma*, and you as an electrical system. Let's begin with somatids.

Plants, animals, and people are meant to be supremely healthy. In the same way that a mother cat will kill an unhealthy runt in her litter, or that insects will attack and take down plants that are unhealthy and emitting out-of-tune frequencies because they do not have a full spectrum of minerals and other forms of nutrition, humans are subject to the same kind of natural law. The work of a French-born scientist truly brought this home in a powerful way.

Gaston Naessens was a scientist living in Quebec who developed a powerful microscope capable of magnifying things more than 30,000x, Using this tool, Naessens discovered a "hitherto unknown sub-celluar, living and reproducing ultra-microscopic form, which he christened a *somatid* (tiny body)." [29]

He found that these tiny, living forms could be cultured in vitro and were observed to be indestructible! In addition to resisting 200° C temperatures, 50,0000 rems of nuclear radiation, and all forms of acid, they also exhibited a hardness that foiled all attempts to cut them with any tool, including a diamond knife. "The eerie implication is that the new

---

29 *The Persecution and Trial of Gaston Naessens*, Christopher Bird, HJ Kramer, Inc.; Tiburon, CA. 1991. p. 4-5

minuscule life forms revealed by Naessens's microscope are imperishable. At the death of their hosts, such as ourselves, the somatids return to the earth where they live on for thousands or millions, perhaps billions, of years."[30]

As it turns out, Naessens was not the first scientist to observe these tiny forms of life. In the 1800s, Pierre Antoine Bechamp, a contemporary of Louis Pasteur, noted "a host of tiny bodies in his fermenting solutions" and called them *microzymas* (tiny ferments) that were able to catalyze strong fermentation reactions, a process that breaks down complex molecules into basic organic compounds.

Bechamp noted that these microzymas "did not appear to exist in chemically pure calcium carbonate made in a laboratory, however, they were abundantly present in *natural* calcium carbonate, commonly known as *chalk*. For this reason, the latter could, for instance, easily 'invert' cane sugar solutions, while the former could not." After studying these tiny forms for many years, Bechamp concluded that they "were far more basic to life than cells, long considered to be the basic building blocks of all living matter." So seemingly indestructible were the microzymas that Bechamp could even find them in "limestone dating to the Tertiary...a period going back sixty million years, during which mammals began to make their appearance on earth." [31]

When Naessens discovered these tiny forms, his microscope was just powerful enough to allow him to observe their behavior closely. What he saw was that in a healthy human, somatids went through successive stages of development – somatid, then spore, then double spore – and these three stages were crucial to life in all organisms – plant, animal, and human. However, when the immune system became unhealthy, the somatids began to degenerate through thirteen additional stages.

The ability of a physical form to change shape, function, and the way it will reproduce is called *pleomorphism*. When it comes to the somatid, as each stage devolves into the next, conditions in the body worsen, creating an assortment of pathological conditions and diseases. In fact, both Bechamp and Naessens found that when conditions in the

---

30 Ibid, p. 5.

31 Ibid, p. 7-8.

body were less than ideal, the somatids became highly active and went to work to disintegrate the body of their host, converting themselves into viruses, bacteria, various forms of yeast, and finally to mycelial (cancer-like) forms.

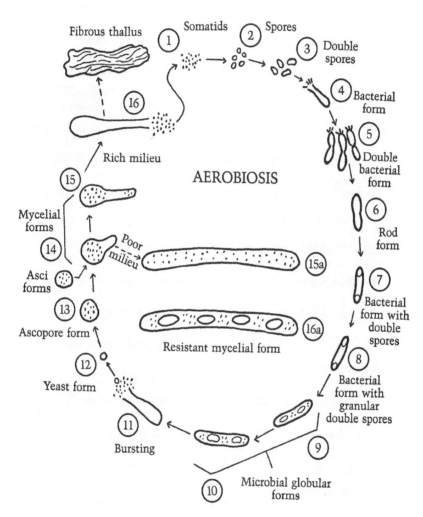

Today we know a lot more about the way somatids degenerate. They create a viral-bacterial-yeast-like fungus that migrates into cells and then into the cell nucleus. Once there, they release acidic waste products called *mycotoxins*. Mycotoxins interfere with the immune system functions, inhibiting both cell repair and tumor-suppressor genes. Without tumor suppressor genes, *proto*-oncogenes will turn into *full-blown* oncogenes, causing cancer.

The key point in all this is that we have been taught to think that viruses and bacteria come from somewhere "out there" and we should try to protect ourselves from these invaders. The truth is that these "invaders" are the results of various stages of physical degeneration and are serving the same function as insects in the world of plants – to destroy the imperfect, unsustainable, damaged, or malfunctioning form of life.

Viruses and bacteria are symptoms of a degenerating human that is disintegrating from the inside. To pretend that they come to us from outside the body and then douse ourselves with chemicals while ignoring the need for superior nutrition is utter ignorance of how things really work. Viruses and bacteria are warnings to us that we are not healthy and resilient enough to sustain ourselves as living beings.

Here is a statement that I will repeat again later: *the body is a collection of plasmas that exist in an electric universe*. It is important that we understand what this means for healing and health.

Plasma was originally described as a "gas with particles in it." It was probably described that way because scientists could not see the electromagnetic field holding the particles in place. They could see the particles, and since no solid or liquid was present, they assumed that the particles were floating in a cloud of gas. When they disturbed the particles, they observed that the particles kept returning to their original configuration. What they did not yet understand was that the particles were held in place by a field of electromagnetic energy! So let's have a short course in electricity. When electrons move along a path, you get a current of electricity:

Whenever you have a current of electricity, a magnetic field will form around the current at right angles to the direction the electrons are moving:

Once a magnetic field forms, it will tend to develop filaments. We call these filaments "magnetic lines of force." Particles then collect along these filaments and are held in place because the particles have an electric charge and so do the filaments. That is why the particles return to their original configuration if someone disturbs them. It's a matter of electrical charges being in effect. Here is a picture of plasma in the raw and its filaments:

Here we see that plasma also forms spirals, sheets, and intricate patterns, all of which are very common:

Here are some common patterns that appear in plasma:

It is plasma that determines the shape of our physical stuff:

Everything in our world and our universe is made of an assortment of plasmas, and the arrangement of these plasmas holding our particles in place is what determines the shape, coloration, and function of the physical matter that forms in the 3-dimensional world.

The conclusions you can draw from all of the above are;

- When you have motion, you will have wave action, also known as frequencies.
- When you have wave action, you will have particles.
- When you have particles, you will have electric currents caused by moving particles.
- When you have electric currents, you will have magnetic fields that form and wrap around the current.
- When you have the formation of magnetic fields, you will have the development of filamentation.
- When you have filamentation, you will collect particles along those filaments.

- When you have particles held along filaments, you will end up with plasmas of varying patterns.
- When you have particles held in patterns by electromagnetic relationships, you have the basic framework for the construction of a unique form of matter.
- The basic framework of all matter is plasma patterns formed by the interactions of the electric charge of particles and the electric charge of filaments.
- All frequencies interact in dynamically constructive, destructive, or reproductive ways. Constructive interactions enhance and support one another. Destructive interactions cause one or both frequencies to decay. Reproductive interaction creates new or novel frequencies known as binaural frequencies, or even trinaural or quadnaural frequencies and beyond.
- All things from the tiniest microbe to the biggest galaxy are collections of currents, their magnetic fields, their interactions, and the plasmas that result from such.
- You and I are collections of currents, magnetic fields, and plasmas.
- Consciousness and intelligence are embedded in frequencies and particles and become more complex as the pattern becomes more complex.
- As demonstrated in the lab of Dr. Wm. Levengood, plasma responds directly to consciousness.[32]
- Because we are constructed of various configurations of plasma that respond to consciousness, we are self-organizing, self-repairing, and self-directed. [33]

Dr. Wm. Levengood discovered that the human being was a set of plasmas with each organ and type of tissue having its own frequency signature. The total set of frequencies in an individual is called their "frequency signature" or "frequency print." The overall signature of each individual is unique, like a thumbprint of sorts.

---

32 *Consciousness and Energy, Vol. 2: New Worlds of Energy*, Penny Kelly, Lily Hill Publishing, 2012. p. 198-202.

33 Ibid, p. 107-110.

Dr. Mehran Keshe, another scientist studying and working with plasma, defines plasma very simply as a "house of fields." In other words, it's a region of space that is chockful of currents and their electromagnetic fields.

Since the body is a collection of plasmas, you can think of your body as a house of electromagnetic fields created by the numerous electrical currents that run through and maintain it. There are many different kinds of matter that make up the body: skin, hair, heart, muscle, bone, liver, kidney, lung, pancreas, stomach, teeth, fascia, eye, fingernail, brain, glands, fluids, colon, spleen, nerves, valves, and more. Each of these types of matter is the result of a unique plasma...which is a unique arrangement of frequencies, fields, filaments, and the particles they collect.

When a frequency is missing or you have extra frequencies courtesy of viruses, bacteria, parasites, or toxins, important biological and chemical reactions may not occur or may occur only partially. When your frequencies get "out of tune," you will not feel well. When your frequencies get seriously out of tune, you will age. When enough of your frequencies die out, so will you.

Healing and the ability to become an eternal being is based on the ability to reset your frequencies to their original rates. The understanding that every individual human is a small electric universe explains many things. In the future, the ability to restore individual frequency signatures will allow us to bring someone "back to life."

All chemical reactions are the result of changes in the electrical and magnetic forces. A change in your electrical currents, fields, or frequencies causes changes in the plasma that makes up the chemicals. *Chemistry follows frequency.* This means that frequencies are primary. Frequencies control chemical production and reactions.

Using frequencies and plasma we can erase a disease by erasing the frequencies that produce the disease. Dr. Todd Ovokaitys, M.D. is using frequencies to restore enlarged hearts to normal size and function, ending their congestive heart failure. He pairs two complementary frequencies that wrap around one another forming a cable. Then, in the open spaces created between the intertwining frequencies, he embeds a third frequency that brings the heart back to good health.

Using frequencies to restore or reorganize plasma, we can erase tumors, stimulate the natural rebuilding of missing arms and legs, change the mindset or consciousness of an individual, find an individual signature of someone anywhere in space and time.

Understanding plasma and frequencies makes it possible to reverse the aging process in a plant, animal, or human. We can enhance the germination process in seeds, and increase plant health, vigor, rate of growth and productivity. We can also make a copy of the plasma frequency signature of any food or substance, then infuse that signature into water and use that water to nourish or to heal.

Using frequencies and plasma we can manufacture materials out of "thin air" by duplicating their plasma structures and configurations in ways similar to the ways we now duplicate chemical structures.

As mentioned above, research has shown that plasma responds directly to consciousness. Why is this possible? Because consciousness is a characteristic of moving energy, and moving energy consists of currents, fields, and frequencies. Consciousness *is* the energy in motion that makes up our world. This means that everything in our world is alive, conscious, and intelligent.

❖

Taking what we have said so far about somatids, plasma, and the fact that everything is based on frequencies vibrating in an electric universe, a non-negotiable aspect of healing is exercise. You NEED to exercise if you want to get well or feel energetic, calm, and centered. Why? Because *exercise produces electricity in the body* and this electricity not only maintains the electromagnetic fields that hold your particles in place, it drives the millions of chemical transactions that define your body and who you become.

As pointed out above, chemistry follows frequency and this means that if you do not have a given frequency in your energy body, you are not able to produce a specific plasma and its resulting physical material or processes that the frequency makes possible. The result is that the chemical transaction does not take place and you end up with a disease, a dysfunction, or disability of some kind.

There is an informative video that I think everyone should have to watch. It is a lecture by Dr. Jerry Tennant MD, ND who explains voltage in the body, how the body produces and stores electricity, and why you can't function or even begin to heal without it. The title is *Healing is Voltage* and can be found at the following link:

https://www.youtube.com/watch?v=pm-Ia6vI4PA&t=1750s

Says Tennant, "The big muscles are the body's battery packs, and the fascia (connective tissues) are the transmission lines." When an organ or part of the body develops a problem, it is almost always because the muscle that supplies that organ cannot hold a charge. The task then is to find out why. All too often it's because of lack of movement. There is not enough stretching, walking, lifting, etc. Or maybe there is suddenly too much movement resulting in too much electricity and you blow a fuse, so to speak, which doesn't get reset. How do you know if you have too little or too much electrical activity? Your pH will tell you.

Your pH is a measure of electrical conductivity and is a scale of measurement that runs from 0 to 14. If your pH measures somewhere between 1 and 6.5, not enough electrical activity is going on. We say 'you are too acid' or you're 'running too cold'. The result is that there will be too few chemical transactions happening because there is not enough electrical energy to make them happen. All of the necessary nutrients can be present in a system whether you are talking about a physical body, a soil system, or a petri dish, but without the necessary electrical activity, not much happens.

If your pH is somewhere between 7.5 and 14, you have too much electrical activity going on. We say 'you are too alkaline' or you're 'running too hot'. The result is that the production of chemicals may not have time to form, or that their transactions are occurring so rapidly that the structures these chemicals are meant to sustain or renew cannot get the benefit of the transaction because the transaction is over too quickly. A good analogy might be the ability to smell the food, but that is not enough to restore you. When you want to heal quickly, bumping yourself into alkalinity with its barrage of transactions can be a good thing, but as an ongoing state, it creates its own difficulties in the form of weak systems and lack of stamina.

The electrical flows through the body can create enough pressure to blow or short the transmission lines and create a blackout in an area of the body. The organs, tissues, and glands will try to carry on for awhile, but eventually a problem appears because something in that area is starving for information and the electricity that carries the waveforms that then shape the physical matter. We are finely tuned human beings and the best range of pH is between 6.8 and 7.2.

As mentioned above, good electrical flow is created and maintained by exercise. The exercise need not be excessive. A pair of 6-pound hand weights lifted into the air above your head 7-8 times once a day are enough to make a big difference. Add a few "arm curls" in which you move the weights back and forth from hip to shoulder and there is enough upper arm electricity generated to rebuild the muscles in your arms.

Walking has an extraordinary effect on the entire body. Bending to touch your toes 7 or 8 times, or stretching to reach toward the ceiling – each of these is extremely helpful in generating electrical activity that regenerates your battery packs – the big muscles. Anything that twists the spine from head to hip is going to maintain youthful movement for life, including being able to move the head and neck freely.

In closing this section on exercise, I want to point out something about aging that many people don't know or think about until it's too late. Imagine your body and its bones as a structural framework similar to a modern day skyscraper. When building the skyscraper, builders put together a framework of steel I-beams and then hang all of the walls, ceilings, floors, plumbing, and electrical systems on that framework. The result is a modern building that is comfortable to work in.

The body is very similar. All of your organs, muscles, glands, and connective tissue are hung very artfully on the framework of your bones. This is a living framework that depends on you to maintain it through high-nutrition food, water, exercise, regular elimination, and a good supply of electricity. If you do not eat and drink what the body needs, there will be an inability to continuously rebuild, restore, and regenerate. If you do not eliminate or detox wastes, you will poison yourself from the inside out. And if you do not move pretty continuously, you will not generate the electrical activity that maintains the body structure and its energy.

If you stop moving, muscles deteriorate to the point that they are no longer able to hold the organs, glands, and other tissues in place. Everything sags and the organs and inner structures begin to fall toward the bottom of the body bag, causing numerous problems, cutting off one another's circulation and breathing room, and interfering with all function.

In a woman, the sagging and piling of tissues and organs in the bottom of the body can cause them to fall out through the vagina or anal opening. I remember my surprise when this happened to my mother. In a man, the same thing happens as tissues fall into and around the scrotum and anal opening. This is not good. I also recall the day of one of my children came home from work as a new hospital employee saying, "Mom, his junk was hanging in the toilet! How does that happen??" It happens because we do not continue to exercise enough to keep muscles strong and hold the electrical energy that keeps our system healthy with everything in its proper position. Once you lose muscle, it's difficult to maintain anything else. Why? Because muscles are the batteries that supply you with a steady flow of electrical energy. Once the energy body goes, the physical body will be right behind it.

We are part of an intelligent system of life, and this includes our planet and the entire cosmos. Mother Earth has systems, cycles, and processes of her own that keep her healthy and functioning. The soil, the atmosphere, the oceans, the mountains, the shift of seasons from cold to hot and back again, the electrical storms bringing rain and the cleaning effects of lightning, volcanoes, earthquakes, the sun, the wind, the rotation of the planet – all play important roles in the maintenance of our world and our health.

Remember Victor Schauberger's statement that water was intelligent and sought to build itself into ever more complex and intelligent systems of life? This is true of all living things from suns to planets to plants to animals to humans.

We take shape and form in an ocean of currents, fields, and frequencies that, all together, help us to maintain ourselves. We cannot remove ourselves from them without experiencing the effects of that withdrawal. We cannot introduce foreign currents, fields, and frequencies into our environment without experiencing the effects of those insertions. The last thing we want to do is cause traumatic effects that destroy or severely alter the human energy system. We cannot tolerate or generate destructive interference of the fields of plasma that hold us together, or that trigger the somatids to begin moving through the thirteen stages of degeneration that are designed to disintegrate the human body when it moves too far from good health.

Your entire body, indeed, the entire cosmos, is a vast living system of intelligence that is based on cooperative communication with an end goal of creating superior beings, forms, systems, and processes that can sustain themselves and reproduce life forever. In the next chapter, we will go a little deeper into the connections between body and earth. ❖

8
Building the Human Body

YOU HAVE PROBABLY HEARD THE PHRASE, "Thou art dust and unto dust thou shall return." What dust are we talking about here? We are talking about mineral dust – the fine dust of calcium, magnesium, potassium, copper, manganese, nitrogen, sulfur, phosphorus, and many other earth elements. We are made of the same stuff Mother Earth is made of and this is the reason we are known as "earthlings". We are subject to laws of nature that do not care about things like cost, logic, or what is currently fashionable. If we violate nature's laws, we will pay the price in pain, depressive moods, and early death.

To get healthy again, it is helpful to understand at least a little about how you are constructed. I have tried to include as much of this kind of information as possible because it is especially helpful as we talk later about what steps to take to begin rebuilding your body to a state of good health.

Let's revisit what we discussed in an earlier chapter – the fact that the human being is an electric being. The question is, *How do we go from an electric being to a material being?*

The electrical currents that flow through the body are accompanied by electromagnetic (EM) fields that surround the currents. These EM fields develop filaments, and then particles tend to collect along the filaments. It is this combination of the electric currents keeping the EM field in place, the EM field developing filaments, and the tendency of particles to collect along these filaments that creates a basic pattern for the development of physical matter. The number of currents, their frequency, the strength of their EM field, the number and arrangement of filaments, and the collection of particles along these filaments creates a soup of extraordinary possibilities because the variety of arrangements is exponentially huge and the number of interactions between and among these particles is even greater. You can get some idea of the immense diversity of the primordial soup when you consider the immense numbers of currents, fields, filaments, and particle line-ups that exist and give rise to whole galaxies, solar systems, humanoid beings and the millions of cells they are composed of. They are all constructed following the same principles and laws.

To get a better sense of how these amazing fields are translated into a physical human, imagine a couple of currents that are moving through space and that spiral around one another like the double helix.

Then imagine that the space between those currents creates an electromagnetic field that is fairly strong and stable. There is actually an electromagnetic field all around the spiraling pair, but the field that is directly between the two spiraling currents is the most stable. The filaments in this area end up attracting and holding elements like carbon, hydrogen, nitrogen, and oxygen that arrange themselves in a variety of patterns to form the 5 bases: guanine, cytosine, adenine, thymine, and uracil.

Guanine, cytosine, adenine, and thymine are the four bases used in DNA.

Guanine, cytosine, adenine and uracil are the four bases used in RNA.

One base, plus one sugar molecule, plus one molecule of phosphoric acid combine to form a nucleotide. A sequence of three nucleotides then come together to form a codon. The codon contains an initiation codon, a function codon, and a termination codon. Together these three form a unit of genetic code that makes up a DNA or RNA molecule. Each codon codes for one specific amino acid. The code determines the order in which amino acids are put together to build a protein chain during protein synthesis. Simply put, the genetic code dictates the sequence of amino acids in a protein.

Initiation codons signal the first amino acid to be used in the synthesis of a protein chain, which is simply a string of aminos. Either AUG (adenine, uracil, guanine) or GUG (guanine, uracil, guanine) is used as a "start" codon. Termination codons tell when to stop assembling the amino acids in a protein chain.

Codons use minerals freely and if a specific mineral or trace mineral is not available, the start and stop codons will not work. The needed protein is never built, or once started, the chain continues to build in a chaotic manner and becomes nonsense with the result that the protein does not work correctly.

> ### *From Element to Matter*
>
> *1. A base (G,C,T,A, or U) + sugar + phosphoric acid = nucleotide*
> *2. Set of 3 nucleotides =*
> *3. Codon =*
> *4. Set of 3 codons made up of an Initiation codon, a Function Codon, and a Termination Codon = a piece of genetic code called DNA or RNA*
> *5. To be noted: EM fields, minerals, and amino acids are critical ingredients in the process of building bodies.*

I think it is some very interesting symbolism that the body is made of a lot of chains – long chain fats, short chain fats, peptide chains, polypeptide chains, amino chains, protein chains, and many other chains. The reason they all have different names is based on how long they are. For instance, a peptide chain has from 2-50 amino acids linked in a chain. A polypeptide chain has more than 50 amino acids linked together. A protein is composed of very long chains of amino acids. All of your cells are made up of various kinds of proteins. Proteins make up the basic structures of the body, for example, muscle, hair, collagen, enzymes, antibodies, etc.

An amino acid is a highly active organic compound containing an amino group (NH2) on one side of the structure and a carboxyl group (COOH) on the other side. These two groups are then paired with any of a number of what are called function groups (CHR), each one responsible for a specific kind of action in the body.

Basic Structure of Amino Acids

Amino group
NH$_2$

Carboxyl group
COOH

Function group, where **R** can be any of a number of elements or another group, making the amino acid unique.

Why is all of this important? Several reasons.

1. Because you need to know how you are built and how you operate.

2. Because when I say there is a priority of order in taking supplements, it helps you to understand why aminos and minerals are so critical, and why it is useless to spend money on vitamins if you're not getting the basic aminos and minerals.

3. Because when I say that exercise is absolutely critical in regenerating yourself, you will understand that it is movement that generates the electrical currents that help you get well again.

4. Because I want to emphasize the pathway that takes us from electric current to electromagnetic field to filamentation patterns, to a collection of particle elements that then gather along the filaments and organize into nucleotides. The nucleotides then form codons, the codons group themselves into start, stop, and function codons...the codons dictate the sequence of amino acids...that make up the peptides and polypeptides... that then make up the proteins...that then become your cells.

Each of us is a tiny electric universe! ❖

*Part 2*_____

Real Food

9
Food for the Masses

FOOD, THE MOST BASIC OF NECESSITIES, seems to be everywhere in America. Everywhere you go, you see it, or at least the suggestion that you can get it quickly and easily, with little work or distraction. This illusion of plenty is exactly that, an illusion, existing mostly in First World countries. In the entire history of humans upon the earth, no other single factor has commanded such continual reckoning with as the issue of food.

For thousands of years, we were pulled to the soil, anchored by it, yoked to it. Favorite plots of ground were chosen along big rivers that flooded every spring, depositing an annual dose of natural fertilizers in the form of silts that left the soil rich and fertile. If the river changed course or the land became exhausted, we moved on to a fresh place, leaving the old location fallow and allowing it to renew itself.

Back then, we did not have complex scientific descriptions of what went on in the soil, but even in our less scientific stages we knew the soil was alive. We sang to it, danced over it, sweet-talking, coaxing it to produce, and it did because it was alive and healthy!

Early men and women learned quickly that healthy, nourishing food brimming with nutrition was the key to survival and their ability to reproduce without problems. Food wasn't just something to put in the stomach or titillate the tongue. Those without superior nutrition did not survive. Without high levels of nutrition, babies were born weak or deformed, young people became irritable and unwilling or unable to participate in the work that was necessary to keep the group alive. Adults succumbed too soon to difficult conditions, illness, or infections. Whole settlements arose then disappeared when high quality nutrition was unavailable.

Those who survived followed daily routines designed to assure themselves of the best nature had to offer in terms of nutrients. The goal was to maintain radiant health. No tribe could be hampered by a child that needed constant doctoring. Nomadic families could not afford to haul around members who couldn't keep pace with them, and no group could afford to constantly support members who did not contribute to the group itself. More importantly, no one wanted to *be* the sick one, the cripple, or the incapable one. It was frustrating to be unable to keep up with the group and perform like everyone else.

A huge difference between those early families and the families of today is that the early ones knew the power and importance of good food, and we do not. They knew which foods were needed to create and maintain superior health, and they knew where and how to get that food regardless of the terrain they lived in. Much of this wisdom has been lost over the past several hundred years with the rise of the Industrial Revolution.

By the time the 17th century had come and gone, machinery and other laborsaving devices were proliferating rapidly across Europe, luring us away from the soil. Perhaps we were attracted by the endless amount of work the machines could do, by their tirelessness, or the sheer power they exhibited. Maybe we were bored after thousands of years of plowing and planting. Whatever it was, we were fascinated with things that tick and click or whirr and pound. Because of this, machine culture began to flourish side-by-side with agriculture, and the idea of an easier life was probably as mesmerizing as it was naïve.

Early pilgrims who came to America were looking for spiritual freedom – but the rich, fertile soil they found was a nice bonus. Perhaps it never occurred to them that the famines following crop failures and the miserable health conditions in European cities were deeply connected to the decline of soils and falling levels of nutrition in the foods that were available there.

Neither has it occurred to anyone today that America's Founding Fathers were able to imagine a place like America, then come up with the strength and energy to build such a place because they were eating food grown in the living soil that was everywhere here, at least in the beginning. Today, we barely have enough energy to change jobs let alone envision, start, and win a revolution.

The Real Costs of Poor Health

If you don't want to bother learning to feed yourself differently, then you don't really want to heal yourself. Expecting someone to give you a pill or cut out your parts and make you magically better is childish, irresponsible, and doesn't get to the source of your problem. This kind of expectation is like demanding that others do for you what you are unwilling to do for yourself. The medical doctors I know well would love to have patients who would take responsibility for doing those things that will enhance the body's efforts to heal itself *and* who are realistic about what the M.D. can offer. To start a true healing process, it's almost a given that you will have to change your diet to real, whole, organic food.

If you think you cannot afford whole, high-nutrition, organic foods, get out a piece of paper and pencil and add up the monthly cost of the following items:

What you spend on groceries each month	_____
Eating out: breakfast, lunches, and dinners	_____
The cost of your medical insurance	_____
The cost of your dental insurance	_____
Orthodontic work for you and your children	_____
The cost of your vision insurance	_____
Glasses, contact lenses, lens cleaning supplies	_____
Co-pay amounts not covered by insurance	_____
The cost of specialists you must see	_____
Alternative health practitioners you visit	_____
Prescription medicines & drugs you must buy	_____
Over-the-counter cold and flu medicines	_____
Over-the-counter arthritis medicines	_____

Over-the-counter allergy medicines   _____

Over-the-counter asthma medicines   _____

Over-the-counter digestive upset medicines   _____

Psychological counseling   _____

Special education/tutoring for ADHD children _____

Sick days off – due to fatigue or illness   _____

Vitamins and minerals you buy   _____

Herbal supplements you buy   _____

The cost of enzymes and digestive aids   _____

Aspirin, dry skin lotions, toothpaste, deodorants, and make-up to cover up your headaches, bad skin, bad breath and poor body odor   _____

The cost of poor productivity that results from irritability and tension in family relationships   _____

The cost of nursing home services for your elderly parents   _____

The cost of special shoes, clothing, chairs, canes, braces, walkers, beds, stairs, showers, tubs, toilets, etc.   _____

The cost of special diets for allergies, illness, weight loss, etc.   _____

The cost/membership fees of weight loss centers or groups   _____

The cost of extra clothing that must be maintained as weight goes up and down   _____

The cost of physical therapy programs   _____

The cost of gyms, aerobic programs, or exercise programs to lose weight   _____

The cost of gasoline to get to doctors, clinics, gyms, and therapies of any kind   _____

The cost of hotel and motel rooms or alternative sleeping arrangements for family during hospital care   _____

The cost of days lost at work so you could
stay home and take care of a sick family
member   _____

      TOTAL COST OF POOR HEALTH   _____

Now, take a really good look at these costs and the total. This should do several things. First, it should give you a fair idea of what you could really afford to spend on *good* food.

Second, it should make you see the amount of time, energy, and money you spend compensating for mediocre-to-poor health. We could carry the argument for high nutrition food even further by adding in the costs of a job that you take just so you can have medical benefits that you know you need because of poor health. In that case, you could legitimately add the cost of special work clothes, a car to drive to the job, gasoline, mileage, insurance, the need to hire someone to clean, cook, or cut the grass because you no longer have time, the cost of child care, the potential increase in food costs because of a greater reliance on convenience foods, and anything else associated with the job.

Third, ask yourself, "To what degree do the costs and activities in this list seem normal?" The more normal they seem, the more caught you are in the thinking produced by our current food system. What could you be doing with that same time, energy, and money if you were perfectly healthy and free to do whatever you wanted? Would you read more… tinker in your workshop…take swimming lessons…make love…sew, knit, quilt, or crochet more…invent things…go hiking…have a child…build something…take a trip to a place you've always wanted to visit…write a book…go dancing…cook gourmet meals…grow roses…visit antique shops…sit in the back yard and enjoy a peaceful afternoon…attend the theater or a rodeo…see a live basketball game…join a yoga or meditation group…work one job instead of two…allow one spouse to quit work and stay home?

Lastly, can you even imagine being supremely healthy – or would this leave you feeling left out of the circle of family, friends, and coworkers who are struggling with illness, fatigue, the effects of degeneration, and catastrophic disease? What would you talk about if you didn't have your own complaints and physical difficulties to add to the general conversation that goes on around you every day?

The important lesson in all of this is: don't tell yourself that you can't afford good, whole, high-nutrition food because I'm going to turn that around and tell you emphatically that you can't afford *not* to buy good food! If you can't afford to buy it, then grow it. It is the absence of this kind of food that leads to illness or disease in the first place. Bacteria and viruses are not at fault; they are important members of the physical family with the job of breaking down old carbon-based matter and recycling it for further use. When there is a fall-off of high level immune function, our cells devolve into lower forms of expression that we call bacteria or viruses, and we appear to have a disease with specific symptoms. Bacteria and viruses are the *result* of disease, not the cause of it. [34]

Your genes are not at fault. Genes are triggered into action – or fail to be triggered into action – by the subtle frequency waves given off by molecules of vitamins, minerals, and enzymes in your food. Those who blame our genes for illness are akin to those who blame rape victims for being raped. Genes are not the problem. Genes that do not work properly are the result of poor nutrition.

This is not to say that those doing research into our genes are misguided or wasting their time, for there is much to be learned; and if you step back far enough to get a bigger picture, you will see a definite civilizational goal among human beings to recognize and understand the hidden details of life and creation.

We are extremely creative beings searching for new and exciting yet practical applications of the Source Energy from which we all come. We know there is a Source. That is not in question. But what are the possibilities of that Source? What can we become? Who knows what we can learn to do, to correct, to create, refine, and re-create if we understand the fine points of what makes us tick? I love science, I love the physical world we live in. I love the *meta*-physical worlds of spirit and energy, and I love having a creative life myself. My concern at this point is that we may not survive as a group to continue exploring and creating if we do not correct the way we feed ourselves.

---

34 Christopher Bird, *The Persecution and Trial of Gaston Naessens* (Tiburon, CA: HJ Kramer Inc, 1991) p. 4-11.

Chemical Agriculture is Born

In the same way that Weston Price and his peers were struggling with the deluge of degenerative diseases that appeared in humans between 1900 and 1950, difficulties in animal breeding and crop production caught the attention of veterinarians and agricultural scientists. Animals were also suffering from a host of degenerative diseases, and plants were being attacked by insects and fungus everywhere.

A few men, like Dr. Charles Northern and William Albrecht, Professor of Agronomy at the University of Missouri, had been seriously encouraging farmers to put great effort into re-mineralizing and restoring soils to once again become living soils. However, by the mid 1950s they were working against the rising tide of big business and chemical corporations that entered the world of agriculture after World War II.

During the war, a number of chemical engineering companies had produced and stockpiled tons of chemicals for making bombs. When the war ended, they were left with no markets for these chemicals. Then they discovered agriculture. People were leaving farms and moving to the cities, looking for jobs and big money. As farm families fractured, there were not enough hands to do the work. With falling crop production, increasing pressure from pests and diseases, rising numbers of people in the world who expected someone else to grow the food they needed, and an American self-image as a sort of "food savior" to the world, agriculture was ripe for an influx of chemicals.

Within a very short time, chemical companies were using the stockpiled bomb chemicals to make NPK fertilizers. Use of these fertilizers caused further imbalances in soils and plants, which then necessitated pesticides, herbicides, and finally fungicides. Soon these chemicals were being developed by the thousands. Chemical salesmen went out across the country, peddling these potions to farmers and convincing the agriculture departments of many universities that they needed to recommend these chemical concoctions to the farmers in the area. When department heads showed resistance, large sums of money were given to the university to "help" with research that would prove the usefulness of the chemicals.

Before long, a whole new generation of young farmers – all university trained – began using chemicals for everything from plant growth to insect, weed, and disease control. The traditional wisdom of constantly restoring the soil was abandoned as old-fashioned.

Once NPK fertilizers were in widespread use, farmers no longer needed animals for the rich manure that had been composted and applied to soils. The animals were sold off. Once the animals were gone, the animal barns were no longer needed and fell into disrepair.

The new, young farmers bought big tractors and big equipment, plowed under the pastures, orchards, and gardens once used to grow a variety of healthy feeds for cows, horses, and chickens, then planted everything to a single crop. The farm, once a closely related community of plants, animals, and people that was self-sufficient and self-maintaining, began to disintegrate. Instead of tending a lot of little crops whose incomes and losses served to balance each other over the course of a year and prevent a catastrophic loss, the farmer now went into high-risk debt, gambling that he could make enough money from a single crop large enough to sell in the world export markets. However, once into the export markets, he lost control of what he could charge. Instead of going up, the farmer's income dropped, and now he had huge debts whose payments had to be deferred "until harvest."

Trying to make a few more dollars, he sold every ounce of grain he had produced, failing to hold enough seed in reserve for the next year. It was easy to believe the chemical salesman's claim that he could purchase better seed the following year, seed that would supposedly germinate faster, resist more diseases, produce a bigger crop, and make him more money.

Instead, caught up in corporate-style agriculture, many farmers couldn't make the payments and lost the entire farm, which was then bought up by corporate-style managers who were not interested in restoring soils, and who knew little or nothing about raising high-nutrition foods. They were interested in getting a crop to market in the cheapest, quickest manner possible, and getting paid.

Today, many farmers use chemicals and poisons because they don't know how to raise food any other way. They are doing what *their* fathers did, and since their fathers were the early chemical farmers, that's all they know. The old ways of maintaining healthy livestock in order to continuously restore the soil have been lost. Many farmers no longer know how to take care of animals, barns are expensive to build, physical labor is no longer fashionable, and families no longer live and work together, partly because no one knows how to get along with one another and partly because the lure of big money in other careers entices the young ones away to the cities.

Specialization has become the way of most farming today. Some raise beef or hogs, some raise wheat, some raise fruit, others raise cabbage, or chickens. As farming fractured into hundreds of specialty practices, it became more and more difficult to see the whole picture.

When a single farmer is raising corn, beef, chickens, fruit, and everything else he eats and needs, he isn't interested in doing something that will be bad for one part of his operation even if he thinks it would be good for another part of the operation.

When you can't see the whole, it's easy to let go of the little practices that maintain balance. They no longer seem important or necessary or related to what you're doing. Today, we have a situation in which it's every man for himself, and the wheat farmer doesn't care what the beef farmer needs, nor does the beef or pork farmer pay attention to what the chicken or the fruit farmer needs. And none of them seem to know or understand what the human being needs.

Real farming has long been one of the most demanding professions there is. Among other things, it requires you to be a scientist, keenly observant naturalist, animal breeder, weatherman, veterinarian, animal mid-wife, plant breeder, machine operator, machine repairman, carpenter, bookkeeper, manager, entrepreneur, and physical laborer, as well as your own source of self-discipline, motivation, and ongoing self-education. Few people are interested in farming to begin with, and when they discover how many diverse skills and talents are required, they go elsewhere looking for easier jobs.

Today, foods and farming have gotten caught up in the mass-market mindset of industrial production and competition. Foods are now handled in ways similar to clothing and fashion design. Every year new "food concepts" are carefully created, designed, packaged, and presented at big conventions attended by salesmen who buy for the big grocery store chains, mini-marts, gas station chains, and small independent stores. The hope is always that something in this year's line-up will be a hit, become a fad, and then move into the category where it is thought of as a staple in American kitchens. The problem is that these new foods are not really foods. They contain a few skeletalized or chemicalized remains of what might have been food at one time, mixed up with sugar, food coloring, and artificial flavoring agents. They have pretty boxes or wrappers presenting pictures that look like food, and sometimes they smell like food. You can eat them as if they are food, but they aren't *real* food capable of rebuilding and restoring bodies. They are pretend foods used to make money in the annual money-making competitions of the industrial markets.

Competition implies a lack of caring for the other guy. When we stop caring for others, society shatters. When the goal is to make money, that's one thing. When the goal is to feed yourself, that's another thing. And when the aim is to feed yourself in ways that sustain you in excellent health, that's something else altogether.

❖

A Little Food Education

I grew up in the thumb area of Michigan in a large family. My grandmother lived to be 100 years old, and her father – my great-grandfather – lived to 101 years old. Grandma gave birth to 14 healthy children, raised them all, and until she was in her mid-80s, she continued to live on her farm and raise or grow her own food. She took chicken, beef, butter, milk, and vegetables to her friends in town who were 20 years younger and already confined to beds or wheelchairs with poor health, giving them "heck for thinking they were old and useless." When she left the farm, she traveled the world for some years, then settled down in her house in town, where she stayed until her mid-90s.

For a long time, I expected that my parents and I would live to be very old, just like my grandparents and great-grandparents. Then my father discovered he had cancer. He survived that, but died at the age of 69 from congestive heart failure, a complicating factor of emphysema. I was already suffering from rheumatoid arthritis before he died. My husband was suffering from severe asthma and had long ago been diagnosed with chronic obstructive pulmonary disease. For five years, he was barely able to drag himself to work during the winter because it was almost impossible for him to breathe in cold weather.

My husband and I were in our mid-40s at that time, and it was clear that at our present rate of deterioration, we might not make it any further than my father. I looked at the extraordinary good health of my immediate ancestors and felt I had to begin learning how to heal myself. What I have learned came too late to help my father, but it was not too late to help myself or my husband, the rest of the family, and many others as well.

When I ask people who attend my classes what they know about food in general, the answers they give are excellent examples of the extreme misinformation and confusion that most people have about food today. They try to tell me that "meat is taboo, especially red meat…and vegetarianism is in…soy is good…fat is the culprit in heart disease…milk is the cause of sinus problems, asthma, allergies, mucus, and ear-nose-and-throat infections…eggs, cheese, and fat are the source of both high cholesterol and heart problems…whereas milk, wheat, beans, and peanuts cause life-threatening allergies or gastrointestinal upsets..." They never mention sugar or inflammation from poor nutrition!

When I started studying nutrition and came across the work of Weston Price, I stacked my grandmother's good health and life-long diet on top of Price's information and asked myself, "How is it that our ancestors were as healthy as they were when they ate all kinds of meat, fat, milk, cheese, eggs, and grains without cancers, heart disease, allergies, high cholesterol, and numerous forms of food intolerance?"

I had been mostly vegetarian and had not been drinking milk for over ten years at the time I came down with rheumatoid arthritis. I was also keeping up with all the latest articles on what we should be eating and was diligently applying these guidelines to my life. But observations of my grandmother's life and the things I was learning about real nutrition were lining up in direct opposition to what was being printed in popular magazines. Real food seemed to be a complete contradiction to what was advertised on television or announced on the boxes and labels of the many foods I purchased.

If you are getting your education about food from the magazines that fill grocery store shelves, you will end up going in circles and not knowing what to eat and what to avoid. Someone says eat lots of this, and someone else says eat lots of that, while someone new contradicts both of them. If you are basing your decision of what to eat on the information circulating in the popular culture, you are going to end up in a physically degenerated condition because no one is writing or talking about real food or the fact that there is not enough nutrition in whatever food is out there. Everyone is grasping at straws.

To make matters worse, researchers are hired by companies to "validate" certain products and are paid handsomely to come to specific conclusions that help marketing and advertising departments sell the new foods by creating false beliefs.

In some cases, early researchers drew erroneous conclusions that did not hold up over time. A good many doctors, as well as scientists and researchers, looking through the original research of their peers barely glanced at the methodology and numbers. They read only the abstract or conclusions at the end of the research, adopting these conclusions without ever evaluating the actual research methodology and numbers, thus spreading the misinformation. Everyone was assuming that others had read and carefully evaluated the actual research, which was not the case. [35]

People writing for magazines were also not reading the original research that had been done in various studies; they were only reading what other popular press writers had written. Everyone was perpetuating the circle of misinformation until it became entrenched as dogma. Food processing industries grew up based on the demands of people who had been supplied with serious misinformation.

I ran into this dilemma when I decided to try writing articles for the popular press. Pieces that focused on what I had learned about food and health were quickly rejected. Finally, I was told by one editor, who wanted to use part of one article and cut out all the relevant pieces, that they did not want to print something that would make their advertisers look bad, and that every health magazine had doctors, nutritionists, and advisors on their boards who were vested in the present system.

❖

---

35   Sally Fallon, *The Oiling of America*, a lecture given in 1998.

There is no more destructive idea in the culture today than the idea that you can live, thrive, and stay healthy on "manufactured" foods. You may get by for a while, you may survive for a time eating foods that are empty of nutrition, but you will not feel well during that survival, you will not perform well, and you will not last very long before something in the body/mind system gives out. Certainly, the last thing you want to do is trigger your family weak spot. For some families the weak spot is multiple sclerosis, for some it is high blood pressure, cancer, or a weak heart. In others, it is schizophrenia or manic-depressive disorder, perhaps a tendency toward weak lungs or kidney disease.

Once you trigger the illness that runs in your family, it is not a simple case of eating better, taking a few vitamins or herbs, and expecting to recover. You must literally embark on a total rebuilding program in which you constantly supply yourself with top-quality nutrition at a rate of about four times the normal rates until all the poorly built cells that were constructed under the old nutritional program have died off and been replaced by new, healthy ones. My own personal experience has been that a big improvement can be made in one year, but if you stick with it for three to five years, you will end up rebuilding your entire body/mind system to the point that some people may not recognize you.

You are not destined to be sick, ill, or suffer from degenerative disease. If you give the body what it needs to constantly repair and rebuild itself, then good health is the normal state of affairs, healing is a natural process, and high energy and longevity are the results. Your body knows how to heal itself. You just need to know how to support its efforts to do so. Good food is the foundation of any healing program.

You have a choice between feeding yourself with mass-produced, factory food, or *real* food. Real food has been taking a bashing, and a great deal of misunderstanding has been circulating in this country for years. Real foods seldom cause diseases and allergies. After all, we thrived on these foods for 10,000 years and are supremely adapted to them.

For example, lots of people in this country will tell you they are allergic to wheat. But what we are eating is not really wheat. It is a highly over-processed, skeletonized, bleached-out version of what was once whole wheat. Almost all of the vitamins, minerals, amino acids, natural oils, subtle metabolic co-factors, and digestive enzymes have been removed. The result is a useless substance that irritates the body, thus, the apparent "allergy to wheat." When you add in the destruction of the microbiome in millions of people due to antibiotic use and failure to eat the kinds of things that maintain the correct bacteria in the gut, the results are tragic. This tragedy also extends to many other foods and are made worse by heavy metals and a an assortment of other hostile substances that are sprayed on our food.

Real food is whole and full of living enzymes. Science has never been able to synthesize enzymes because it has never learned to synthesize life. Living food is full of organic vitamins and minerals. The key word here is *organic*. Lots of manufacturers are fully aware that food processing strips food of important nutrients, so they add a few vitamins and minerals back into the foods they process. But the vitamins and minerals that a manufacturer puts into a food item are *inorganic* and not at all the same as the vitamins and minerals that the processing took out.

When a food plant such as a green bean produces sulfur (a mineral) or a cantaloupe produces retinol (vitamin A), these minerals and vitamins are *organic*, which means they are sized, shaped, and ready for use in a living body. They are *absorbable*. They also have additional subtle co-factors and wave energies in them that work synergistically with all of the other nutrient factors in that food. The body welcomes these food nutrients immediately and uses them easily. Our ancestors lived to advanced ages in a healthy condition on all kinds of meats, fats, milks, cheeses, eggs, grains, along with a huge variety of vegetables and fruits.

The body has a great deal of difficulty utilizing inorganic minerals and chemically synthesized vitamins because these molecules are too big, or are oddly shaped, or they do not have the subtle frequencies and electromagnetic energies that produce the dozens of secondary effects that help coordinate the full power of the metabolic reaction the body is trying to organize and carry out. A good analogy here might be the difference between trying to build a fire with dry, seasoned wood, and trying to build a fire with wet wood. The wood is still wood whether wet or dry, and it will burn eventually, but in the meantime the warming effect of the fire is greatly reduced. You may have to use a lot of paper, cardboard, or kindling to keep it going, and there is a lot of smoke that clouds the air, as well as creosote that clogs the chimney with unused combustible products.

The body *will* try to use artificial foods with their inorganic minerals and synthetic vitamins – not to mention the food coloring, chemical preservatives, flavoring agents, pesticide residues, and heavy metals, but the results are less than optimum and there are a lot of wastes and lost energy that clutter up the system.

A few people in my classes have tried to insist that our ancestors did not live to advanced ages in a healthy condition. They have tried to tell me that life expectancy has never been higher than it is today here in the U.S. and a few other First World countries. They have tried to get me to accept the idea that our ancestors were ignorant primitives that lived to the age of 35 then died miserably. The truth is that there *have* been periods of time when we died too soon *and* periods of time when we have lived to ripe old ages. When the Industrial Revolution began, we set forces in motion that played havoc with our health. Those who stayed on the farms or close to the land did not suffer the poor health of those in the cities where life expectancy dropped and the misery index skyrocketed.

If you have been narrowly educated in public schools and believe that the only history that counts is the Western white man's version…if you think that First World countries have the best way of life and Third World people are ignorant savages…if you believe that you know more and know better (rather than knowing *differently*) than those who came before you….if you are looking only at the last few hundred years of the Western white man's history…then learning more and more about real food will probably cause some serious perceptual upsets.

As our European ancestors were coaxed off their land to work in the first factories, the need arose to provide them with food. As people began moving into cities to be near the factories of the Industrial Revolution, their diets suffered and so did their immune systems. As the Industrial Revolution spread, physical, mental, emotional, and spiritual health plummeted along with longevity.

Gone was the high resistance to disease and infections. Bubonic plague, known as the Black Death, accompanied this transition from country to city, from good food to poor food. The plague swept across Europe and wiped out half of the population. Many others died early, miserable deaths from measles, smallpox, cholera, tuberculosis, and pneumonia. We have been trying to recover our health security ever since.

People like to say we are living longer than we were two or three hundred years ago because it makes them feel better. But before the Industrial Revolution, before the days of big machinery, large cities, and gigantic factories, those who evolved stable cultures, good food supplies, and cooperative societies tended to live very long, useful lives, healthy and alert to the end. It was a frequently observed fact that old European women who emigrated to America in the early 1900s, but kept their former ways of raising food, cooking, and eating, often ended up healthy and strong to the age of 100 or more while they nursed and then buried their much younger daughters who had adopted the white-flour/white-sugar diet of the New World.

Somewhere along the line, in an effort to keep food flowing into the cities, Europeans began adopting a diet of white flour, white sugar, canned vegetables, jams and jellies, alcohol, and sweets. Perhaps remnants of such a diet survived from Rome to blossom once more in the courts of Marseilles and London. And who knows where Rome may have gotten such haute cuisine, maybe from Egypt or even Babylon? Diets live and die along with the people who adopt them as eating habits.

European missionaries carried the white man's diet around the world, becoming a potent wedge between people and the healing lifestyles they had evolved over thousands of years. Everywhere they went, disruption of indigenous lives followed. People who lived in close relationship to the land, who loved the land, who depended on the continuation of their feeding traditions for maintenance of their high immunity, were suddenly forced out of their sustaining routines, into schools and churches, and onto barren soils. They were fed Western foods right along with Western culture and religion. The result was confusion, disease, psychological malaise, and death everywhere the missionaries went.

Today we do not have missionaries to contend with, we have marketing departments. A great deal of misinformation has been generated by over-enthusiastic marketing programs designed to get sales moving for a product that just isn't selling. Once the misinformation gets out there, we build on it, creating a labyrinth of wrong turns in terms of our diet. If we do not correct this, we simply will not survive. ❖

10

Real Food

AS I WRITE THESE WORDS I am 73 years of age, which is still on the young side in my view! I do not take any kind of medication, I have recovered from arthritis, a variety of cysts and skin cancers, repaired my eyesight to an extraordinary degree, and stopped or at least slowed thinning hair. I still maintain excellent hearing, my ability to run or jump, and the same degree of flexibility I had when I was a kid. I work 12 to 16 hours a day, seven days a week, doing a wide range of physical, mental, emotional, and spiritual work, and seldom experience fatigue.

I eat a base diet of whole, organic foods, many of which I have grown, collected, or raised myself. I have not had fluoridated water for 33 years, take supplements as needed, follow regular detox routines as a form of healing and maintenance, and exercise as part of the daily work routine. Yet, I am not a purist in what I do here. Some days have no exercise. Some months are too busy for detox procedures. Some days include cake or cookies, potato chips and salsa, perhaps wine or beer, and I have not been willing to give up ice cream entirely. Yet, the mainstay of my base diet is so nutritious that I do quite well with an occasional excursion into the world of goodies and junk food.

I have come to expect that I will have prodigious amounts of energy, that I will feel good a majority of the time, and that colds, flu, or other illness and disease will pass by without affecting me. When I do eat foods from "the outside," I can tell by the immediate dip in my energy and mood that I have eaten empty food. If I keep it up too long, I may have a blunt reminder of one of the weak points in my physical system. Since I know how to recognize the very early signs of a problem and also know how to correct for that problem, I am willing to risk eating a few things that I know are not very good for me. Perhaps I might do even better for much longer in life if I was more purist in my eating, but humans do not live by bread alone.

I have family, friends, and visitors that do not understand why I work as long and hard as I do to produce my own food. Many have asked me why I don't just take it easy and go to the store. The fact is that I do go to the store for lots of things, but I have several reasons for growing my own food.

First, I learned from an old chiropractor who was a great healer, "Sometimes the easy way is not so easy after a while." The grocery store may be easy when you're young, have money, and are healthy. But if you drink fluoridated water and continue to eat manufactured foods without nutrition, you will age quickly, suffer serious degeneration, and soon life is not so easy any more.

Second, I want *real* food, the tried-and-true kind that our ancestors depended on, and you can't get that from the junk-food or even the grocery store. Real food is food that comes straight from the garden, the field, or the animal without a lot of processing.

Third, vegetables and fruits are grown in soil where many kinds of bacteria live, including staphylococcus and streptococcus organisms. Since plants must defend themselves against these bacteria much like we have to, they produce factors called *pacifarins* as their protective defense. When we eat the food grown locally and in our own gardens, these pacifarins are passed on to us and help protect us against the unique forms of staph, strep, and other antagonistic bacteria that exist in our local environment. Thus eating local foods is better for you than eating foods from half way around the globe.

Fourth, real food that is whole and unprocessed contains factors called *auxones*. These are factors are grown by Mother Nature and help you digest and absorb the specific vitamins, enzymes, co-vitamins, and co-enzymes that are contained in any given kind of food. In other words, foods that contain Vitamin A will have auxones that help you absorb and utilize that vitamin in the body. Foods with lots of Vitamin D will have auxones that help your body absorb and use that vitamin. The same is true of the other vitamins and minerals found in whole, unprocessed food.

For years, I grew, made, and baked as much of my own food as possible. I raised pasture-fed beef or bought it from someone who raises pasture-fed cows. I drank whole, unpasteurized milk and cream; churned my own butter; made my own yogurt and a few cheeses. I bought organic wheat directly from a farmer in North Dakota, ground the wheat and baked my own breads, muffins, and rolls before the natural oils in the flour turned rancid. My daughter and I raised our own chickens and enjoyed their eggs regularly. I grew corn, broccoli, peas, potatoes, tomatoes, celery, cabbage, cauliflower, Brussels sprouts, kohlrabi, radishes, onions, turnips, carrots, beans, beets, cucumbers, summer squash, butternut squash, pumpkins, zucchini, okra, ten different kinds of lettuce, cantaloupe, honeydew melon, watermelon, strawberries, and raspberries. I made my own catsup, vinegars, jams, jellies, pickles, and juice. I also grew almost two dozen culinary herbs, and collected a dozen other medicinal herbs that grew wild on our property.

What I didn't or couldn't grow here, like grapefruit, spelt, or lemons, I bought from other farmers across the U.S. who knew the value and power of real food and who made an effort to grow the highest quality food they could.

Then my life changed rather drastically, taking me with it! I no longer had the time, the help, or the support that is necessary to grow my own food. While this seemed like a terrible problem at first, I soon realized that it was an opportunity to experience the same kinds of challenges that most of the rest of the population was facing – where to get food offering the best nutrition! This forced me to fall back on what I knew about food quality.

The thing that is important to note here is that I don't always choose organic food. Instead, I look for signs of mature food that is fully developed. This will offer the best nutrition, and if it comes with the unwanted payload of chemical residues and heavy metals, I depend on my regular detox procedures to get rid of these.

You can tell quite a bit by the size, color, smell, and texture whether the nutrition is decent. When something has been picked too early, it will not reach its full nutritional potential or a mature color. The more intense the color, the better the quality of the nutrition. In addition, color also indicates the kinds of nutrition that will be found in something. Purple indicates proanthocyanidins. Yellow indicates Vitamin A, beta carotene, and iron, green often indicates sulfur, and all vegetables contain certain nutritional oils. The color difference between fully ripe and almost ripe is subtle, but if you know what to look for, you can spot the difference immediately. Another good indication of nutrition level is how heavy the food is. A bushel of top quality, nutrient-dense wheat weighs 62 lbs. A bushel of deficient, low nutrition wheat weighs 60 lbs; what seems like a minor difference makes all the difference in the world.

Another indicator of nutrition level is how much natural sweetness the fruit or vegetable has. How sweet something is can often be assessed by smell and sometimes by its outside texture. Again, something picked too early will never develop the natural sugars, scents, thin skins, and high-level nutrition it should have.

Knowing the natural size of produce is also helpful. Finding a gigantic peach on the grocery store shelf may impress you, but it may be just a bloated, dry, tough, and tasteless mass. If it doesn't have good color and you can't smell its perfume, it will probably be a very disappointing peach. If you paid a premium price because of its size, you have allowed yourself to be cheated.

A local butcher shop is a godsend as far as I'm concerned. I almost never buy meat from a grocery store because they can't tell me where that meat came from or who raised it. Farmers who are devoted to raising the best grass-fed beef, chicken, or pork can be found all across the U.S. They often sell to old-fashioned butcher shops in their area, and here in southwest Michigan, some will sell beef or pork "on the hoof." You can buy a whole, half, or quarter beef, or split it with someone you know who appreciates the low price and fabulous meat. You then specify how thick to cut the steaks, how many pounds of roast or hamburger to a package, whether you want the bones and tallow or not, and you will be notified to pick it up all cut, wrapped, and frozen.

Once in awhile, I get something at the grocery store that proves to be very low in quality once I get it home. Examples might be oranges or lemons that are almost completely dried up inside when I cut them open or a cucumber that turns moldy the day after purchase. If this is the case,

I take it back and ask for my money back. Most people don't think you can do this with food, but you can. And the message it sends to the buyer at the store is: "Don't try to sell me garbage. I'm not settling for that. Find better produce."

Really good stores go out of their way to find the things their customers love. If they are going to do this, however, they need to know what you like. Tell them! Communication is essential. If grocery stores are going to become suppliers of real food, they need to hear from you. When they respond to your requests, thank them.

When people discover that our food supply has almost no nutrition in it, they often feel angry, outraged, confused, or helpless. They begin blaming the government and various organizations for trapping them in an economy that does not value or understand the soil, agriculture, or the importance of high-nutrition food. They feel they're on a conveyor belt that will deliver them to the realms of poor and degenerating health where they will then be trapped by the pharmaceutical companies who demand outrageous prices for the drugs that will keep them alive. This attitude is not really helpful unless you consider the fact that anger is really "change energy" – the way we feel when we want something to change right now!

What is helpful is to realize that the government is run by a lot of people who are just like you and me. They're mostly trying to do their best, they don't want anyone to get sick from eating something "bad," and many actually believe that the best way to prevent this is to process the heck out of the food substance until there's absolutely nothing left in it that might cause a bad reaction in anyone. Unfortunately, there is then nothing left in the food in terms of nutrition – and the plan to make our food supply safer is now backfiring. People have degenerated so dramatically that immune systems are extremely fragile and can no longer handle irritants of any sort. By removing all the factors that might cause a reaction – the vitamins, minerals, fats, oils, and enzymes – the food becomes tasteless, colorless, and lacks texture. To restore the taste, color and texture, food processors add artificial vitamins, inorganic minerals, chemical colors and texturizers, white sugar or corn syrup to sweeten, and sometimes vegetable fats in the form of polyunsaturated oils. Since the body has no use for these, it simply does the best it can, but over time, the result is disaster.

A couple of years ago, I was teaching a class in *Getting Well Again, Naturally,* and a young woman in her late-20s was attending. For years, she had slowly begun avoiding one real food group after the next because everything she read in the popular press talked about how each was bad for you in one way or another. Now, she was having trouble with her weight, menstrual periods, headaches, irritation, depression, fatigue, constipation, and difficulty with concentration and focus.

As we talked about real food, about meats, milk, eggs, and cheese, about fats and cholesterol, grains, beans, nuts, vegetables, and fruits, she began to grasp the truth about real food.

At lunch, everyone from class was involved in animated conversation when I noticed her sitting in her chair, ignoring her food and staring off into the distance for some time.

"Are you all right?" I asked her, wondering if she was ill or somehow uncomfortable.

"My god…" she exclaimed, "…the vastness of the illusion around food…"

I knew instantly that she was seeing the misinformation, seeing straight through the myths and poor advice that had taken shape around food. All at once, the widespread ignorance about real food and the continuous marketing campaigns that push artificial, manufactured foods at us from every direction were clear and in perspective for her.

If you truly want to heal, one of the most important steps you can take is to return to real food. ❖

11
Meat

WHEN I FIRST STARTED to raise cows and chickens, it was because I wanted the manure for my vegetable garden. As was typical for those who have lost their connection to the soil and the food chain, it never occurred to me to think of these animals as food at first. When I ended up with 13 roosters in the first batch of chickens, and the cow I bought gave birth to a calf only three days after I brought her home, an old-time farmer across the road suggested I think about raising my own beef and chicken. I shied away from the idea for a while, but finally, with considerable trepidation, decided to learn how to kill and dress my own meat. I prepared long and deeply for the day, my tears falling freely. Yet nothing prepared me for the extraordinary differences between this meat and the meat I had purchased at the grocery store.

What I had raised with great love produced such tender, tasty, melt-in-your-mouth meat that I could hardly believe the difference. I hadn't done anything exotic or unusual with my animals. I just made sure there was plenty of pasture to run in, good grass and grazing for both cows and chickens, freedom to mingle, a few grains, and supplements to keep them healthy. I also refused to use hormones or antibiotics.

Asking an animal to give the gift of its life so that I could eat was a powerfully humbling experience that deepened my awareness of the value of life and made me acutely conscious of my interdependence with all things. It taught me to make sure that my animals had a good life while they were alive and to honor them and their needs because in the end, filling their needs filled mine. I have learned much.

The chickens run around their 1½ acre yard freely, scratching up crawling bugs, chasing flying insects (bugs and insects are high-protein foods), eating grasses and weeds (grasses and weeds are really herbal foods), and watching out for predators such as raccoons and chicken hawks. They come and go from the chicken coop, rest in the shade of the big hickory tree, mate freely, and defend their place in the pecking order with gusto. Every day I replenish their grains (usually corn, oats, and wheat) and water, sprinkling a little montmorillonite clay in both food and water to prevent salmonella in their wonderful eggs, which have bright, fluorescent-orange yolks.

When it is time to cull the flock, I kill them as quickly and cleanly as possible. With great care, I remove the oil sack back by the tail, then the intestines, being careful not to break them open for this would release bacteria and e-coli into the cavity of the bird. Then I scrub and rinse them, putting them into the freezer or the stockpot immediately.

In contrast, chickens raised in a commercial operation often spend a very short, miserable life in a wire cage that is roughly 5" x 8". They can't even turn around let alone run around. They eat synthetic feeds with low quality synthetic proteins in them. Their feed is supplemented with estrogen-based hormones to plump up their breast for market and antibiotics to keep them alive long enough to get to market. Their manure is carried off by one conveyor, and their pale, tasteless eggs are carried off by another. Often they are riddled with disease and cancers by the time they are sent to the food processor.

The processors kill the sick, stressed birds and put the carcass on a moving assembly line. There, a mechanical reamer will ream out the intestines, breaking them open and spreading bacteria all over the inside cavity of the bird. The processors think that any bacteria will be taken care of by rinsing the carcass in antibacterial solutions and irradiating the meat. But sometimes the antibacterial rinses kill only the most susceptible bacteria, leaving the more persistent and deadly to flourish and grow, and irradiation is very destructive to humans who eat the meat.

The meat itself is tough, rubbery, and tasteless. Besides the absence of nutrition, there are residues of whatever chemicals, heavy metals, antibiotics, and hormones the chicken ingested. The result is difficulty for us in digesting it. Food sensitivities and allergies appear in us; not because of the meat, but because our bodies do not like the chemicals or heavy metals in the meat. As for the estrogen-based hormones used to make chicken breasts nice and plump, I suspect that the white meat fad that spread across the country over the past decade has added more than a little pressure to the wave of estrogen-based breast cancers that began appearing in record numbers of women across the country, not to mention the early maturation of many young girls.

When you buy meat today you are never sure what you are going to get. But the chances are quite good that you will be buying something that was raised in a feedlot or cage and whose nutritional deficiencies were severe. Any animal raised in a nutritionally deficient environment is going to be nutritionally deficient food and will unbalance your own health and physical system.

Cows and pigs do very well living in the open on good grasses and pasture that has a wide spectrum of weeds (herbs) in it so they can doctor themselves by going after what their system needs. And they do a great job of this!

If you buy beef that shrinks by a third when you cook it, you have purchased meat from a cow that got too little calcium and too much potassium. Many farmers keep their cows in feedlots and buy feed that was fertilized with NPK fertilizers. Since calcium is so easily chemically-bound by other mineral factors when the soil is out of balance, newly growing grain will uptake potassium from the N-P-K in the soil, using it as a substitute for calcium.

When the cow eats this kind of grain, it gets heavy doses of potassium instead of the necessary calcium. This is especially true if the cow is already deficient in magnesium, selenium, and boron. For the cow, the result of too much potassium is a lush, watery, bloated body that looks like a solid weight gain. It makes the cow look big and healthy. This is a dangerous illusion because the cow is actually much more disease-prone than normal and very susceptible to insects and pathogens, which is why antibiotics and other drugs are routinely administered.

In the old days, before we started trying to rush the process, farmers raised cows on pasture grass, vegetables, hay, and plenty of mineral salts. This way of feeding created meat with great flavor and texture.

After slaughter and dressing, the sides of beef were allowed to hang in the cooler for two or three, even four, weeks. During this time, living enzymes (mainly cathepsin) in the muscle and tissue of the beef would go to work breaking down the tough muscle fibers. The longer these enzymes were allowed to work, the more tender the beef would become. The goal was to allow the enzymes to do a good job of breaking down fiber and tenderizing without allowing total disintegration of the meat. By the second and third weeks, someone would have to go into the cooler or ice house every day to wipe off the thin layer of fine bluish-white mold on the outside of the carcass. This simple care step prevented the meat from going bad while it tenderized. When the process was complete, the meat was melt-in-your-mouth tender, had retained the rich flavor of grass-fed beef, and was ready for your body to digest without undue exhaustion of digestive juices or enzymes.

Nowadays, cows are kept in small pens and feedlots where we try to fatten them quickly with corn and other grains. Cows that eat grain suffer from acid stomach, which upsets their digestion in the same way it disrupts ours. This also interferes with mineral absorption, and thus, the meat lacks texture and flavor. When the corn is potassium-laden instead of rich in calcium, their tissues swell with water.

When the cow appears to have gained enough weight, it is sent off to market where it is killed and then hung in a cooler for perhaps only a week before carving. During this period, the hanging beef loses quite a bit of water through evaporation. Meat packing companies won't let the meat hang long enough to really tenderize because it loses too much weight through this evaporation of water from tissues. Every pound of water loss cuts down the financial profit because beef is sold by the pound. Thus, ready or not, it is cut, wrapped, and sent off to market. When you buy it and cook it, the rest of the water evaporates, the meat shrinks, and what remains in the pan is tough, leathery, and tasteless. It is also difficult to chew, difficult to digest, and without the payload of nutrition that it should have had.

❖

In a human population, the shortage of calcium and an excess of potassium in our grains and meat has the same effect on us as it does on a cow. We get heavy and bloated-looking. That swollen, bloated look is one of the first signs of malnutrition, the later signs being a severely swollen belly while the rest of the body looks like a skeleton. At present, the entire U.S. population is swollen, bloated-looking, and bears considerable resemblance to the proverbial Pillsbury doughboy.[36] The result is that we think we need to go on a diet. As soon as we start dieting, we get even less of the nutrition our body needs, and the downward degenerative spiral continues. The real truth is that we need high-nutrition food.

Long ago, it was a tradition that when a cow was killed and dressed, almost every part of it was used for something. People ate the muscle meats along with the glands, the organs, the brain, and other parts. The hides were tanned to make leather, the hooves, tail, and bones were scrubbed and put into stockpots to make gelatin-rich, mineral-rich beef stock, and the fat was rendered into tallow.

Some of these parts, especially the glands, had to be used right away, and as the grocery store system grew, buyers hesitated to buy anything that wouldn't keep for at least a week or two. Gradually, people shopping for their food in grocery stores forgot about the old ways of eating. They tended to be mesmerized by the thick, red steaks and roasts from the muscle portions of beef.

As people got further and further from the soil, had less and less time to cook, or no longer knew what to do with the odds and ends that came from a cow, the demand for things like tongue, thymus, or heart dissolved, and these items disappeared from the grocery store shelf altogether. As we stopped eating glandular and organ meats, we stopped getting the subtle and specialized support nutrients that these parts of the animal offered.

Today many people turn their noses up at gland and organ meats. They would rather take supplements that supply at least some of these important nutritional factors, even though the real thing from the cow does a much better job of supplying usable nutrients. Meats are a great way to get high quality amino acids, Vitamins A, D, E, and B-12, along with many major minerals such as zinc and magnesium, and trace minerals.

---

36 *Pillsbury* is a registered trademark of the Pillsbury Corporation.

Overall, meats are an excellent source of minerals that are organic. By "organic" I mean that the minerals come from living systems and are ready to use by the body. When the nutrients in meat or any food are ready to use as well as easy to absorb, we say they are "bio-available." Many minerals are also part of a matrix of powerful yet subtle nutritional factors, some of which we probably haven't even discovered yet. .

In year past there was a lot of bad press about Creutzfeld-Jacobs disease (CJD), also known as mad cow disease. Some people blamed the agricultural industry for spreading this disease because of its practice of grinding up already diseased cow parts and processing them into feed proteins for other cows. But evidence kept well hidden from the mainstream points to another very likely origin of the disease.

The most telling evidence is from a man named Mark Purdey who was raising organic beef in England. When cattle in the local area were being attacked and infested with a pest known as the warble fly, the UK government issued a court order that all cattle had to be treated with a pesticide. The pesticide chosen was Phosmet, a powerful organo-phosphate, which was applied along the spine of the cows and allowed to run down their bodies. Mark Purdey refused to comply with the court order to douse his cows with Phosmet as this would have ruined his organic status. He was taken to court but won his case and did not apply the pesticide to his cows.

A short time after the Phosmet baths began, CJD turned up everywhere on farms surrounding the Purdey farm. Although the British government tried to push the theory of a strange new infection somehow rooted in bad feed, Purdey's cows had eaten some of that same feed and showed no signs of coming down with mad cow disease.

Having something of a scientific nature himself, Purdey began to research the problem. He learned that CJD almost always began in the retina of the eye and proceeded from there into the brain. Prions, a form of protein in the retina and spine of mammals, worked as shock absorbers for damaging ultraviolet rays and other oxidizing substances – unless they were damaged by exposure to organophosphates. Once damaged, the prions tended to react with manganese, which turned them into rogue molecules and set off a chain-reaction of tragic destruction in the eye and brain.

Says Fintan Dunne in *Acres, USA* news, "Once this prion defense system is rendered ineffective by organophosphates (the same chemical used to get rid of head lice or scabies in people) there is…an unmediated impact on tissues. Eventually, UV radiation damages the retina, and oxidative stress (goes on from there to) destroy the brain tissues of CJD patients. This theory would expect to find higher CJD incidence in mountain regions, where UV radiation levels are elevated. That prediction holds true." [37]

Cambridge University prion bio-chemist David R. Brown is dismissive of the science behind the "strange new infection" model of CJD, also known as Bovine Spongiform Encephalopathy (BSE), and insists there is "no evidence an infectious agent is present in either meat or milk." And in the U.S., the "Center for Disease Control has conducted experiments on mice that confirm the organophosphate risk."

"The pharmaceutical industry is all the more determined to hide the chemical source of BSE and CJD because a spotlight on chemicals would expose the role the insecticides have in Alzheimer's – another neurodegenerative disease – that might lead to claims which would dwarf those from BSE and CJD litigants." [38]

The message in all of this is that mad cow disease is not some mysterious, vicious infective agent with no known cause. It is the result of a pesticide that damages, then disables, an important defense system in the body, creating mutations that then go on to become very destructive.

Many years ago, not long after Louis Pasteur had discovered bacteria and declared it to be the cause of disease, he, Bernard Claude, a physiologist, and Pierre Antoine Bechamp, another chemist, began to argue. Pasteur believed that the bacteria had to be killed or they would invade and create illness. Bernard and Bechamp believed that bacteria were the *result* of disease, not the cause. Bernard declared that the conditions existing in the terrain where the bacteria lived were the all-important

---

37 *Acres USA News*, March 2001.

38 *Acres USA News*, March 2001.

determining factors and that the bacteria would not appear if the tissues of the body were healthy.

For the rest of their lives they argued back and forth, Pasteur declaring that the bacteria reigned supreme, whereas Bernard and Bechamp kept insisting that it was the terrain that mattered most.

Although Pasteur won most of the public sympathy during his lifetime, it is said that on his deathbed, he suddenly sat up and said to his family in attendance, "Bernard was right. The microbe is nothing, the *terrain* is everything."[39]

And it's true. Time has proven Bernard, Bechamp, and now Gaston Naessens to be right. The terrain has to be kept at a certain level of health or we start to disintegrate from within. Gaston Naessens and his discovery confirming the existence of what Bechamp called microzymas and what Naessens calls somatids is just the latest in a line of scientists pointing in the right direction. That direction contradicts the entire "military model" of medicine that tells us we are being attacked by invaders who want to destroy us and therefore we have to resist and kill them off. Any cells, tissues, or organs that are lost in the process of administering the medicine are merely collateral damage, unfortunate but unavoidable. We kill the messengers – the viruses, bacteria, and tumors – and lose the message completely. What is the message? There are several. The body is an entirely cooperative system. We could not exist as human bodies if this were not the case. Learn to cooperate with your body. It's your home while you're here in this life. *It's time to stop the degeneration and start a rebuild...take care of your terrain!* ❖

---

39 Walter McQuade and Ann Aikman, *Stress* (New York, NY: Bantam Books, 1975) p. 18.

12
Milk

WHEN I WAS A LITTLE GIRL, the milkman used to deliver milk to our house two or three times a week. He put the milk, which came in one-quart glass bottles, in a covered metal box on the front porch. The bottles had a thick glass lip around the top edge and a thick layer of cream floating on the milk. I thought having a milkman was extremely modern and sophisticated compared to my grandma, who had to go out and milk her cow, then separate the milk from the cream before putting it in a pitcher in her refrigerator.

Much later, when I was about 12, a large, modern grocery store opened in town. We began to buy milk in wax-coated cardboard cartons that declared the milk inside to be both "pasteurized" and "homogenized." The milk didn't have any cream floating on the top, and at that time, I thought how convenient it was that we didn't have to take time to shake the bottle every time we wanted to pour a glass of milk.

Years later, after buying this farm, I kept at least one or two cows who would produce a calf each year. Every day I milked the cows, then put the fresh, raw milk in a pitcher in the refrigerator.

"Why bother when you can just go to the store and buy it?" people often asked. Why? Lots of reasons. I wanted raw milk with all of its enzymes still in it. I wanted butter made from raw cream. I wanted fresh, unpasteurized cream on my blueberries and raspberries. I wanted the prodigious amounts of vitamins and minerals in raw milk. I wanted the raw, saturated, animal fat in my diet. And I wanted access to the Wulzen

Factor (Vitamin K), an anti-stiffness factor discovered by Weston Price that is destroyed during pasteurization. [40] [41]

The process of pasteurization started back in the early 1900s when many people were looking for answers to the unsolved horror of tuberculosis and believed the disease might be coming from cow's milk.

When Louis Pasteur claimed that bacteria were the source of disease and that high temperatures could destroy many forms of bacteria, the authorities suggested that everyone should heat milk to a temperature somewhere between 140 and 180 degrees, a process that came to be known as *pasteurization*. Although milk is pasteurized to kill harmful bacteria, the process also kills the enzymes that are necessary to help digest and absorb all of the nutrients in the milk. In addition, heating anything to high temperatures denatures proteins. Denaturing changes the shape and structure of the protein molecules in milk as well as many other foods, rendering them unusable by the body and reducing the nutritional value of the food.

As it turned out, milk was not the root cause of TB. The real culprit was degeneration caused by a drop in nutrition in both people and animals. The result was the appearance of bacteria that appeared in one individual, but would quickly spread to others, both animals and people. In a weakened individual, the bacteria overwhelmed the immune system.

As most of us know, the immune system is responsible for protecting us against bacteria and viruses. However, it is also responsible for destroying poorly-built cells that developed under less-than-optimum conditions and become inflamed or dysfunctional. This is why we have autoimmune problems like arthritis, Hashimoto's syndrome, celiac disease, Crohn's and irritable bowel syndrome, psoriasis, and more than 100 other autoimmune conditions. The body is not attacking itself; it is the immune system doing its job of getting rid of poor quality cells.

❖

In the days before pasteurization began, a six-month diet of raw, healthy milk was a powerful *healer* of tuberculosis, and those who could

40 Price, p. 437-458.

41 Sally Fallon, *Nourishing Traditions* (San Diego, CA: ProMotion Publishing, 1995) p. 15.

afford it went to spend six months or more at "health farms" out in the country where they rested and drank plentiful amounts of milk, cream, cheese, and yogurt. Called "the milk cure," this method of healing disappeared after pasteurization began because pasteurized milk just didn't heal anything. In fact, it creates constant mucus problems in the sinuses and disturbing amounts of gas in the intestinal system.

Today, we know that tuberculosis is just another degenerative disease resulting from poor nutrition. The moment there is a drop in nutrition, degeneration in the body accelerates. This is followed by a sharp increase in the production of viruses and bacteria, and a fall-off of immunity to other bacteria and viruses that may be around. People and animals are all susceptible to TB if the quality of the nutrition they receive falls below a certain level. In cows, tuberculosis is called *brucellosis* or sometimes Bang's Disease. In our typically aggressive and shortsighted way, we have gone after the disease with chemicals in an effort to suppress the bacteria, instead of correcting the problem of poor nutrition.

Today, cows are tested regularly for bovine tuberculosis, and there is not much need to worry about developing the once-mysterious TB. However, by the time the true cause of TB was discovered and a test for it was developed, an entire industry had sprung up to pasteurize milk. The government did not want to put people out of work, and no one really knew the harm that pasteurizing caused, so the processing of milk became a law and continues today, except in California and a handful of other states where a very health- and beauty-conscious population demand that raw milk be made available, and thus it is sold in the stores there.

The tragic loss for the rest of us is that during the heating process the natural enzymes in the milk are destroyed. These are the very enzymes that Mother Nature designed and developed in milk to help our body digest and absorb the nutrients in it.

Without the help of the natural enzymes in raw milk, not only does the pancreas have to work much harder to digest it, it is much more difficult to find anything nutritionally useful in it. Instead of being a healing food, pasteurized milk becomes another irritant, causing allergies, sinus problems, digestive troubles, and mucus in the body. This is why you will so often hear or read the argument that cow's milk is only for calves and is bad for adult humans. The truth is that real (raw) milk is *very* good for you.

❖

Before pasteurization and homogenization began, it was common to sell milk as a whole and unprocessed food. Some cream was removed for making butter or sour cream, but the rest of the milk was consumed whole.

Not long after pasteurizing became common, the milk industry started homogenizing milk. I suspect that those who processed and packaged milk for sale realized that they could separate the cream from the milk and sell a single cup of cream for more money than an entire half gallon of milk. However, the remaining bit of cream that would rise to the surface of the milk was a clear indication that most of the cream had been removed. Old-timers who knew the power of cream objected to this because they used the amount of cream sitting on top of the milk to assess the quality and value of the milk. The more cream, the higher the quality. With homogenization, the fact that there was very little cream sitting on the milk was obscured because homogenization prevented the cream from rising. Marketers and salesmen *said* it was "whole milk" and that's what they printed on the carton, but it wasn't, and there was no way to easily know the truth unless you were a chemist with access to a laboratory.

Another factor in homogenization may have been the move away from the old breeds of dairy cattle – Jersey, Guernsey, and Brown Swiss – that produced milk with 5-7% cream content, to newer breeds like the Holstein that produce milk with only 2-3% cream. In the old days, this would have been an unacceptable level of cream, and no one would have been able to sell such milk. Again, homogenization allowed us to disguise the low cream content, and today, 2% and lowfat milk are purchased and consumed without a second thought.

Homogenization is a simple process of shaking or forcing the milk through small tubes so violently that many of the large enzyme molecules present in the milk are shattered into tiny, irregular pieces. People drink the milk and take in the shattered enzymes. These tiny pieces of enzyme then manage to pass into the blood stream where they irritate the walls of veins and arteries. One of the body's responses to this irritation is to produce cholesterol. This is only one of the reasons for cholesterol buildup, but it adds to the difficulties the body must contend with.

In the old days, cows were fed and fattened on pasture grass, herbs, and vegetables. Nowadays, cows are fed and fattened on corn and soybean crops containing the residues of toxic chemicals and heavy metals. These toxins have a great affinity for fat cells, and the fat in cows' milk picks up these toxins, passing them on to the humans who drink the milk. Worse, cows that do not have access to pasture and are raised only on grains will develop a gassy, acid condition and dairy farmers must feed them baking soda to help ease their discomfort and the slow-down of milk production.

When milk causes digestive upsets, allergies, gas, and sinus problems, it *may* be because an individual does not produce the specific enzymes necessary to digest milk and milk fats. But more often, it is because pasteurization has destroyed its protein structures, homogenization has shattered a key enzyme that then becomes an irritant, and the whole mess carries a load of toxins and chemicals because pesticides and heavy metals that came in with the corn and soybean diet are drawn to the fat in milk.

When a farmer milks cows, the milk is picked up from the bulk tank and delivered to a milk-processing factory. Once there, it is broken down into its basic constituents – water, milk solids, light cream and heavy cream. Next it is pasteurized, then homogenized and put back together using carefully controlled recipes depending on whether the goal is skim milk, 2% milk, or whole milk. When the milk has been reassembled, a few synthetic vitamins and minerals may be added, and sometimes a little instant milk powder to give the milk a little more body and color. Once milk has gone through this process, it's hard to consider it as milk at all anymore.

The loss of the nutritional powerhouse that milk used to be has contributed to the subtle processes of degeneration in millions of people. With increasingly poor nutrition, bile production in the liver and gall bladder is reduced. Without plenty of bile to emulsify fats, we are unable to utilize these fats, and without fats you will be unable to absorb and use vitamins A, D, E, and K – the fat-soluble vitamins that are the necessary basics for any kind of healing.

For a long time, I drank almost no milk. Today, I know the healing power of milk in its whole, raw, unprocessed forms. *Raw*, unpasteurized milk, cream, butter, sour cream, and cheeses do not cause allergies, asthma, ear-nose-and-throat problems, high cholesterol, heart disease, or many of the other difficulties blamed on dairy products. These problems are the result of degenerative processes in the body caused by poor nutrition. Pasteurized milk will aggravate these conditions by clogging up the body, the sinuses, the lungs, ears, nose, and throat with mucus, which becomes a perfect breeding ground for bacteria. The lactic-acid-producing bacteria that keep you safe from certain pathogens is destroyed when milk is pasteurized. Over half its water-soluble vitamins are lost, proteins become much less available, and minerals, which are many, are changed structurally in subtle ways that make them inorganic and more difficult to assimilate.

Real, raw milk does not create these problems. Whole, unpasteurized, unhomogenized milk comes complete with high levels of nutrition plus all the enzymes and digestive factors that are necessary for you to digest that milk.

My granddaughter cannot drink commercially processed, store-bought milk at all. When she does, her eyes swell and dark circles – the telltale "allergy bull's-eyes" – appear under them. After a week on the pasteurized stuff, her sinuses are swollen, her nose is plugged up; she sneezes, wheezes, and suffers. However, these problems disappear when she drinks the whole, raw milk our cows produce here at the farm. Not only do problems disappear, but her good health and high energy reappear.

The definition of good health is not just an *absence* of symptoms; it is the *presence* of high energy, endless stamina, creative intelligence, an interest in work, and a peaceful disposition.

A cup of raw milk on my oatmeal in the morning, a couple of tablespoons of butter on my muffin at noon, a dish of homemade yogurt, and a chunk of cheese as an afternoon or evening snack have brought a smoothness to my skin, a shine and fullness to my hair, firm strength to my fingernails, stable weight loss, the disappearance of cravings, and a tremendous sense of well-being. ❖

13
Fats and Cholesterol

NOTHING IS MORE MISUNDERSTOOD in the modern diet than fat. Although it is slowly changing, the popular press still prints warnings about the dangers of eating fat. Everywhere you look you are urged to eat non-fat or low-fat foods, to use polyunsaturated vegetable oils, and if possible, to eliminate fats. Animal fats and saturated fats are expressly named as the culprit in all manner of diseases from heart attacks and high cholesterol to cancers, obesity, and atherosclerosis.

I have had some people nearly faint away when they hear the truth about fat. They think they have been doing everything right to maintain their good health…eating no meat, drinking no milk, avoiding fat, eating lots of whole grains and soy products. When they end up with a catastrophic illness and have done everything they can to no avail, they often find their way to my classes and are shocked to discover that what they thought was the correct way to eat has greatly contributed to, or even caused, their illness.

The facts of the matter are that you not only *need* fat in your diet, you need saturated animal fats and *mono*unsaturated and *super*unsaturated fats, and you should avoid polyunsaturated fats in almost all forms. When you think of fats, think in terms of what you need to take in for your body's sake, not in terms of what you need to avoid. One of the worst things you can do is eliminate fats from your diet.

Fat molecules are made of carbon atoms strung together in a chain, with one or more hydrogen atoms along the length of the chain. Fats come in a variety of forms and each form has different uses in the body. Short-

135

chain and medium-chain fats create quick energy. They also have anti-microbial, anti-fungal, and anti-tumor properties, as well as an ability to enhance growth and improve the function of the immune system.

Long-chain fats and extra-long-chain fats are needed for building tissues and cell membranes as well as producing hemoglobin, cholesterol, and other hormone-like substances. Long-chain fats are also necessary for absorption into the lymph system, for velvety skin, vitality, and fast healing power. They can lower blood pressure if it is high and raise it if it is low, create a sense of stamina and calm, and help generate needed electrical currents that drive chemical transactions in the body.

Butter contains mostly short- and medium-chain fats, as does coconut oil, both of which are good for you. Olive oil, a *mono*unsaturated fat that is somewhat usable in the body, is mostly long-chain fats, as are fish oils, while flaxseed oil and hempseed oil are *super*unsaturated fats. Beef and pork both contain saturated fats having a range of short- to long-chain fats, but are mostly long-chain.

Your brain is 55-65% fat, and you need fats in your diet to help your brain run smoothly and well. Mother's breast milk is 50-55% saturated fat and is critical for development of the brain and central nervous system in the newborn and young child. [42]

Researchers have found that putting children on low-fat or soy milk diets not only interferes with brain development, it results in allergies, learning disorders, attention deficit disorders, hyperkinetic behaviors, and other mental, emotional, and social problems in children. One of several problems with soy is that it does not have the fat so desperately required by the developing human brain. Another is that soy deranges the endocrine system. [43] [44]

Several years ago, pediatricians of America issued a statement saying they believed that soymilk formulas were not appropriate for infants, and that such formulas had contributed to the epidemic of ADHD

---

42 Udo Erasmus, *Fats that Heal, Fats that Kill* (Burnaby, BC, Canada: Alive Books, 1993) p. 50-51.

43 Gary Null PhD, *Nutrition and The Mind* (New York, NY: Four Walls Eight Windows Press, 1995) p. 225.

44 Fallon, *The Oiling of America,* 1998.

children. I heard this on a National Public Radio (NPR) news program and was thrilled that the truth was now out in public. But that was the last of that subject! The whole topic disappeared and we are still not paying attention to what we are doing with food.

Saturated Fats

Adults have come to believe that eating saturated animal fats will cause high cholesterol, high triglycerides, atherosclerosis, and similar diseases. But these problems are not caused by eating fat; *they are the results of eating sugar and skeletonized foods with no nutrition in them coupled with high stress.* We will talk about stress later.

The belief that fats cause heart disease, cancer, and other diseases is known as *The Lipid Hypothesis*. This theory started back in the 1950s when a researcher named Ancel Keys not only did some very poor research, he also came to an erroneous conclusion. Once published, however, others jumped on the bandwagon and began to undertake biased, lopsided, already-prejudiced research. Some of this research was funded by the budding vegetable oil producers who needed a reason backed by "scientific research" to convince people it was a good idea to switch from traditional fats – the butter, lard, and tallow that we had used safely for thousands of years – to the new, factory-made, imitation fats known as margarine and corn oil. Once this faulty research was published, the food factories began serious marketing campaigns and succeeded in getting millions to change their diets to the "new and improved" foods they were producing. [45] [46]

Fortunately, we are beginning to wake up in terms of our need for healthy fats. Even the famous Framingham Study in Massachusetts, which tracked thousands of people for 40 years, reversed its position recently, saying, "The more saturated fat one ate, the more cholesterol one ate, the more calories one ate, the lower the person's serum cholesterol (was). We found that the people who ate the most cholesterol, ate the most saturated

---

45 Uffe Ravnskov MD, PhD, *The Cholesterol Myths* (Washington, DC: New Trends Publishing Inc, 2000) p. 15-16

46 Fallon, *The Oiling of America,* 1998.

fat, ate the most calories, weighed the least and were the most physically active." [47]

Numerous other studies indicate that when saturated fats and cholesterol are reduced, there is only a *very* marginal reduction in heart disease, whereas deaths from all other causes go *up*, including cancer, stroke, suicide, brain hemorrhage, and even violent deaths.[48] [49]

Another thing that simply must be understood about fats is that when you eat sweets and processed grains or foods made with either of these, for example white and whole wheat flour, white rice, pasta, many common breakfast cereals, or any kind of sugar, whether in candies, cookies, cakes, syrups, soft drinks, shakes, or some other food, *these foods will be turned into saturated fats by your body*, however, these versions of saturated fats are not well-constructed or usable by the body. [50]

Udo Erasmus, who studied fats intensely after being dangerously exposed to carcinogenic chemicals and knew their affinity for fats states bluntly, "Killer saturated long-chain fatty acids, which are sticky and therefore increase our chances of stroke, heart attack, clogged arteries, and diabetes, are produced from refined sugars." [51]

The important, enzyme-rich, saturated fats needed by the body and found in such foods as whole raw milk, raw cream, raw butter, and meats have all been cast into the category of forbidden foods that are likely to kill you, while the real culprits – processed foods and refined sugar – are ignored and continue to be advertised as something that will make you feel good, sexy, or part of the "in crowd."

Our entire population has been seduced into eating boxed, canned, fast foods, and food-look-alikes composed of tasteless chemicals and white flour, which have been made palatable by the addition of sugar. The result is rampant atherosclerosis, heart disease, high blood pressure, diabetes, and a long list of other diseases.

---

47 Fallon, *The Oiling of America,* 1998.

48 Ibid.

49 Ravnskov, p. 30-31.

50 Erasmus, p. 31-32.

51 Erasmus, pg. 34.

Cholesterol

Cholesterol, another supposed bad boy, is actually a very important healing agent in the body. Cholesterol is manufactured in the liver, and the body uses it to protect tissues and manage the fluidity/hardness of cell membranes, thus controlling what gets into or out of your cells. Most male and female sex hormones are made from cholesterol, as are other hormones that regulate conditions such as water balance in the kidneys, the stress response, the strength of artery walls, and many other functions. Vitamin D is made from cholesterol. So are bile acids. Cholesterol is part of a light covering on the skin that keeps it from drying out, and it even works as an antioxidant when the body is short of these.

Problems with cholesterol arise when you do not have enough of the right materials available for the body's continuous rebuilding needs – especially the right kinds of saturated, monounsaturated, and superunsaturated essential fats (essential fatty acids are often called EFAs) that work hand-in-hand with proteins.

When the body does not have enough building materials to build good structure, it will begin to skimp on body structures such as bones, teeth, organs, and artery walls. If these structures get too thin, the body will then produce extra cholesterol to temporarily "plaster" the insides of thin or weak artery walls, veins, or organs, shoring them up in an effort to strengthen them. In the case of arteries, this helps prevent them from leaking, breaking, or bulging out to form aneurysms, but it also prevents the normal and natural expansion and contraction of the arteries and veins. The result is a rigid cardiovascular system, creating a condition that we call hypertension or sometimes high blood pressure."

In addition to low nutrition and high sugar, the other dangerous factor in raising your cholesterol is a constant level of physical or emotional stress. Too much cholesterol will also be produced whenever you take in more calories than you can burn off, regardless of the source of those calories. The bottom line is that you need to manage and balance the fats in your diet. Too little fat is worse than too much. Too little cholesterol is worse than too much because true research – not the fake, manipulated kind – shows that, as cholesterol goes down, the incidence of heart attack is lowered minimally while the incidence of cancer goes up. [52]

In her book, *Nourishing Traditions,* author Sally Fallon discusses cholesterol saying, "When thyroid function is poor, often the result of a diet high in sugar and low in nutrients, the body floods the blood with cholesterol as an adaptive and protective mechanism, providing a superabundance of the materials needed to heal tissues and produce protective steroids. Just as a large police force is needed in a locality where crime occurs frequently, cholesterol is needed in a poorly nourished body to protect the individual from a tendency to heart disease and cancer. Blaming coronary heart disease on cholesterol is like blaming the police for murder and theft in a high crime area." [53]

Fallon also illuminates Dr. Nathan Pritikin's famous fat-free Pritikin Diet and the results for those who followed it. "Those who possessed enough will power to stay fat-free for any length of time developed a variety of health problems including low energy, difficulty in concentrating, depression, weight gain, and signs of mineral deficiencies. Pritikin may have saved himself from heart disease, but his low-fat diet did not spare him from cancer. He died, in the prime of life, of leukemia." [54]

Fallon points out that if you step back to look at the bigger picture surrounding the issue of fat intake, you will see that as consumption of animal fats went down and the consumption of polyunsaturated vegetable oils went up, heart disease, cancers, depression, suicides, and violence in society went up right along with the increase in polyunsaturated vegetable oils. When you put several statistical curves next to each other, one showing the increasing use of vegetable oils, one that shows the increasing heart disease, and one for the increase in cancer, the curves run almost parallel to one another. [55] [56]

Saturated fat and cholesterol are so important in the diet that it is difficult to see and hear them get beaten up in the popular press again

---

52 Ravnskov, p.145, 208, 210, 218.

53 Fallon, *Nourishing Traditions,* p. 11.

54 Fallon, *Nourishing Traditions,* p. 4.

55 Fallon, *The Oiling of America,* 1998.

56 Erasmus, p. 111.

and again. Many people, even scientists, confuse saturated animal fats with *hydrogenated* fats. A natural, saturated animal fat like beef tallow or lard is solid at room temperature and fairly stable even at high cooking temperatures. Lots of people think that shortening is saturated animal fat. It is not. Shortening is vegetable oil that has been turned into a solid, hydrogenated fat. The process of hydrogenation is so destructive that I quote a small section from Sally Fallon's *Nourishing Traditions*:

> **"Hydrogenation:** This is the process that turns polyunsaturates, normally liquid at room temperature, into a fat that is solid at room temperature – margarine and shortening. To produce them, manufacturers begin with the cheapest oils – soy, corn or cottonseed – already rancid from the extraction process. These oils are then mixed with tiny metal particles – usually nickel oxide. Nickel oxide is very toxic when absorbed and is impossible to totally eliminate from the margarine. The oil with its nickel catalyst is then subjected to hydrogen gas in a high pressure, high temperature reactor. Next, soap-like emulsifiers and starch are squeezed into the mixture to give it a better consistency; the oil is yet again subjected to high temperature when it is steam-cleaned. This removes its horrible odor. Margarine's natural color, an unappetizing grey, is removed by bleach. Coal-tar dyes and strong (artificial) flavors must then be added to make it resemble butter. Finally the mixture is compressed and packaged in blocks or tubs, ready to be spread on your toast.

> "Margarine and other partially hydrogenated oils are even worse for you than the highly refined vegetable oils from which they are made, because of chemical changes that occur

during the hydrogenation process. Under high temperatures, the nickel catalyst causes the hydrogen atoms to change position on the fatty acid chain. Before hydrogenation, two hydrogen atoms occur together on the chain, causing the chain to bend slightly and creating an electron cloud at the site of the double bond. This is called the *cis* formation, the configuration most commonly found in nature. With hydrogenation, one hydrogen atom is moved to the other side (of the chain) so that the molecule straightens. This is called the *trans* configuration, rarely found in nature. These man-made *trans*fats are toxins to the body. But unfortunately your digestive system does not recognize them as such. Instead of being eliminated, the *trans*fats are incorporated into the body's cell membranes as if they were *cis*fats – and your cells actually become hydrogenated! Once in place, *trans*fatty acids with their misplaced hydrogen atom wreak havoc in cell metabolism. These altered fats actually block the utilization of essential fatty acids, causing many deleterious effects ranging from sexual dysfunction to increased blood cholesterol and paralysis of the immune system.

"In the 1940s, researchers found a strong correlation between cancer and the consumption of fat – the fats used were hydrogenated fats, not naturally saturated (animal) fats. (Until recently, the confusion between hydrogenated fats and naturally saturated fats has persisted not only in the popular press, but in scientific databases, resulting in much error in study results.) Consumption of hydrogenated fats is associated with a host of other serious diseases, not only cancer but also atherosclerosis, diabetes, obesity, immune system dysfunction, low birth weight babies and birth defects, sterility, difficulty in lactation and problems with bones and tendons; yet hydrogenated fats continue to be promoted as health foods. Margarine's popularity represents a triumph of advertising duplicity over common sense. Your best defense is to avoid it like the plague." [57]

---

57 Fallon, *Nourishing Traditions,* p. 12-13.

A Short Course in Fats

Let's have a very short course in fats, putting the facts out there as simply and clearly as possible.

Your body is made of cells. Each cell is enclosed by what is called a cell membrane. The cell membrane is composed of a double layer of fats. This double layer is constructed by weaving together a variety of fatty acid chains, some of them saturated, some unsaturated. Saturated trans-fats tend to be straight and stick-like in form. They pack together very tightly and can create an impenetrable cell wall. The *mono*unsaturated fats have a slight kink in them, which prevents such tight packing. The *poly*unsaturated fats have two kinks in them making them almost L-shaped. The *super*unsaturated fats have 3 kinks in them which makes them almost C-shaped and it is this C-shape which proves to be so important in the construction of cell membranes simply because the C-shaped molecules do not pack together very well. This allows the cell membrane to retain some porosity, respond better to its nutrient environment, open to admit nutrients or eliminate toxins, and close to prevent invasion by bacteria, viruses, pesticides, or other unwanted substances.

The looser packing of *super*unsaturated fat chains is made possible by the kinks in their molecular construction. Those kinks are created by two hydrogen atoms sitting next to each other. (See drawing two pages back.) These adjacent charges create differences in electrical potential and these, in turn, create electrical currents, which help to drive chemical transactions in and around the cell. The more transactions your cells can manage, the healthier you will be.

The bottom line is…

- There are saturated fats, and there are unsaturated fats.

- You *need* both saturated and unsaturated fats in your diet.

- No less than 20% of your calories should come from fats. 30% is better!

- The needed balance between fats in your body is about one-third saturated fats, one-third monounsaturated fats, and one-third superunsaturated fats.

- In the saturated fats category, there are:

- o   Short-chain fats found in butter, known as butyric acid.

- o   Medium-chain fats found in coconut, palm, and palm kernel oils, all known as palmitic acid.

- o   Long-chain fats found in beef, lamb, mutton, pork, butter, and cocoa butter.

- Saturated fats are very stable even at high cooking temperatures, thus the danger of *trans*-fats is avoided.

- The body burns short- and medium-chain saturated fats as a major source of quick, long-lasting energy.

- The body uses medium- and long-chain saturated fats to build protein structures, make some energy, construct cell membranes, and make small amounts of unsaturated fatty acids for its own use.

- Of the unsaturated fats, there are 3 kinds: *mono*unsaturated, *poly*unsaturated, and *super*unsaturated.

- *Mono*unsaturated fats with a slight kink and one double bond are found in olives, almonds, avocados, peanuts, pecans, cashews, filberts, and macadamia nuts, and the oils of all these.

- *Poly*unsaturated fats have two double bonds, thus two kinks, and are found in safflower, sunflower, walnut, pumpkin, and sesame oils.

- *Super*unsaturated fats have three or more double bonds, thus, three kinks, and are found in flax seeds, hemp seeds, flaxseed oil, hempseed oil, walnut oil, and dark leafy greens.

- The most important unsaturated fats for humans are the superunsaturated fats.

- The superunsaturated fats are rich in Omega 3 and Omega 6 oils.

- In the body, the Omega 3 and Omega 6 oils are known as *essential fatty acids*, (EFAs) which means the body cannot make them, they must be supplied.

- Omega 3 oil is sometimes known by its more scientific name, Alpha-Linolenic Acid, and flaxseed oil is the richest source.

- Omega 6 oil is sometimes known as Linoleic Acid, and the richest sources are hempseed oil, flaxseed oil, safflower or sunflower oil.

- Another important form of Omega 6 oil is called Gamma-Linolenic Acid and is found mainly in borage, black currant, and evening primrose oils.

- A third form of Omega 6 oil, called Arachidonic Acid (AA), is found in meats and animal products such as milk, cheese, etc.

- Omega 3 and Omega 6 oils must be supplied to the body in a 1:3 ratio. This means approximately 1,000 mg of Omega 3 for every 3,000 mg of Omega 6. For health maintenance, if you need 3,000 mg of Omega 3 oil per day, then you would need 9,000 mg of Omega 6 oil per day. This would be a balanced ratio of superunsaturated oils in your diet.

- Hempseed oil is the best source of unsaturated EFAs because it contains the correct ratio of Omega 3 to Omega 6 oil.

- All of the unsaturated fats are very unstable and tend to react quickly, making it necessary to keep them refrigerated and to have a good supply of antioxidants in the body at all times.

- Light is the biggest enemy of any unsaturated fats. Any oils you buy should come in cans or dark, light-proof bottles.

- Almost as a matter of course, the fatty acid chains in *poly*unsaturated vegetable oils are seriously damaged during processing, making them useless and harmful to us. They quickly become rancid when exposed to light, oxygen, or heat. Rancid oils *seek and destroy* vitamins A and D in the body.

- If you do not have the correct assortment of fats in your diet, you will not be able to use vitamins A,D, E, and K because these are oil-soluble vitamins. If you cannot use vitamin A, you simply will not heal. And conversely, without vitamin A, the essential fatty acids will not work. Without Vitamin D you will not be able to utilize calcium, which means your bones will degenerate. Without E you will have difficulties with skin, cardiovascular function, eyesight, and slow healing. And without Vitamin K you will not be able to maintain healthy bones, heart function, and resistance to aging.

The point of all of the above is that you absolutely must have good quality fats in your diet, both saturated and unsaturated. What's more, they must be available in the right proportions.

The saturated fats you eat are best for you when they are eaten raw, and the best source of raw saturated animal fat is raw butter, milk, or cream. The richest source of unsaturated Omega 3 fat is flaxseed oil, which also contains some Omega 6. The richest source of unsaturated Omega 6 fat is safflower oil, however, most safflower oil is rancid from processing and exposure to light in the clear bottles it is packaged in. The best source of both Omega 3 and 6 in one oil is hempseed oil, because it carries them in the correct proportions of one part Omega 3 to three parts Omega 6 oil. You can also get some Omega 3 and 6 oils by including *raw* nuts such as walnuts, pecans, cashews, almonds, and plenty of dark green leaves such as kale, collards, dark lettuces, and lambsquarter in your salads.

Hempseed oil can be found at your local health food store. If you have difficulty finding it, use flaxseed oil. A good way to get both the Omega 3 and 6 essential fats into your diet is to put 1-2 TBSP of flaxseed oil on your tossed salad every day, then on top of this pour your regular olive oil-and-lemon (or apple cider vinegar, or red wine vinegar, or balsamic vinegar and oil). If you insist on Italian or Ranch dressing, be twice as diligent in adding flaxseed oil, which is somewhat bitter. Just pour the Italian or Ranch right over the flaxseed oil. Be sure to eat/sip all the dressing in the bottom of the salad plate. If you can get hempseed oil, use the same amount, 1-2 TBSP on your salad and cover the taste with a bit of your regular dressing. If you are in love with Ranch dressing and can't eat a salad without it, make your own using milk or half and half. Even dressings made using an envelope of Hidden Valley ingredients are much better for you than store-bought dressings because you can choose your own oils or milk.

For these essential unsaturated fats to work in your body, you must also be sure to take vitamins A, C, B3, B6, E, beta carotene, and the minerals magnesium and zinc.

*Do **not*** avoid saturated animal fats as if they are the plague.

*Do **not*** use commercial vegetable oils that were produced with high temperatures or in lighted pressing facilities. This is even more important if they are Omega 3 and 6 oils. And anything in clear glass or plastic bottles that exposes the oil to light will be rancid and very harmful to you. Oils react first to light, then to oxygen, and lastly to heat.

*Do **not*** cook with vegetable oils, they are too unstable. As a general rule try not to fry your foods because extremely high temperatures will denature fats and proteins. If you have a hankering for something fried, use bacon fat, lard, beef tallow, or coconut oil because these are very stable. When you fry, use the lowest frying temperature possible.

Do eat butter. If you have access to butter made from raw, unpasteurized cream, enjoy it even more freely. If it is raw butter, try to eat at least two tablespoons per day as a minimum, although four to eight tablespoons would be more acceptable.

Do enjoy ice cream if you make it yourself using raw milk or cream.

Do eat beef, pork, chicken, mutton, fish, and other meats because they are good for you, but don't overdose, especially if you're still eating sugar or if you don't know who raised the animals and how they were fed.

Do use olive oil or peanut oil (both *mono*unsaturated) in small amounts to make salad dressings if they have been cold pressed in a dark workroom and you buy it in a can or dark bottle that the light cannot get through. Otherwise, the body does not have much use for *mono*unsaturated fats, and even less use for *poly*unsaturated fats because it will make its own versions when needed. ❖

14

Organic Vegetables & Fruits

WHEN YOU GO INTO ANY ORDINARY GROCERY store or market today, you will see a large assortment of vegetables and fruits in the produce section. Quite often, they are big, shiny with wax, and tough as shoe leather. When you bite into them, they do not have the rich, velvety taste and sweet juice of healthy, mature fruits. Often they make you pucker up because of this.

The plastic bags that hold lettuces and other vegetables can have mild fungicides on the inside of the plastic to keep the vegetables from becoming moldy. Even so, all too often, fresh fruits and vegetables rot and turn to slime within days of purchase.

If you were to go into an organic market, the fresh fruit and vegetable section is not nearly as extensive or impressive. The fruits frequently look small, dry, shrunken, and completely unappetizing. They, too, have very little juice inside, and when you buy them and take them home, they don't last any longer than commercially grown fruits and vegetables. They don't taste any better either, and sometimes they taste worse.

The biggest reason for many dry, shrunken foods in the organic world is the failure of organic producers to restore their soil to a living condition. A good many organic growers simply switch from using chemical pesticides, herbicides, and fungicides to using their "approved" and more natural organic counterparts. In other words, the strategy is the same…plant seeds, then just try to keep the plants growing and upright long enough to produce a fruit and get it to market. Nutritional quality is seldom thought of.

Remember what was said earlier about cows getting too much potassium instead of calcium? The same thing happens in plants, especially in big, commercial, food-growing operations. When calcium in the soil is minimal, or present but chemically unavailable because of pH conditions and other bonding issues that interfere with the action of critical minerals, the plant will uptake potassium as a replacement for calcium. In a plant, too much potassium causes the plant to produce lots of big, lush leaves, making it look healthy and green. This appearance is deceptive because without the right minerals, the plants will be sick and their fruits will be weak, bloated, and tasteless.

Overloaded with water, yet without enough calcium and the other minerals needed to build good structure and maintain the energies required for the hundreds of chemical reactions that produce healthy, tasty fruit, these are the plants that need serious propping up with pesticides, fungicides, and herbicides. Often, growers pick the swollen, tasteless fruit early, before the plant succumbs to mold, mildew, or other disease...which adds to the problems of poor taste and low nutrition.

Perhaps you have seen the swollen legs of sick people suffering from heart and circulatory diseases. It's the same thing with plants, except that plants do not have heart attacks. They will continue to struggle with all their might to produce a fruit that will contain at least a few viable seeds so that their existence will go on through their offspring.

When you are buying fruits and vegetables, ask yourself what kind of soil those fruits might have been raised in. Be aware of the following quality scale that goes from lowest nutrition and quality to highest nutrition and quality:

1. **Commercial** – Foods raised in commercial fields or greenhouses with dead soils and using NPK fertilizers. These will often be big, bright, waxy, tasteless, and have the texture of cardboard. Sometimes they will be mealy; almost always they lack the inner juices full of natural sugars. They will carry a load of pesticides, fungicides, and heavy metals, and be low in vitamins and minerals. They will not taste good when you buy them and will not last long after you get them home, even when kept in a refrigerated environment.

2. **Transitional Organic** – Foods raised in fields or greenhouses in which the farmer has stopped spraying pesticides and fungicides, but has not restored the soil. There may be traces of poisonous chemicals used in previous years. The fungicide Captan can be detected at levels high enough to cause rejection in organic markets 17 years after a farmer stops using it. Again, the food will be very low in vitamins, minerals, and brix. They also need refrigeration and do not last or store well.

3. **Certified Organic/No Soil Restoration** – Foods raised in fields or greenhouses in which no poisonous chemicals or NPK fertilizers have been used for at least 3-5 years, but the soil has not been restored or re-mineralized, and therefore the nutrition in the vegetable or fruit is low. Organic veggies and fruits grown in poor soil without the use of NPK fertilizers often look small and shrunken, and the food will often be just as dry, tasteless, and lacking in vitamins and minerals as commercial foods, yet cost much more.

4. **Certified Organic/Some Soil Restoration** – These are foods raised in fields or greenhouses in which there has been an effort to restore the soil to living status. Poisonous chemicals are not used, the use of compost as fertilizer is common along with paramagnetic rock for re-mineralization. Alternative means of managing pests and weeds produces foods that have some vitamins, minerals, and amino acids in them, as well as better taste and much better shelf life.

5. **Bio-Dynamic®** – Organic foods certified by the Demeter Association are the "crème de la crème" of organic agriculture. These foods cannot get certification until the soil has been completely restored and the fruits and vegetables raised in it show certain levels of nutrition in terms of vitamins, minerals, and aminos. They also have excellent taste, high levels of sweetness, and often do not need refrigeration because the level of brix and complex carbohydrates in them preserves them naturally.

The surprising truth is that foods with high levels of minerals and complex carbohydrates in them do not rot when they are not refrigerated. They simply dry out. This is why refrigerators were not really needed until the early part of the 19th century. As soon as we started mass-producing the empty foods of the modern era, the development of the icebox and then the refrigerator was needed to help preserve worthless produce.

When you buy a cucumber and it becomes a pile of slime in the refrigerator within two or three days, you will know it was seriously deficient in minerals. When you buy a bunch of broccoli and find a hollow core going up the stem...when the radishes you slice look like grandmother's lace doilies...if peach pits split open when you try to slice the peach...when strawberries and blueberries are rubbery...when apples are mealy...when lettuce turns to thin, green papery mush...when cauliflower is tough and stringy...when pumpkins, grapefruit, or oranges are spongy or lack juice...these are all foods that are hardly worth the eating because they are seriously deficient in minerals, vitamins, and good nutrition. ❖

15
Grains & Legumes
(aka Pulses)

IF YOU ARE LIKE MANY PEOPLE, you don't think about grain as grain, you think of it as bread or cereal, pasta or pumpernickel, chips or granola. We know legumes as baked beans, pea soup, or something else. Although grains and legumes have many vitamins and minerals in them in their natural, unprocessed state, once the food processing industry has turned them into the breads, cereals, and other foods that you are familiar with, they have been almost completely stripped of their nutrients.

When you eat anything made with white flour, not only do you *not* get the vitamins, minerals, wheat germ oils, and enzymes that Mother Nature put in the wheat, your body has to supply many chemical and nutritional elements from its reserve stock in order to digest and metabolize these over-refined grain skeletons. In other words, your body has to spend a little of its energy in the hopes of being able to replace this energy and get the bonus of whatever was in the food. When there is nothing in the food, the body comes up short. It's like putting money in a savings account and then discovering that, not only did you not collect any interest, the bank charged you a recurring fee for holding your money.

Nowadays, the most common grains include wheat, oats, rye, and rice. A few less common are barley, spelt, millet, amaranth, and kamut. There are others, but unless you're really a health food store devotee or highly allergic to the common grains, you may not know that other grains are out there or what you might do with them.

Birds are the only creatures that can actually eat, digest, and benefit from grains in their whole, natural, dry state. Some mammals have three or four stomachs to allow for proper fermentation processes in digesting grains. However, if humans wish to benefit nutritionally from whole, unrefined grains, the grains must be soaked or sprouted, and breads must be made with old-fashioned sourdough. Otherwise, substances known as phytates, or phytic acids, in the whole grain will bind with calcium, iron, phosphorus, zinc and the other minerals in it, making these important minerals unavailable to you and contributing to physical degeneration.

Someone once asked me if this meant she had to soak her cornflakes and eat soggy cereal every morning, which caused a laugh in class. Cornflakes and other cereals on the grocery store shelf are not whole; they are highly processed. Soaking grains that have already been made into something like corn flakes or a boxed cereal is not necessary…but then eating these highly refined grains does not get you the nutrition you need either. This includes many forms of crackers, corn chips, and other grain-based snack foods. Add rancid, polyunsaturated, and hydrogenated oils, along with a little refined white sugar, and you have a real witch's brew.

One way to enjoy grains with *all* of their vitamins, minerals, oils, and enzymes is to make and eat 14-Grain Cereal. To make a batch of it, you will need 1 lb. (approximately 1 cup) of each of the following grains. Keep in mind that whole grains are often referred to as "berries."

14-Grain Cereal

Whole wheat berries	Flax seeds
Whole oat berries	Popcorn
Whole rye berries	Buckwheat
Barley	Millet
Mung bean seeds	Lentils
Alfalfa seeds	Brown rice
Sesame seeds	Almonds

Put these grains into a large bowl or pot that will allow you to mix the dry grains without spilling them all over the place. Stir to mix evenly and store in quart jars with lids. You will need about four quart jars for one batch of 14-Grain Cereal. Put three of the jars in your freezer for later use, and put the last one in your refrigerator.

After supper each night, put 2-4 TBSP of the mixed grains into a small grinder. Small grain grinders can be purchased for about $20 at a discount store. Popular brands include Salton and West Bend, and there are probably others.

Grind for about 30 seconds, then stop and look at the grains. If the popcorn is still fairly large, grind for another 30 seconds. Repeat once or twice more until the popcorn grains are smaller and less discernible. Don't grind too long and hard or the heat generated by the grinding will destroy the enzymes in the grain.

Then pour the ground grain mix into a cereal bowl. Pour about 1 cup of organic apple (or peach, or grape) juice over the ground-up grains and stir. Set a saucer or piece of plastic wrap over the bowl and put in the refrigerator overnight or for *at least eight hours*.

In the morning, just stir and eat. You can add a bit of fresh or frozen fruit to it, if you like. In the winter, you can warm it up a little in a larger bowl of hot water, but don't heat too much (don't go over 117°) or you'll destroy enzymes. There are lots of variations on this cereal. Some people just soak the grains in water, some soak them in raw milk with a couple tablespoons of yogurt added, some use water, yogurt, and salt. In the morning, they add maple syrup or raw honey and fruit. If you can't handle the fruit juice because of diabetes, try the yogurt combination. Eating 14-Grain Cereal three or four times a week will provide you with a tremendous boost in nutrition. If you had to survive on this cereal for a long period of time, it would supply all the vitamins, minerals, and amino acids your body needs!

Everything your body does is based on being able to get a steady supply of glucose. Your body needs these *natural* sugars in *whole* forms that break down slowly and don't suddenly overdose your system with sugar, which upsets the balance between your liver, pancreas, and adrenals. Whole grains and legumes are good sources of carbohydrates that break down slowly into sugars and starches for the body to use in making its glucose.

Refined white sugar, brown sugar (which is really white sugar sprayed with a little molasses), corn syrup, sucrose, fructose, dextrose, and especially sucralose are some of the common names for what is really a very dangerous substance as far as your body is concerned. Sugar deranges your endocrine system and unbalances body chemistry. It was originally used as a tranquilizer and sedative.

About one hundred years ago, smoking opium was acceptable, whereas eating refined sugar was considered to be a despicable addiction.[58] People went to jail or were run out of town for adding sugar to beer or bread, ruining what were considered to be two important staples of daily life.[59] Today's beer and bread are nothing like their counterparts of a few centuries ago. Back then, these foods contributed to good health; today, they ruin good health.

A few centuries ago, a pound of sugar cost a year's worth of wages and only the very rich could afford it. Sugar is so highly addictive that those who first tasted it immediately craved more of it, and soon the rich, along with their servants who had sneaked a bit from the pantry, began to suffer from the strange disease called diabetes, along with physical, mental, and emotional difficulties that had never been seen before.

Today, you will sometimes hear doctors and other medical people say that there is no known cause of diabetes and that even Hippocrates was puzzled by the disease. They then go on to point out that this was back in the days before the use of sugar. However, this is not only untrue, it is shortsighted and misleading. Sugar addiction and its diseases were rampant among the Arabic and Islamic peoples of the Middle East. [60] Hippocrates was famed for his healing abilities and likely saw the wealthy people from around the Mediterranean who could afford both the high cost of sugar and the trip to his healing clinic. *If* he was not able to discern the cause of diabetes, it may have been because he was not as familiar with sugar in his own culture.

Sugar, one of the sweet spoils of war, was brought steadily westward by a series of invading armies and their conquests. It is widely believed that Christian soldiers were able to stop the Islamic invaders simply because the Turks, Moors, and Saracens had become tired and lost their ferociousness through use of sugared drinks and candied foods. In fact, the 14th century Crusades were planned and carried out with a mission of

---

58 William Dufty, *Sugar Blues* (New York, NY: Warner Books Inc, 1975) p. 41

59 Dufty, p. 51.

60 Dufty, p. 30.

capturing the sugar technology of the Muslims in order to get a piece of the market in sugar trade and the taxes on it. Christendom did not enjoy obvious military successes with their Crusades, but they succeeded in getting their hands on sugar processing and its lucrative potential, and that was enough to satisfy them. Thus, sugar was introduced into European society over the 14th and 15th centuries.[61]

Today, sugar is a major culprit behind many of our worst difficulties because of our ignorance about real food and because people keep choosing sugar-laden, factory-made foods over the simple, natural foods grown by Mother Nature. Without top quality nutrition to maintain high immunity, we end up with heart disease, diabetes, anorexia, depression, dental cavities, multiple sclerosis, poor eyesight, allergies, headache, chronic fatigue, inability to concentrate, alcoholism, obesity, tuberculosis, high cholesterol and triglycerides, digestive problems, atherosclerosis and arteriosclerosis, arthritis, a tendency toward violent behavior, osteoporosis, and especially cancers. Tumors of all kinds love sugar.

Powerful sugar cartels are happy to leave the blame for heart disease, high blood pressure, cancers, and their accompanying disorders at the door of fats. In an effort to market their wares more broadly, the vegetable oil processors inadvertently aided the sugar cartels by advertising their oils as the answer to "the saturated fat problem" when, in truth, rancid vegetable oils and sugar make a lethal combination. By refusing to look honestly at our diet and what has happened to food, we blame many diseases and disorders on genes – and the sugar-based diet is completely ignored.

For all of these reasons, the pharmaceutical and supplement producers are doing some brisk business these days, and no one is looking at the fact that every single food we eat is processed to death before it reaches grocery store shelves. During the processing, everything we need to survive and thrive in a long, healthy, productive life is removed from the food. Some food processors try to fortify the dead food with a few vitamins and minerals that are just as useless as the food they are added to because they, too, were synthesized in a laboratory and are inorganic and therefore not bio-available when it comes to living systems.

---

61 Dufty, p. 31.

It is difficult for people to get off of sugar when so many of today's foods are simply an unpalatable mix of chemicals whose taste is covered by sugar. You would not even consider eating this stuff if the sugar didn't cover up the taste of the chemicals, making it so addictive and attractive to your tongue.

When you think about the fact that very little of what we call food today actually has the nutritional supplies that the body requires to keep repairing and rebuilding itself, it's a wonder we are all still walking, breathing, and working.

Compounding the "non-food" food problem is the fact that very few people really know how to cook from scratch anymore. Those who do know how have difficulty finding the time for it. We have been duped into working for money in order to buy the necessities of life instead of just making or growing our own. Caught up in glitzy marketing campaigns that create an ever-expanding set of needs, we work, work, work, then shop, shop, shop in a rat's maze of consumerism.

Someday our civilization may be known as the people who became extinct because they insisted on turning everything into a business and money-making venture. Then, when they couldn't afford their own system, they collapsed and died because no one knew how to grow their own food or fiber any more! ❖

*Part 3*_____

The Major Detox Routines

16
Introduction to Detox

WHEN WE GET SICK HERE IN AMERICA, the first thing we think of is taking some kind of medicine or pill. We focus on putting something *into* the body, usually pills. Seldom do we think of getting well in terms of taking something *out* of the body, like metabolic wastes. The word *detox* means to eliminate something toxic. Although the word was formerly used in terms of alcoholics who went to a hospital to "dry out" or "detox," it has now come to refer to the process of helping people heal by eliminating the waste products that pile up in the body as a result of bad food, sedentary lifestyles, consuming careers, stressful relationships, or other situations in life.

Most of us live in a house or apartment that needs regular cleaning and sometimes a major repair, upgrade, or rebuild. Imagine what it might be like to live in your house for 30 or 40 years and never do the dishes; sweep or vacuum; never clean the closets, the basement, or the garage; never replace flooring; never repair the roof.

If brushing your teeth and washing your armpits are equivalent to picking up your socks and putting them in the laundry, most of us could probably say we try to do a decent good job of keeping ourselves presentable. However, this is only keeping up appearances. Picking up socks does not help when the kitchen sink backs up or the roof starts to leak, and it is the same in terms of our body. Brushing teeth does not help when diabetes shows up, a cancer appears, or you suddenly discover you have osteoporosis. When any of that happens, you have already missed a lot of messages from your body that something more is needed. If you start supplying your body with what it needs, it will immediately begin to tear out the old structures that are not up to par and this alone can overload the major elimination systems – the liver, kidneys, skin, lungs, colon, and sinuses. This can create serious problems because the body absolutely must get rid of what it can't use and doesn't need.

Let's say that keeping your colon clean and dissolving plaque in your arteries is equivalent to cleaning out the basement or the garage once or twice a year. How would you rate yourself in this area of personal housekeeping? Do you do this regularly...or do you put it off and just try to get by?

Let's say that clearing your liver of fatty deposits, cellular wastes, and heavy metals is akin to replacing the carpeting, installing a new furnace, and putting on a new roof. Do you attend to these tasks when needed, or do you put them off, sometimes for years, or even sell the house because you don't know how to take care of it?

In a well-known story, the famed scientist, Dr. Alexis Carrel, wanted to find out how long the cells of the body would continue to live and divide because he wanted some clue as to how long the natural, normal, healthy human being should live. He put some cells in a Petri dish, fed them correctly, and rinsed away their waste products every day. To his surprise, they continued to thrive for years. After a while, he realized that it wasn't just the correct nutrition he was providing, it was the fact that he was continually removing their waste products. The experiment only came to an end when Carrel went on a trip and a lab assistant forgot to rinse away the wastes and the cells died.

There are eight major steps in a program of full detox:
1. Removing Parasites
2. Chelation & removal of heavy metals
3. Fasting
4. The Liver Flush
5. The Colon Sweep,
6. The Purge
7. The Castor Oil/Olive Oil Sweat Bath
8. The Coffee Enema.

I learned these processes from Dr. Wm. Kelley DDS, and Dr. Nicholas Gonzales MD. To some extent, they are similar to some of Edgar

Cayce's healing techniques. Each is a powerful procedure used to restore the body to healthy function and to support its efforts to heal and rebuild itself. Each one does a different kind of clean-up in the body.

Parasites are insidious and very common. You cannot heal if you have parasites. They take up the nutrition you are trying to provide to your body and they leave tremendous amounts of waste in your system that then over load your liver and cells. Removing parasites is a first step in serious healing efforts.

Next is chelation and removal of heavy metals from the body. Heavy metals have very powerful frequencies that they give off and that interfere with normal frequencies. Not only do they create a cascade of negative conditions in the body, almost nothing you do to heal yourself will work until the metals and their frequencies are removed.

Fasting, whether it is intermittent fasting or a long-term water fast, puts the body at rest, lets the immune system focus on fighting bacteria, viruses, and other invaders, allows the body to break down and eliminate widespread, unwanted wastes and tissues, and speeds up repair and rebuilding.

The Liver Flush cleans out the liver, gall bladder, and kidneys and removes plaque from arteries. The Colon Sweep cleans out the small and large intestines. The Purge alkalinizes the entire body and coaxes cells all over the body to dump their toxic wastes. The Castor Oil/Olive Oil Sweat bath cleans out the skin and the lungs. And the Coffee Enema accomplishes a small daily miracle by forcing the liver to dump its wastes regularly, preventing any toxic build-up. The following chapters detail these and other detox procedures that are extremely powerful in healing our bodies.

If you do not take the time to clean and heal your body on a regular basis, you will eventually find you are falling apart as a physical, mental, and emotional system that is unable to maintain any kind of spirit for life. You end up spending your fortune trying to repair the essential parts and systems. Worse, sometimes you discover that they cannot be repaired and you are left with a body you can no longer live in comfortably at all simply because nothing works correctly any more. ❖

17
Parasites and Fasting

WHEN YOU GO TO SEE A REALLY GOOD NATURAL HEALER, the first thing they will often tell you is, "You should begin with a parasite program because you can't heal if you have parasites...and everyone has them." Parasites are an amazingly common visitor in the human body. Even if you do not have the kind that produce immediately awful symptoms, you will almost certainly have them.

Years ago, when I was in my 20s, I went to Florida where I picked up a very bad case of parasites just walking barefoot in the sand. I didn't know it until two months later when they had multiplied to the point that I began to have skin rashes that started with a bit of itching and progressed to the point that I was covered with raised, angry red patches of skin itching so badly that I literally shook from the effort to refrain from digging holes in myself to relieve that itch. The itching was waking me at night and was everywhere, on the roof of my mouth, the inside of my ears, inside my chest or foot.

I finally went to a dermatologist who said I had a bad case of parasites and asked if I had been traveling recently. I replied, "Only to Florida," and he nodded and said "Yup, not surprised. You can pick up a lot of problems as soon as you get down into the more tropical areas, even in the U.S." He prescribed a heavy dose of Flagyl to be taken for a month, which I immediately began taking. However, a week later I could not walk and was losing my sight! I called him to report what I was experiencing and he frantically cried, "Stop! Stop the medicine immediately!"

Of course, I did stop, and thankfully, my ability to walk and to see gradually returned. The good doctor then suggested we try a very weak dose of Flagyl for a much longer period of three months. That worked, and I thought I was done with parasites. Thus, when I first went to see Dr. Nicholas Gonzales MD and he said I had parasites, I was surprised.

Since I live on a farm, it is easy to pick up parasites in the warm summer months when I am outside a lot and walking barefoot or subject to insect bites. This may be even more true if you live in the city and go barefoot, eat finger food, or put your fingers in your mouth after having your hands on public equipment, doors, railings, etc. If you have pets – cats, dogs, birds, mice, cows, horses, sheep, gerbils, whatever – you are very likely to have parasites because they just go with the territory! As mentioned, if you travel to warm climates, whether in or out of the U.S., you can easily pick up these unhelpful critters. And it is worth noting that other countries whose soils and water are full of strange parasites, often grow food in that soil and water the plants with that water, then send that food to us. There are all sorts of rules and chemicals and radiation to kill incoming critters and parasites, but the "cure" can sometimes be as bad as the problem, and there's no guarantee that we have stopped the incursion of these nuisances. It is much more realistic to know that some parasites will make it through our defenses and end up causing us a variety of problems.

When parasites get into your system, they begin to multiply quickly, and they need the same kind of nutrition that you need. The result is that they suck up whatever nutrition you happen to be putting into yourself, leaving you with scraps, and as they multiply, there will not be enough good nutrition to go around for both you and them. They then burrow into tissues and help themselves to whatever minerals and substances those tissues are made of! On top of this, they excrete their wastes into your bloodstream, polluting you from the inside out. Left to multiply, they can destroy you in a myriad of ways from malnutrition to severe autoimmune disease to other problems too numerous to mention.

To keep myself and my gastrointestinal tract relatively free of parasites, I have three practices that I follow. Over the summer, I regularly take a tablespoon of liquid Bentonite clay in the morning, followed by a 1/2 glass of warm water. Indigenous tribes of long ago used to take wet green or red clay, roll it into small balls, and let them dry in the sun. When completely dry, the clay balls went into a pouch and were later taken as medicine to ward off parasites, provide minerals, stop diarrhea, or be re-wetted and applied to burns, insect bites, and cuts or scratches, especially when they had to travel. Clay, whether bentonite or montmorillonite, is an amazing, powerful substance!

My second practice is to do a parasite cleanse every November when the weather gets cold and I stop going barefoot. As autumn arrives and the year draws to a close, I have two choices. I can go to Progressive Labs (www.progressivelabs.com), get a bottle of Paradex, and take four capsules a day until the bottle is gone. Or I can go to Hulda Clark's online store (www.drclarkstore.com) and buy one of her parasite kits. My favorite is Dr. Clark Clove, Wormwood, & Freeze-dried Green Black Walnut Hull. Then I just follow the directions she includes with the 3 bottles of what are very powerful herbal supplements that clean out parasites.

Be aware that when you start a parasite program, there will be a die-off that can leave you feeling awful. For the first 3-5 days you may have any or all of the following: headache, nausea, vomiting, fatigue, body aches, sinuses that overflow or plug up, even a slight fever or serious night sweat. This is called a Herxheimer Reaction, or sometimes simply a healing crisis. It is caused when the dead bodies of the parasites fill your blood and overload your liver. Keep this in mind as you choose when to start your parasite program. If you go to work in an office every day and are home on weekends, you might want to start your parasite program so that your first three days fall on Friday, Saturday, and Sunday. That way you won't miss any work if you feel too awful to do anything but lay on the sofa.

Any time your blood is carrying something the body can't use, the liver will filter it out. If your liver gets overwhelmed and cannot take anything more out of the blood, that waste will continue to circulate in your system and you are going to feel miserable. For this reason, it is extremely helpful to know how to do a set of coffee enemas. The coffee enema is a detox procedure we will talk about a little later in this section. For now, just know that a coffee enema is a godsend because it forces the liver to dump its load of toxins into the gastrointestinal tract where it can be quickly eliminated. This leads to nearly immediate relief of the misery or at least a great improvement.

My third practice is the use of a BCX frequency generator to keep parasites from multiplying and taking over. This handy little machine is not cheap (about $2500), but it's not astronomically expensive either. It is one of many versions of Royal Rife's technology and I think every home should have one because it is useful for a host of problems that arise in the form of viruses, bacteria, a variety of infections, inflammation, and chronic conditions.

I originally bought the BCX because I wanted to get rid of cold sores caused by Herpes Simplex 1, a virus that acts like a parasite by burrowing into your nervous system tissues. When I first got it, the instructions walked me through a range of protocols having to do with various healing strategies and parasite programs. I had no problem with any of these because I am generally quite healthy and have long been careful to keep up my annual parasite program.

When I got to the point that I was ready to address the various cold sore programs, I thought I would be careful by not going directly for the Herpes Simplex 1 virus. Instead, I chose a frequency I thought would have a small effect and would clean up fringe versions of the herpes virus. The frequency I chose was Human Herpes Virus #5, also known as cytomegalovirus. I ran the program and when it was done, I went about my day. But within 24 hours, I felt like I had been hit by a Mack truck! I went down like a stone and it took me over two weeks to clear the massive congestion triggered by the die-off of the dead virus. It turned out that this little tool was far more effective than I expected.

My perspective of the BCX is that it is invaluable because it can be set to correct almost anything, it doesn't require a trip to the doctor, doesn't require expensive prescriptions and refills, doesn't have debilitating side effects (at least not once you get past the initial die-off) and a one-time investment lasts a long time, perhaps even a lifetime.

A few people have said they thought it was too expensive for them, but my view is that we all have cars to carry us around town that cost ten times the price of a BCX. We all have refrigerators to keep our food fresh, computers to manage our businesses, expensive televisions to provide us with entertainment and information. These items are not cheap; they are necessary in our day-to-day living. So why don't we have something as powerful and useful as a frequency generator to keep us healthy? I think the frequency generator is a gift straight from the future that we will learn to use to regenerate ourselves in ways we never dreamed possible.

Fasting

There is an old story told over many, many years about a middle-aged man who was not feeling well. He had turned gray, gained a lot of weight, was tired and cranky, argued often with his family and friends, had lost interest in sex, and eventually lost his job. The day he was fired from his job, he went home early and discovered his wife in bed with another man.

This was too much for him, and feeling suicidal, he ran out of the house and into the depths of the forest, abandoning society, his wife, his family and friends, intending to stay in the forest and starve to death.

However, as the days without food went by, he began to feel better and better. He lost weight, his energy returned, he felt peaceful inside, and discovered he loved being out in nature. He had accidentally discovered the benefits of fasting.

Eventually, he returned to his village where people were amazed at the trim figure and calm disposition he had developed. He took a new job in a nature sanctuary, found a new, healthy, interesting wife, and spent a long, happy life doing what he loved to do. Every year for the rest of his life he went into the forest, alone and without food, for a period of time. There he renewed himself by fasting.

Hopefully, this little story will help make clear why the most basic rule of thumb in naturopathic healing is: If you get a cold, sinus infection, bronchitis, strep throat, or any other problem – STOP EATING! The need to digest food creates a huge energy drain on the body, energy that the body should be using to heal itself. Do not eat until you feel better and it is obvious that you are on the mend.

Over the course of any given day or night, your pancreas and entire endocrine system put a great deal of effort into producing enzymes that will *repair* and *rebuild* your physical system. Whenever you eat, your body must temporarily stop producing these repair-and-rebuild enzymes in order to produce *digestive* enzymes. Many foods in their undigested state would be poisonous to the body, so your body breaks these foods down into their most basic components, hoping to extract whatever nutrients might be useful for the ongoing work of repair and rebuilding.

If you don't feel good, the worst thing you can do is eat, especially if you consume sugar or corn syrup. As soon as you eat, you end up feeling worse because the work of healing must be suspended during digestion. If you stop eating, your body is free to concentrate on healing and repairing things. In a relatively short time, you'll feel much better.

Well-meaning parents often coax their child to eat when the child doesn't feel good, thus violating the child's natural wisdom, which is to refrain from eating when he's not well. Even animals know better than to eat when they're hurt or sick. They withdraw and sleep, allowing the body to heal itself and not burdening it with the work of digestion.

The unconscious fear that most of us carry is that we will die without food. Although this is true if we are left without food for months, the truth is that we can go quite a long time without something to eat and still do quite well.

One Wednesday night in December of the early 2000s, a good friend of mine who lived here on the farm was not feeling well. It was the night of his son's birthday, so in spite of his malaise, he went out to dinner with his boys, where he ate a large prime rib steak, baked potato with all the trimmings, and plenty of birthday cake and ice cream. Although he felt even worse after this, the next night he went to a party where he again ate and drank heavily, disregarding his body's signals.

By Saturday, he was experiencing severe gastrointestinal cramping and pain that doubled him over every time he tried to eat something. I suggested he stop eating, but he did not seem to hear this and continued to try to eat various things or take medicines he thought might make him feel better. It didn't matter what he tried to take, even a sip of water caused severe pain and cramping that lasted for two or three hours.

Finally, late on Monday night, he asked for a ride to the emergency room of the hospital. He had now been ignoring the signals from his body for five full days and was no longer able to stand the pain. At the hospital the doctors checked him over, looking for an obstructed bowel or food poisoning. They ran a few tests, told him they couldn't find anything wrong and said he could go home. He did not feel fine, but he sat up and said, "What should I eat?"

"Eat anything you want," the doctor replied in an unconcerned manner, obviously not understanding that this was not going to work for his distressed patient. My friend and I looked at each other. Until that moment, he wanted to believe that our medical system knew more than his body knew. He was a trained respiratory therapist and very familiar with doctors and hospitals.

My own assessment was that he had severe gastritis, and on the way home I asked him if he had really considered not eating.

"Don't I need a certain amount of nourishment in order to give my body enough energy to heal?" he asked.

"It *takes* energy to digest food, leaving less energy for healing. You won't die if you stop eating for a while…you'll *heal*. Your body is talking to you and you're not listening. It's telling you it can't be bothered with food right now," I replied.

When we returned to the farm, I gave him a book to read titled, *Fasting Can Save Your Life.* He read it and was amazed. For eight days, he didn't eat or drink anything except sips of water. On the ninth day, he said, "I think I'm ready to try a little something to eat. What would you recommend?"

I suggested some homemade beef broth since we were in the process of making the potent, highly mineralized broth at that time. Good broth takes three days to make, and there is an old saying that holds much wisdom, "A well-made broth will resurrect the dead." [62] He began with a teaspoonful, increased gradually, and within a few days was eating without pain or difficulty.

I first began personally experimenting with fasting many years ago, but became pretty serious about it when I was diagnosed with rheumatoid arthritis. Every time I stopped eating, the pain was gone or greatly relieved within 24 hours. The problem was that I was already thin and couldn't afford to fast for more than ten days at a time. (I'm sure there is a lesson here for all those people who refuse to eat for fear of getting fat. They might think

---

62 Fallon, *Nourishing Traditions,* p. 113.

they're nice to look at, but sometimes you need a little reserve weight.) After becoming a patient of Dr. Nicholas Gonzales, I resolved some of the problem by alternating ten-day periods of detoxification through fasting with ten-day periods of nutrient-dense, easy to digest foods like beef or chicken broth, homemade yogurt, carrot/apple/beet/celery juice, 14-Grain Cereal, or homemade, whole wheat bread with raw butter, and a carefully designed supplement program.

Fasting is so powerful that it's hard to believe it isn't utilized more. When I first began using fasting to heal arthritis, my granddaughter, Stephanie, was about nine-years-old and subject to constant strep throat and ear infections because of her allergies at that time. One day, my daughter asked me to babysit for Stephie who was home from school with another infection. I had been fasting for three or four days and didn't have the energy to look after a sick child, but I agreed. That morning, I got the idea that maybe Stephie could heal without antibiotics if she fasted as well. I called her mother, a registered nurse, and suggested that Stephie join me in the fast so we could see what would happen. She agreed, and with some caution mixed with adult authority, I explained the situation to my granddaughter.

Being only nine years old, Stephie didn't have much to say and didn't feel good enough to argue. We spent her first day (my fourth day) of fasting by drinking water with a bit of lemon juice in it. The rest of the time we slept. Several times throughout the day, I checked her swollen throat and noted the huge tonsils, which were almost covered with white patches growing on them.

The second day we continued to drink water and rest. Her tonsils were still coated with white, the throat still swollen, and her eyes still droopy and watery looking, but her fever was down a little.

The third day started out much like the first two days. I continued to monitor her condition carefully, aware that I didn't want to be irresponsible with something as serious as a strep infection. I was fully willing to back down and run for antibiotics if she got dramatically worse or if anything really frightening should develop. But around two o'clock that afternoon, when I checked her throat, it was much less swollen, and there were only a few white patches left on her tonsils. I was amazed!

By that evening, her fever was almost gone. She wanted to get up and play, and she began showing an interest in food again. With some difficulty, I refused to let her eat, offering only water. We both went to bed early, and the next morning there was a definite improvement.

By noon of the fourth day, the rest of the white patches disappeared from her tonsils, along with the last of her fever. She began asking for something to eat. Uncertain about what to do, but jubilant about the fact that her body had overcome the infection without antibiotics, I continued to insist that she have only water, but promised we would have a little fruit the next morning.

Gradually, offering only fresh, raw fruit and water for two days, then graduating to salads, then her favorite cooked vegetables – potatoes and peas – we returned to eating, adding meat last. That was the last time we ever put any of the children on antibiotics.

Fasting is really quite simple because it requires that you do nothing instead of doing something. You simply stop eating. For the first couple of days, you may be hungry, headachy, and tired. Doing a coffee enema helps these miserable symptoms immensely. By the third day, the hunger stops, and you begin to experience deep changes in your energy system. Often, your inner quiet becomes profound, perception expands, and your physical body starts to relax, slow down, yet heal quickly.

Two things are helpful when you're fasting. The first is to rest a lot. Don't try to do all the things you normally do. If you must do anything at all, use the time to put together a complete and well-thought-out healing program or change of diet.

The second thing is a coffee enema once a day for at least the first two or three days to help the liver dump the toxic wastes your body has stored and which the body will immediately begin getting rid of during a fast (see the chapter on *Coffee Enemas*).

Don't be surprised if your skin breaks out, hair seems dull, tongue gets coated, and your breath is awful for a while. These are clear indications that you are getting rid of a lot of inner garbage.

There are many kinds of fasts – water fasts, raw fruit juice fasts, raw vegetable juice fasts, herbal tea fasts, and others. The kind of fast you choose should be somewhat dependent on your goal. Water fasts are fabulous for healing infections or losing weight. Raw fruit juice fasts are powerful for breaking down old, dead, or diseased tissues. Raw vegetable fasts are superb for helping heal after surgery or for building new, healthy cells and tissues. Herbal tea fasts are as varied as the number of herbs on the planet, and each one accomplishes something different. For instance, red clover tea cleans the blood, corn silk tea cleans the bladder, raspberry leaf tea nourishes the reproductive system, and other herbs have other effects, all too numerous to mention here.

Fasting can be practiced for as little as one day, or you can go three days, five days, eight days or more. I have experimented with fasts up to 38 days and found them to be extremely powerful in correcting conditions in the body. When it is time to break the fast, I make a batch of popcorn – no butter or salt – and eat one cup of it slowly, chewing thoroughly. An hour or two later, I eat a second cup, and an hour or two after that, a third cup. This provides enough bulk to get the gastrointestinal tract moving nicely again. If you are allergic to popcorn, you could break the fast with oranges or apples, eating two or three of them over a span of 6-8 hours. It is important to re-introduce foods slowly and in small amounts over the first day and not return to eating full meals too quickly.

If you were eating poorly before the fast, do not return to your former diet. Instead, find and incorporate as many real, whole foods into your diet as you can…real milk, butter, eggs, meats, homemade broths and soups, steamed vegetables, breads made with freshly ground whole wheat flour, fresh vegetable juices, and a few good-quality fruits.

If you can get your hands on an older book titled *How To Get Well* by Paavo Airola PhD, ND, it is an excellent guide to conducting a variety of juice fasts, among other things. I'm sure there are many good books that are newer and easier to get than Airola's book. You just have to do a little research to find them. In my humble opinion, there is no better reference on fasting than *Fasting Can Save Your Life* and most of the later books are based on it or draw from it. Read it while you do your first water fast. It is truly an eye opener, and the title says it all. ❖

18
Chelation

I AM NOT AN EXPERT ON CHELATION THERAPIES, but I have had to learn the basics about them for my own healing and will pass this on to you because the truth surrounding this technique is very important.

There are two kinds of chelation therapy: EDTA and DMPS.

EDTA (ethylene-diamine-tetra-acetic acid) chelation is an intravenous procedure used to remove plaque and sclerotic material from arteries and veins, thus improving circulation and eliminating the need for heart bypass surgery, reducing the risk of heart attacks and strokes, and improving oxygen to the brain which, in turn, improves memory, brain function, and clarity of thinking.

This kind of chelation also helps to speed healing over a very broad spectrum because improved circulation improves delivery of nutrients to all areas of the body and delivers oxygen to all parts of your system. Oxygen is the most potent antibiotic known to man and promotes healing of all tissues.

EDTA chelation is done at a clinic where a patient or client sits in a chair while the EDTA chemical is introduced into the body intravenously for about an hour. The therapy works best if the patient goes for treatment about three times a week for roughly ten to twelve weeks every two years. A good, high nutrition diet, regular exercise, avoidance of sugar – which makes the blood sticky and more prone to heart attack – and the practice of routine detox, especially the liver flush, should accompany chelation. When it does, veins and arteries are cleared, the risk of heart attack or stroke is greatly reduced, and the body begins to rebuild a strong, healthy circulatory system.

There has been a great deal of misinformation about EDTA chelation, and stories alleging quackery have attempted to discredit this important healing technique. Some say the medical profession is attempting to protect the high incomes made by doctors who are in the business of bypass surgery. While this may hold some truth, it is just as likely that most doctors are acutely aware of the dangers of heart attack and do not want to take the risk that someone may have a serious heart attack while they are responsible for that individual.

Of course, when there's an emergency and a heart attack is in progress, chelation is not appropriate and the techniques and surgeries that characterize "rescue medicine" are invaluable. Also, since doctors have it drilled into them again and again that they are responsible for their patient's lives – and they pay exorbitant malpractice fees to protect themselves while taking on this responsibility – they don't like to utilize therapies that don't provide the instant fix that relieves their own worries about a patient's condition. Remember, when you visit an MD, he becomes responsible for your health – not you.

In addition, since many doctors know almost nothing about nutrition and detox, they don't understand chelation, and therefore can't use it effectively. Neither can they use the fasting, foods, and supplements that create such powerful effects in the human body/mind system. This is changing, albeit slowly, and in the future, I suspect more and more doctors who are interested in real healing will begin to include chelation, detox, and high nutrition in their practice and will come to trust these in helping to heal the human body/mind system.

DMPS (dimercapto propanesulfonic acid) chelation is used when it is necessary to remove heavy metals and toxic chemicals from the body quickly. Over the last 50 years, we have been poisoning our world and ourselves in thousands of ways, with heavy metals such as cadmium, mercury, lead, arsenic, aluminum, nickel, cobalt, and many others. Over 63,000 different chemicals, various nitrates and nitrites, aspartame, aflatoxins, glyphosate, MSG, antibiotics, DDT, BHA, PCBs, chlorine, cyclamates, diazinon, dozens of preservatives, and a host of "natural" flavorings and colorings are accumulating in our bodies where they derange hormones, cause serious degenerative diseases, and interfere with our blood's capacity to carry many nutrients and oxygen. [63] [64]

Let's take mercury, since it is quite common in our mouths in the form of mercury-silver amalgams (50% mercury/30% silver) used to fill cavities in teeth.[65] Research has shown that mercury oxidizes from the average person's amalgam fillings at the rate of 150 mcg. per day![66] When dentists order, store, and dispose of the mercury-silver compound used to fill teeth, they must follow strict federal guidelines for the handling of hazardous, toxic materials.[67] Yet, once it's in someone's mouth, the claim of the American Dental Association is that it's harmless.

Unfortunately, this is not true. When molecules of mercury oxidize and break away from the filling, they are breathed into the lungs, absorbed into mucus membranes in the mouth, or combined with food and swallowed into the gastrointestinal system. From these points of entry, the mercury gets into the brain, the blood, and even crosses the placenta in a pregnant woman and can do its damage within minutes.[68] Once in the blood, molecules of mercury either sit on the docking sites that would normally hold oxygen, or the mercury causes hemoglobin molecules to swell and twist out of shape. Once twisted, oxygen cannot dock on the molecule of hemoglobin. Since a shortage of oxygen immediately creates a shortage of energy, you will suffer from fatigue. Since oxygen is also a powerful antibiotic, you are more susceptible to colds, flu, and other diseases going around your community. [69]

---

63 Paavo Airola PhD, *How To Get Well* (Sherwood, OR: Health Plus Publishers, 1993) p. 167-177.

64 *Acres USA News,* Acres USA Publishing.

65 Hal Huggins DDS, MA, *It's All in Your Head* (Garden City Park, NY: Avery Publishing Group, 1993) p. 23-24

66 Huggins, p. 35.

67 Huggins, p. 36-37

68 Huggins, p. 33.

69 Huggins, p. 105-106.

Heavy metals that get into your gastrointestinal system wreak havoc there as well. Staphylococcus and streptococcus organisms live naturally in your gut because their job is to break down the remains of the food you eat and prepare it to be eliminated. When a staph or strep molecule meets mercury, they are immediately aware that their existence is under threat from the frequencies and effects of that metal. So they run to a neighboring cell and steal or "borrow" the DNA from that cell! They then have enough DNA to out-maneuver any antibiotic by mutating with astonishing rapidity. The result is an infectious "super bug" that can resist anything we can throw at it.[70]

When you consider that staph and strep bacteria also live in the soil where we spray all kinds of toxic pesticides, herbicides, and fungicides, all of which have been stabilized with heavy metals to cut down their activity and volatility until they can be sprayed on that field, you can see why super bugs have become a real threat in our world.

In my opinion, this is why we have so many antibiotic-resistant drugs. I'm sure there is some truth to the idea that too many antibiotics are being given to fix things that the immune system can and should take care of by itself, and this contributes to the problem of bacterial resistance. However, the real culprit is the use of heavy metals in pesticides, herbicides, fungicides, and the thousands of other chemicals in our world today, which we then ingest and suffer the effects of.

If you are not healing properly after doing all the right things, including exercise, good nutrition, the right supplements and herbs, and a good detox routine, you may need chelation therapy to remove heavy metals. You cannot heal if you have too many heavy metals in you because they so powerfully distort your cells, interfere with cellular processes, and hinder the repair efforts of the body. There are good clinics around the country. They often don't advertise because they don't want to draw unwanted attention to themselves. But if you ask around, you can find a good one. ❖

---

70 Huggins, p. 55.

19
The Liver Flush

WHEN I DEVELOPED RHEUMATOID ARTHRITIS, I became a patient of Dr. Nicholas Gonzales MD in New York, who taught me the great value and power of regular detox in the body. I also followed up my visit to Gonzales with several telephone conversations to Dr. William Kelley, the man who taught Gonzales and who agreed to share what he had learned with me. Although Gonzales has made a few changes to the detox program he teaches, and Kelley insists on a few things of his own, the detox programs that follow in the next three or four chapters are a combination of what they teach, plus what I have learned over the past twenty-seven years.

There is no organ in the body, with perhaps the exception of the colon, that is as critical as the liver in keeping you healthy and free of toxic waste. When the liver is clogged, you will develop all kinds of problems. These include such things as liver spots, a red nose, intestinal gas, headaches, insomnia, bad breath, poor vision, swollen legs and feet, skin diseases, sterility, appendicitis, allergies, bronchitis, and the more dangerous diseases like cancer, TB, or cirrhosis. Says Raymond Dextreit, "… (you) must realize that there is no cure of any disease, no true health, without a healthy, well-functioning liver." [71]

The liver *is* the key to starting any kind of healing. The job of the liver is the minute-to-minute detoxification of your entire body as you

---

71 Raymond Dextreit, *Our Earth, Our Cure* (Secaucus, NJ: Carol Publishing Group, translated by Michel Abehsera, 1993) p. 31. This is a great book to have in your natural healing library because it's full of uses for something so available.

go through your day-to-day and especially as you begin to break down poorly built or diseased tissue. Thus, this detox procedure is an age-old way of making sure this powerful and important organ gets cleaned out and renewed regularly so that waste materials do not pile up throughout the body simply because the liver is overloaded with wastes it has already filtered out.

LIVER FLUSH INSTRUCTIONS:

To do a Liver Flush you will need:

1 gallon of organic apple juice or apple cider

1 oz of ortho-phosphoric acid (order a 2 oz bottle of *Phosfood* from Standard Process Inc, or *O.P.A* (OrthoPhosphoric Acid) from www.progressivelabs.com)

Cal-Amo capsules (from Standard Process or a local chiropractor)

Epsom salts (from your drug store)

Heavy whipping cream and berries (blueberries or strawberries)

Bentonite liquid (32 oz bottle from Sonné or Progressive Labs)

Olive oil and a fresh lemon

1. **It takes about five days to do a liver flush**. The first four days are fairly simple, but a little planning is required. If you work outside the home, you should plan your liver flush so that you are finishing the fifth day on a day when you don't have to go to work. Planning to take the next day off is also a good idea. You can work over the first four days, but the fifth day, which is the day of the actual flush, you will want to be at home, at least from 2 pm through the wee hours of the morning. Also, don't schedule your liver flush to end the day before a big party. Party foods and drinks will undo what you just worked so hard to achieve – a clean, unplugged, well-working liver.

2. **To begin**: On the morning of the first day, **add one ounce** (which is 2 TBSP or ½ bottle) of **ortho-phosphoric acid to the gallon of apple juice** and shake well. (*Note: you will have to find a chiropractor*

or nutritional consultant who sells Standard Process or order from Progressive Labs. You can't buy it from a health food store.) Over the next four to five days, **drink** the entire gallon of apple juice at a rate of **3-4 full (8 oz) glasses a day.** Generally, it takes four days to drink the majority of the apple juice, with usually 1 or 2 glasses left to be finished on the morning of the fifth day. Drink the juice between meals rather than with meals, and *be sure to brush your teeth with baking soda or thoroughly rinse out your mouth with baking soda water after the juice,* using about 1 tsp of soda to a glass of water. This is critical because the two acids in the juice (malic and phosphoric acid) will damage your teeth if you do not use the soda to counteract it. Over the days that you are drinking the apple juice and phosphoric acid mixture, eat normally.

3. When you begin a liver flush, you should also begin a series of coffee enemas. On each day of the liver flush, **do two coffee enemas** (I call this a "set of coffee enemas") one immediately after the other, **preferably before 7 pm.** Be aware that coffee introduced rectally does not have the same effect as coffee ingested by mouth, and it is not likely to disturb your sleep. However, it's still a good idea to do the coffee enemas early in the day if you are home all day, or in the earlier part of the evening, so it doesn't keep you awake in case you're really sensitive to it. The instructions for the coffee enema can be found in a chapter titled *The Coffee Enema,* further along in this book.

4. On the fifth, and last day, of the liver flush, which is the day that you finish the last glass of apple juice, **take 2 capsules of Cal Amo right before breakfast** and take **another 2 capsules right before lunch**. Eat a normal breakfast and lunch on this day, and be sure you finish your lunch by 12 noon. If you are still drinking your apple juice, try to finish the last of it before 12 noon.

5. **At 2 pm, (or 2 hours after your lunch if you're on a slightly earlier or later schedule), drink 1-2 tablespoons of Epsom salt dissolved in a half-glass of warm water.** You can add a bit of fresh orange, grapefruit, or lemon juice to cover the taste if you like. I follow the Epsom salt drink with a glass of plain water, which is incredibly sweet and delicious after the Epsom salt. After drinking this little concoction, you may want to stay near the bathroom. Your stomach will rumble, your

bowels will loosen, and you may or may not have a bowel movement or two.

6. **At 5 pm, or 5 hours after you ate lunch, again drink 1-2 tablespoons of Epsom salt dissolved in a half glass of warm water.** Add juice if desired, and follow with fresh, cool water. Your intestines will rumble even more, and staying near the bathroom becomes more important!

7. **Between 6–7 pm, or 6 hours after your lunch, take 1 capsule of Cal Amo and eat a dinner that consists of heavy whipping cream and berries.** Any kind of berry is acceptable, but it's the cream that is important, so eat as much as you want. I put frozen blueberries in a bowl and pour a cup of the cream over them. Usually, I eat two bowls of this delicious mixture. You can also put the blueberries and cream in a blender to make a blended shake, just be careful not to leave the blender on too long or you'll have butter instead of cream with your blueberries.

8. **At 10:30 pm, (or ½ hour before you go to bed) drink ¼ cup of Bentonite liquid,** which is actually clay in a liquid suspension. It doesn't taste bad, in fact, it doesn't have any taste, just a creamy texture, but it performs small miracles in your intestinal tract. It attracts to itself both parasites and the silty, toxic wastes dumped by the liver, helping to carry these out of the body later.

9. **One-half hour after drinking the Bentonite clay, at approximately 11 pm, drink ⅓ - ½ cup of olive oil.** The juice of one fresh lemon can be added to the olive oil, and this makes it much more palatable. I squeeze the lemon juice into the olive oil, shake vigorously or blend briefly with a stick blender, and put it in the freezer for 15-20 minutes. This is much easier to drink than straight olive oil! It may take you 10-15 minutes or so to drink the entire amount, but immediately after finishing the oil, **go to bed and lie down on your right side with knees drawn up. Stay in that position for at least 45 minutes.** You might even fall asleep and stay in that position for a couple of hours, which is all right.

10. **Between 1-3 am, the liver enters its most active period of the day, and you may waken feeling nauseated.** This is because the liver has dumped all of its stored toxins into your gastrointestinal tract.

If you are quite toxic, you might experience more than a little nausea. You may vomit, have diarrhea, or a serious "night sweat" alternating with chills. ***To avoid all this, get up by no later than 2:00 am and do a set of coffee enemas.*** This not only aids the liver in dumping even more of its toxins, it helps move them out of the body before they can make you ill. In actuality, it is a very good sign if you feel nauseous or have other symptoms of toxicity because it means that the liver and gallbladder are actually flushing themselves out and the healing procedure is working. When you have finished the set of coffee enemas, go back to bed and to sleep for the rest of the night.

11. **The next day, eat normally and take two (2) Cal Amo with breakfast, two (2) Cal Amo with lunch, and one (1) Cal Amo with dinner**. You may feel a little low the next day, although many people have no aftereffects at all.

❖

Now...what is this procedure about, and why is each step very important?

First, when you put the ortho-phosphoric acid into the apple juice, you now have a drink containing two acids: the malic acid found naturally in apple juice, and the phosphoric acid that you added. These two acids work together to dissolve plaque, calcium deposits, and other "stony" deposits in the arteries, liver, kidneys, and elsewhere. They soften and dissolve gallstones and kidney stones, reducing them to sand and gravel.

There are two kinds of aging. One is chronological aging, the other is biological aging. One of the criteria for determining your biological age has to do with how soft, flexible, and deposit-free your organs and tissues are. Some authorities consider aging to be due simply to hardening, also known as *sclerosis*, of the body tissues. A baby's tissues and organs are soft, pliable, and free of waste deposits, which is why they often have such good health. By removing sclerotic material in your body, you free your arteries and organs to work better and reverse your biological age.

Drinking the apple juice with its two acids over the course of five days dissolves a lot of this sclerotic matter. The liver filters this toxic material out of your blood until the day of the actual flush process when it is flushed out of your body altogether.

On the day of the actual flush, the two doses of Epsom salt, which contain high levels of magnesium, relax the openings of the gallbladder, the bile ducts, and the ducts in your liver. Ordinarily, the mouth of the gallbladder is like a pair of tight, firm, rosebud-like lips with a small, rubbery opening. When you drink the Epsom salts, those tightly pursed lips relax, soften, and open.

Then, along comes a good dose of cream with a few berries in it! And what happens to the liver and gallbladder? The job of these two organs is to emulsify fat, and cream is pure fat. So the liver and gallbladder immediately and vigorously contract, squirting out bile *along with the softened, shrunken gallstones, stored wastes in the liver, and any sand- or gravel-like material that has accumulated in them.* All of this passes easily into the small intestine, which is why you may waken in the night feeling nauseous.

The clay you drink around 10:30 pm not only helps to bulk up the wastes, some of which will be quite silty, so you can excrete them more easily. Clay is a powerful healing agent in its own right, as is the olive oil, which is a known as a *specific*. A specific is something that is generally known and used for a specific kind of healing and that works the same in a majority of people. Olive oil is a specific healing agent for mucous membranes and tissues in the digestive tract.

Be aware that each step in the liver flush performs a key role in the sequence of events that lead to a clean, healthy liver. Do not skip any of the steps or try to substitute procedures or you will not get the results you are working for.

A simpler version of the liver flush was first used during the 1920s as a way of improving liver function. The procedure outlined above is an improvement and refinement of the original technique and serves the healing process in the important ways in which it acts, as outlined above.

All in all, the liver flush is a simple yet powerful way of removing gallstones without surgery, cleaning out liver deposits, removing plaque from arteries and organs, all of which helps to end everything from hot flashes and insomnia to depression and fatigue. It helps improve eyesight, eliminates the side-effects of chemotherapy, and dispels numerous other problems while improving function throughout the body. Since the liver is the organ that produces your cholesterol, a liver flush also helps to normalize cholesterol metabolism. I have had people tell me that the liver flush dropped their cholesterol level by 35 points almost overnight.

A number of people have asked if they can do a liver flush when they don't have a gall bladder or perhaps have had a colostomy. The answer is "yes" in both cases. You may not have a gall bladder, but you still have a liver.

An even greater number of people have also asked about doing a liver flush while undergoing chemotherapy. It is best if you complete one or two liver flushes before chemo. Doing so makes it easier to handle the side-effects of chemo. In addition, sometimes chemotheraphy makes the tissues on the inside of the mouth so inflamed that eating fruit, especially citrus fruit becomes impossible. Whether you do a liver flush before chemotherapy or not, this particular detox procedure is a very powerful way to begin clearing the chemicals from your system once chemo is over.

Perhaps sharing a story will illustrate this best. Some years ago, a woman named Kristin had just had surgery for colon cancer and was undergoing chemo. She heard about these healing methods from a friend and called to register for one of my classes. On the day of class, she arrived, terribly thin, with huge dark circles under her eyes, tired, and adamant about not putting her body through any more difficulty. For the entire weekend, she listened carefully, asked really tough questions, and left at the end of the weekend still uncertain as to whether or not she should try the liver flush. I had encouraged her tentatively, based on the reports from other people who had done remarkably well with this kind of detox after chemotherapy, yet I felt this was a decision she had to make for herself. A few days later she returned to buy the few specialty things she needed, then went home to start.

A week later I answered the phone to find an ecstatic voice on the other end of the line. It was Kristin. She had finished the liver flush a day or two earlier and said, "I can't believe the difference in how I feel. It's like a black, oppressive cloud has been lifted from my mind, my heart, and my body!" She went on for a few minutes, excitedly sharing how glad she was to have done the liver flush, about how uncertain she had been because she'd already been through so much, and what a wondrous sense of life and good feeling now filled her.

Others have shared similar things, whether they were healing from cancer, dieting to lose weight, struggling with congestive heart failure, or trying to recover from some other illness. The liver flush is meant to be used about three times a year, an average of once every fourth month (e.g. January, May, and September). Get a calendar, mark off the five days needed to complete this detox procedure, then keep that date with yourself and your health. If you do, you will be amazed at the results. You will look and feel younger and will keep your body in good working order. ❖

20
The Colon Sweep

IF YOUR GASTROINTESTINAL TRACT BECOMES CLOGGED with layers of thick, sticky wastes, your ability to absorb the nutrients needed to constantly rebuild and repair your body goes – no pun intended – right down the tubes. It is only in the last decade or so that scientists and medical people have come to realize the importance of what they call the *microbiome,* colonies of beneficial probiotic bacteria that absolutely must be maintained in the gut in order to have and keep good health. The beginning of a healthy microbiome is the colon sweep

You have about 35' of small intestine and 5' of large intestine. When your intestines start to plug up with waste matter, they don't necessarily become blocked in the sense that nothing will pass through. They become lined with gunk that gets in the way of your ability to digest and absorb nutrients.

The small intestine begins at the lower end of the stomach, and the entire 35' of it reminds me of a big pile of spaghetti piled up inside of you. The walls of the small intestine are lined with what are called intestinal cilia. These cilia are thin, filament-like fingers that line the inside walls, and when clean and healthy, they wave back and forth like grasses in the wind, filtering the ingested food through their fine fingers, mixing enzymes and important bacteria with the food to make it digestible while extracting and absorbing vitamins, minerals, and other nutrients that pass over their surfaces. When gunk piles up on the walls of the small intestine, these cilia become mired in it and unable to move. The cilia fall out leaving bald patches. When this occurs, the tiny enzyme-producing structures that operate at the base of these cilia stop working and food is neither broken down properly nor absorbed. It just passes through without leaving its nutrients and we begin to degenerate.

The large intestine, also known as the colon, is a long tube that begins in the lower right quadrant of the abdomen and rises upward (the ascending colon) to about your waistline where it makes a 90° turn and goes across the abdomen (the transverse colon) to the left side of your body. From there, it slants upward a little, passing under the left ribs, then turns and runs down the left side of the body (descending colon) toward the anal opening, making something of an S-shape right before the rectum.

For a moment, picture the transverse colon like a rope bridge suspended across a chasm. Then, imagine that someone comes along and starts loading boxes onto the bridge. It may hold up for a while, but as the load gets heavier, the bridge starts to droop seriously. When this happens, the heavy colon begins pulling other tissues down from above. The colon ends up in a "U" shape that lays on top of the tissues below it, interfering with normal function in surrounding organs and tissues. Intestines, bladder, sexual organs, and rectum can all have great difficulty going about their daily business with the heavy colon sitting on top of them. Over time, the build up of this layer of gunk tends to have a paralyzing effect on the ability of the colon to move, thus bowel movements slow down, get farther apart, and not all the waste matter is removed, making the problem worse.

As the heavily stuffed colon stretches and droops, it ceases to work effectively at all and constipation sets in. Food goes in, drops to the bottom of the loop, and the colon is neither strong enough nor flexible enough to push it back up and on out. As waste backs up in the system, pockets can bulge out here and there, creating perfect breeding places for infection. Meanwhile, your eyesight gets worse, skin looks terrible, hair falls out, breath gets bad, joints get stiffer, and you succumb to every cold and flu or other infection that comes around.

This thick, gunky layer is also a good place for rogue bacteria to make their home, and as these bacteria multiply and leave their own wastes, the colon can go from irritation to inflammation to a state known as "leaky gut syndrome." This is a condition in which the tissue of the colon is so weakened, it begins to allow waste matter to leak into the body, poisoning you and causing all manner of havoc. This seriously drains the resources of the immune system, which struggles to deactivate the constant invasions of bacteria and other toxic materials coming through the wall of the colon into the sensitive areas of the abdomen. Thus, cleaning the colon on a regular basis is equally as important as flushing your liver.

More than once I have heard the old saying, "Death begins in the colon." If either the colon or small intestine begins to plug up with old waste matter, elimination backs up and absorption of nutrients slows down. I know people who only have a bowel movement every four or five days. A healthy colon will expel some matter after every meal. If you eat three times a day, that would amount to three bowel movements a day.

To do a Colon Sweep you will need:

1 gallon of organic apple juice

1 bottle of Intestinal Bulking Agent II (available from Holistic Horizons)

2 qts of plain yogurt containing live cultures (Do not use any lowfat or sweetened yogurts. Bravo Yogurt is best.)

1 bottle of Probiotic capsules containing at least 20-30 billion live cultures per capsule

1. **It takes ten days to complete the full Colon Sweep**. You may eat your normal meals during the colon sweep, and if you work outside the home you can continue to go to work. However, plan to start your Colon Sweep on a Friday or Saturday because the first day or two, there is often a heavy, crampy feeling in the gut and sometimes a nagging headache, chills, and body aches.

Day 1
2. **On Day 1 at 10 am,** or sometime halfway between breakfast and lunch, put **8 oz of organic apple juice in a shaker** cup or mason jar that has a lid. **Add 1 rounded tsp of Intestinal Bulking Agent II** to the juice, cover and **shake vigorously** to mix well, then **drink immediately**. If you let it sit for even a few minutes, it begins turning to jelly due to the pectin in the Bulking Agent.

3. **Immediately after drinking the juice and bulking agent, drink 8 oz of water**, downing it completely. You may feel a bit full after this, which is normal.

4. **At 3 pm, or halfway between lunch and supper, repeat Steps 2 and 3**, taking a second dose of bulking agent in apple juice, and following this immediately with 8 oz of water.

5. **At 8 pm, or halfway between supper and bedtime, repeat Steps 2 and 3**, taking your third dose of bulking agent and again following with 8 oz of water.

6. Sometime **between 3 pm and 8 pm, do a set of two coffee enemas,** one immediately after the other.

7. **Eat ½ cup of yogurt at bedtime**.

Day 2-5

8. **Repeat Steps 2 through 7 each day for a total of five days until you have taken a total of fifteen (15) doses of Bulking Agent**. This completes part one of the Colon Sweep.

Day 6-10

9. **For the next five days** the procedure consists of the critical step of replenishing your bacterial flora. **Take 2 Probiotic capsules with warm water on an empty stomach between meals and at bedtime. Eat ½ cup of yogurt with each meal and at bedtime. If you prefer probiotic powder, sprinkle a dose of it on your normal meals – breakfast, lunch, and dinner**.

What was happening during the colon sweep, and why do you do this detox procedure? First, the bulking agent can absorb many times its own weight in water and enlarges in much the same way as a sponge does when exposed to water. As mentioned above, you may feel some real discomfort the first day or two due to the expansion of the bulking agent in the intestinal tract. The discomfort is a good sign because it means the bulking agent is stretching the intestines to maximum diameter.

This swollen mass then begins working its way through the small and large intestines, filling every nook and cranny, scrubbing, scraping, and forcing out all manner of stored wastes that would not otherwise be excreted.

Most people doing the colon sweep will pass a variety of exotic particles and substances. Many describe passing long casings, similar to a snakeskin or sausage casing, which is actually the dried mucus and dead cells from the surface of the intestines and colon. These wastes accumulate over a period of many years and seriously interfere with the absorption of nutrients and your ability to expel waste.

This procedure is also the most effective way of removing abnormal bacteria, parasites, worms, candida albicans, and other organisms from the gut that take hold after antibiotics or chemo have killed off the helpful bacteria that form the microbiome in the gut. During the colon sweep, all harmful organisms and bacteria are scraped away, but so are the beneficial organisms, and it is for this reason that the yogurt and acidophilus are so essential.

After a colon sweep, organisms such as candida, staphylococcus, streptococcus, and other virulent bacteria that live in your gastrointestinal tract and whose job it is to finish breaking down the food you have eaten, will grow quickly and replace themselves in a very short time. The beneficial organisms that control these more virulent bacteria are much slower to grow. If you do not eat the yogurt and take the acidophilus for *at least five days* in order to boost the presence of beneficial probiotic bacteria, you can end up with severe gastritis, candida, bloating, gas, and other difficulties related to food and digestion. Save yourself the trouble, and if you are going to err, err on the side of a few *extra* days of yogurt and probiotics, not a few less.

Once you have completed the Liver Flush and the Colon Sweep, you are half way through the first round of detox procedures. At this point, I often hear things like, "I haven't had a single migraine or even a headache… The flu skipped over me this year…I didn't realize how bloated I was until after that Colon Sweep when I had to hitch my belt a notch tighter…It seems impossible, but I think my eyesight has improved…There's still a little stiffness in the morning, but I could swear my arthritis pain has almost disappeared…Even though the weather is cold, I haven't had my usual difficulties breathing…" and other reports of improved function.

At this point in the program, there is a jump in your body's ability to absorb the nutrition in the foods you're eating and the supplements you're taking, and many people begin healing rapidly. This is a critical step in healing because you can put all the good food and medicine in the world into your system, but if it passes through unabsorbed, you won't heal and you will have wasted your money. Sometimes people notice only a slight lessening of the problem that was bothering them at this point, but those who continue to detoxify themselves on a regular basis notice steady improvement in every area of life, health, and energy, as well as the function of the entire body/mind system.

Sometimes you will experience a combination of shock and power. The shock comes from actually seeing an improvement in your condition and an awareness of how low you had dipped in terms of living fully. The power comes from the realization that you can make a real difference in your own life and heal completely. This then raises your spirits and makes it easier to keep going, so let's move on to the next step in the full detox program, the Purge. ❖

21
The Purge

THE PURGE IS ONE OF THE MOST IMPORTANT DETOX ROUTINES, especially for those with serious infections or cancers. Several versions of the technique exist, but the best one is outlined in the original edition of Dr. William Kelley's book, *One Answer To Cancer.* [72]

William D. Kelley DDS, cured himself of pancreatic cancer when he was in his late 30s by refusing to give in to the disease. By understanding nutrition and developing a series of detox routines designed to clean out the toxic by-products of disease, he was able to support the processes of repair and regeneration in his body until full healing occurred. In Kelley's view, the Purge is the most powerful of the detox procedures because it puts the body at rest, which aids the rapid removal of metabolic wastes. In addition, the Purge pushes the body into a completely alkaline state in which repair and rebuilding of damaged tissues occurs very rapidly.

In Kelley's view, people who develop cancers are not doomed to death at all, because it is relatively simple to stop these growths and even their metastases, but it is much trickier to get the body to break down and remove dead cancer tissue. This dead tissue is extremely poisonous and more often than not, it is the poisonous run-off from these tumors that kills the individual by plugging up the liver, lungs, skin, and kidneys, clouding the brain's orders, messing up endocrine function, impeding digestion and

---

72 Kelley's book, *One Answer to Cancer*, is available on the Internet. Simply type the name of the book into Google or your search engine and it will come up. I use **www**.whale.to/a/**kelley**.html**.

other bodily activities, generally making you so sick that you don't care if you live or die. Of course, as soon as you get to that point, your cells know you have given up, and they give up. You become history.

Although the poisonous wastes from asthma, diabetes, or arthritis aren't quite as powerful as that from cancer, there is a continuous accumulation of wastes from these diseases. In addition, poorly built and poorly functioning tissues and cells within the main systems of the body need to be cleared out regularly. If you do not clear toxic debris from your body, you will have great difficulty healing and may only get worse. Thus, the value of the Purge is in its power to remove large amounts of waste from the body, including waste material from *inside* your cells, in a quick and efficient manner.

To do The Purge you will need:

Plenty of fresh fruit and salad fixings

A juicing machine or hand reamer for citrus fruits

12 grapefruits

12 lemons

24 oranges

1-gallon jug or pitcher

Epsom Salt (from your local drug store)

1 gallon of distilled or purified water (from your local grocery store and sometimes known as Reverse Osmosis or R.O. water)

Cal-Amo capsules (from Standard Process)

Yogurt and good quality Probiotic capsules with 20-30 million live cultures in them.

It takes 5 days to complete the medium-length version of the Purge, 6 days to complete the longer version. If you work outside the home, you can continue to work for the first two days. The next two days you will have to be at home and near the bathroom, so plan to start your Purge on Thursday and Friday so you can be at home Saturday and Sunday. The last day of the Purge is similar to the first two days, so you can go back to work without difficulty.

Days 1

Day 1 of the Purge is fairly simple and normal. It consists of eating only **fresh fruit for breakfast and through the morning, a large salad full of raw vegetables for lunch and dinner on both days, and doing a set of coffee enemas in the late afternoon or early evening**. Eating fresh fruit does not mean you eat an apple or a banana and then starve the rest of the morning. It means eating until you are satisfied. If that means two bananas, a kiwi, an apple, and a bowl of strawberries over the course of the morning, then that is what you need to have on hand.

A salad for lunch and dinner does not mean three pieces of iceberg lettuce, with a wedge of tomato and two slices of cucumber. It means a big salad of 30% mixed greens, and 60% chopped vegetables such as tomatoes, fresh parsley, cucumbers, carrots, cabbage, radishes, peas, kohlrabi, green beans, broccoli, cauliflower, and finely diced onion, sprinkled with garlic salt and black pepper, and generous doses of virgin olive oil, melted butter, and flaxseed oil mixed with the juice of a fresh lemon drizzled over the top.

A good dressing is 2 TBSP olive oil mixed with 2 TBSP melted butter (not margarine) and 2 TBSP flaxseed oil with the juice of ½ lemon. For variation, add up to 1 TBSP of dried or 2 TBSP of fresh herbs such as oregano and basil, or parsley and savory, or dill and thyme. Make the dressing early, then leave it in the refrigerator overnight to release the herb flavors. If the butter hardens in the refrigerator, do NOT warm the dressing in the microwave to melt it again. In fact, never use a microwave for anything because it so completely denatures the molecules and frequencies in the food that they become destructive to you instead of nourishing you. Just warm the container briefly in a bowl of warm water. Or, put all the ingredients together except for the butter and flaxseed oil, adding the butter and flaxseed or hempseed oil just before serving.

When I am eating only salad, I start by filling a 1 QT bowl, eat it all, and sometimes refill it. If I get hungry in mid-afternoon, I have another bowl full. You will find you can eat a lot of salad without feeling stuffed. The biggest problem I run into is all the chewing required. I get tired of chewing, yet it's very important to chew the raw foods in your salad very well. Do not eat after 8 pm. If you get hungry, drink a pint of water, then try meditating, doing some gentle stretching exercises, or go to bed early and sleep so you won't know you're hungry. If you're desperately hungry, eat an apple.

Day 2

1. Repeat Day 1

2. At the end of Day 2, **make a citrus punch** consisting of the following:

Juice of 6 grapefruits

Juice of 6 lemons

Juice of 12 oranges

You need a good, sturdy juicer to do this. I use an Omega Juicer. Collect the juice from the above fruits into a gallon jug. When finished juicing, you should have between ½ and ¾ of a gallon of pure citrus juice. Don't worry if it has a bit of pulp in it.

Then add distilled or Reverse Osmosis water until the gallon jug is full. You now have 1 gallon of "citrus punch." Put it in the refrigerator until morning.

It takes about an hour to make the citrus punch, so don't wait until it's time to drink the first glass to start making it; plan accordingly. You could also make the citrus punch in the morning if you don't have time at night, but I like to have it made and waiting for reasons that will become clear shortly.

Day 3

1. On the morning of Day 3, **arise about 6:30 am** and take the citrus punch out of the refrigerator so it begins to warm to room temperature. Do not put it back in the fridge again. Then, dissolve 1 TBSP of Epsom salt in a half-glass of distilled or Reverse Osmosis (R.O.) water, stirring until completely dissolved. **Drink this combination of Epsom salt and water**, following it with a half-glass of plain or purified water. The Epsom salt water is quite bitter, so the plain water will taste delicious by comparison and help remove the bitter taste!

2. **At 7 am**, which is one-half hour later, **take another tablespoon of Epsom salt dissolved in a half-glass of R.O. water**, followed by a half-glass of plain or purified water.

3. **At 7:30 am**, which is one-half hour later, **take a third tablespoon of Epsom salt dissolved in a half-glass of R.O. water**, followed by a half-glass of plain or purified water. You will now have taken three doses of Epsom salt over a 1 hour period.

4. **Approximately two hours after the last dose of Epsom salt, (about 9:30 am) drink an 8-10 oz glass of this citrus punch.** You may want to lay down or rest after the 3 doses of Epsom salt & water. Stay near a bathroom!

5. Thereafter, **drink a glass of the citrus punch every hour.** You are to **eat no food that day** except, if you wish, an orange for dinner.

6. With your **12:30 pm glass of citrus punch**, take **1 capsule of Cal Amo**.

7. With your **6:30 pm glass of citrus punch**, take a **2nd capsule of Cal Amo**.

8. With your **10:30 pm glass of citurs punch**, take a **3rd capsule of Cal Amo**.

9. **Finish drinking the entire gallon of citrus punch in one day**. It will take you 12-16 hours to drink the entire gallon, hence the early start. During the purge, you may feel a variety of symptoms, such as nausea, headaches, muscle aches, and pains. Such symptoms indicate the body is releasing stored wastes, and although you might be uncomfortable, do not be alarmed. If you become seriously nauseous or have a very bad headache, do a set of coffee enemas immediately. If necessary, do another set at night. **Rest a lot during the day.** Stay close to the bathroom.

10. Before going to bed, make the second gallon of citrus punch using the remaining 6 grapefruits, 6 lemons, and 12 oranges. Refrigerate until morning.

Day 4

On Day 4, **repeat the entire set of instructions for Day 3,** including the three doses of Epsom salt, drinking the gallon of citrus punch made from grapefruit, lemons, and oranges, and taking the Cal Amo. You can expect to spend a lot of time running to the bathroom again. You will also notice that what's coming out looks just like what's going in! Dr. Kelley recommends that if you have cancer, you repeat the Epsom Salt and citrus punch routine for a third day, extending the Purge for an extra day because it is so good at removing wastes from ALL your tissues. He mentions that for every gallon of the citrus punch you drink, an equivalent gallon of waste material is removed from body cells and tissues. That's a lot of waste!

Day 5

On Day 5, (or Day 6, if you extended the Purge an extra day) return to the fresh fruit and salads that were eaten on Day 1 and Day 2. At each meal on Day 5, include ½ cup of Bravo Yogurt. Do a set of coffee enemas in the late afternoon or early evening. Take 2-4 capsules of probiotics at bedtime. After that, you are done! You can return to your everyday food, routines, and supplements until the next round of detox.

The Liver Flush, Colon Sweep, and Purge are like tools in your healing toolbox, meant to be used to accomplish certain goals. Hopefully, at this point, you are beginning to get a feel for these healing tools and how or when to use them.

The power of The Purge is its ability to soften and alkalinize cell walls which allows stored wastes, toxins, and other useless material inside the cells and tissues of the body to be removed. It also greatly speeds the rate of rebuilding due to the greater number of chemical transactions taking place inside the body. The great majority of disease in people is the result of being too acid, especially cancers, arthritis, and many forms of auto-immune dysfunction – all problems that develop because not enough transactions are happening and tissues get caught in a stiff stasis.

It bears repeating that the Liver Flush cleans the liver, gall bladder, kidneys, and cardiovascular system by removing gallstones, kidney stones, other stony material, fatty deposits, plaque, the remains of old chemicals picked up by the liver, and sometimes even bone spurs from your system. These things may not be immediately life threatening, but they interfere with your body's efforts to maintain itself and keep working in a normal, healthy way.

The Colon Sweep is used to clear gunky material in both the small intestine and large intestine. In doing so, it removes candida, other yeasts, and unwelcome bacteria, often scrapes away polyps and small growths, and forces a rebuilding of the absorptive surfaces – the cilia – in the small intestine. This greatly improves your ability to absorb the nutrition needed for healing and allows the microbiome in the gut to begin restoring the proper balance of microbes and beneficial bacteria. The material it clears from the large intestine allows the colon to begin returning to its original position, cuts gas, ends constipation, and brings biochemical changes that benefit the entire body. The Colon Sweep also helps avoid diverticulitis, Crohn's Disease, Irritable Bowel Syndrome (IBS), colitis, and even colon cancers, all of which are problems of degeneration caused by not enough nutrition or an inability to absorb what you're putting in.

You use the Purge when you need to heal a serious bacterial infection like peritonitis, staph, or strep because bacteria cannot survive in a completely alkaline environment. It is also used to remove wastes and do some seriously deep cleaning of tissues in the rest of the body that the Liver Flush and Colon Sweep do not specifically reach. Use the Purge to help break down and eliminate cancers whether they are dead or alive, eliminate mucus from lungs, eliminate waste build-up in the skin, and waste products in cells throughout the body. The Purge is so powerful that I have seen it do away with the beginning signs of cervical cancer or cancer of the eye with just one 3-day Purge.

Only a few examples of when to use these three forms of detox might include…using the Liver Flush to get relief from hot flashes, because these are the result of a sluggish, overwhelmed liver. The Colon Sweep is useful for scrubbing the colon and removing small growths and polyps, or clearing away Candida while the yogurt/probiotic regimen re-establishes the correct balance of micro-organisms in the gut. The Purge is extremely good at clearing up colds, flu, bronchitis, or pneumonia. In years past, before surgery became big business, the Liver Flush was used to remove gallstones, kidney stones, and improve digestion. And let me say again that the Purge is excellent in clearing the effects of chemotherapy.

Although there are many forms of detox available to us, the Liver Flush, Colon Sweep, and Purge are the basic tools needed to keep the body clean, youthful, and functioning in a healthy fashion. If they are practiced regularly, you can remain vibrant right to the end of your life. ❖

22
Castor Oil/Olive Oil Sweat Bath

THE BODY USES FOUR MAIN SYSTEMS to excrete waste materials: the liver and gastrointestinal tract, the kidneys, the lungs, and the skin. Too often, we forget that the skin can be used to help seriously detoxify the body and speed the removal of metabolic wastes.

If you begin using the program outlined in this book, or even just change your diet to include more whole, healthy foods, the body will begin taking advantage of these and will make an effort to repair and rebuild itself even more vigorously. As it does so, it will break down old, poorly-built cells and begin mobilizing stored wastes to be removed. The toxic run-off from the breakdown of metabolic misfits and debris, and especially that from cancers or other illnesses, tends to accumulate too rapidly for the body to excrete through the liver, gastrointestinal tract, and kidneys. It will then start to push things through the skin. The result can be all sorts of skin eruptions and blemishes from pimples to liver spots, from rashes to open sores. Such conditions may be worrisome, but should be viewed as a sign that it's time to do a castor oil/olive oil sweat bath.

When I started regular detox shortly after becoming a patient of Dr. Gonzales, my skin began to break out with a dark red, terribly itchy rash. My forehead, eyelids, breastbone, shin bones, and forearms were the places most affected. My eyelids became so swollen that the lid over my right eye split in two places. When I called Gonzales, he told me to "…tough it out!" and asked if I was doing the sweat baths. When I said no, he suggested I start them immediately. I should have listened, but I didn't, and I was sorry. Even though the eyelid healed without trouble, I continued to suffer from an ugly rash with an itch that drove me crazy for another four months.

When I finally found time to do the castor oil/olive oil sweat baths, they turned out to be almost miraculous in their ability to clear up skin.

To do a Castor Oil/Olive Oil Sweat Bath you will need:

2 TBSP castor oil (cold-pressed and organic)

2 TBSP olive oil (extra virgin, cold pressed, organic)

A bathtub with a slip-proof mat in the bottom

1 QT of purified or R.O. (reverse osmosis) water and cup or glass

1 t-shirt, a sweat shirt, a pair of sweat pants, and heavy socks

Several large bath towels

Oatmeal or glycerin soap (no deodorant soaps, please)

A bed with 3-4 heavy blankets or quilts

A clock or cell phone or wristwatch

A rubber sheet, old shower curtain, or piece of plastic (optional)

1. **It takes about one morning to do a sweat bath**. You can also do the sweat bath in the evening if you prefer. Total time is about 2-3 hours. If you do the sweat bath in the morning, **do not eat any breakfast beforehand**. If you do one in the evening, skip supper so that you have an empty stomach. If you are going to do one in the afternoon and you have eaten lunch, wait at least three hours. Your body should not be burdened with the job of trying to digest food when you are asking it to dump toxins. *You will be much more uncomfortable* if you have just eaten a meal. You can get something light to eat afterwards even if it's late at night. And you may feel so wonderful that you might not want to eat anything for a few hours afterwards, since food is a serious disturbance in the body.

2. Let's assume you are going to do your sweat bath in the morning. **When you get up in the morning, brush your teeth with a non-fluoride toothpaste. Drink one cup of purified or R.O. water**.

3. **Prepare your bed** by laying a piece of plastic, a rubber sheet, or an old, plastic shower curtain over the pillow and fitted sheet. This will keep your sheet, mattress, and mattress pad from getting wet and sweat-stained, because you will definitely sweat – a lot. Double up one towel and put it over the plastic on your pillow. Put two heavy towels over the plastic covering your mattress. Lay them end-to-end and try to position them so that they will catch most of the sweat from your body. Be sure they will extend from head to to. Get out extra quilts or blankets and put them nearby so you can cover up with them when you lay down to sweat.

4. **In a small bowl, mix 2 TBSP of castor oil with 2 TBSP of olive oil, stirring well**. Take this mixture to your bathroom, along with the t-shirt, sweatshirt, sweat pants, heavy socks, another couple of towels, the quart of purified water, and the cup or glass. Put the drinking water and the cup on the edge of the tub or someplace where you can easily reach it once you are in the tub.

5. **Turn on the hot water in the tub and begin filling it with water as hot as you can stand it and as deep as you can make it**. If your hot water heater is small and you don't think you will have enough to fill the tub, you may want to heat some water in a large pot on the stove and add it to the tub, then add water from the tap to get as much hot water as possible. The shallower the water, the faster it will cool, and you need it to stay hot enough long enough to get yourself into a good sweat. Just don't burn yourself. We usually make sure the water is at least 108-110°. If it is less than that temperature, you may have to sit longer and add more hot water after 10-15 minutes in order to get the body up to temperature.

6. While the tub is filling, **get completely undressed, and rub the oil mixture into your skin from head to toe**. If you have long hair, tie your hair up on *top* of your head and out of the way. Make sure that you do not have a ponytail or knot of hair at the *back* of your head that will make it uncomfortable for you to lie back in the tub or in the bed once you get to the sweating portion of the routine. You can rub some of the oil into your hairline about an inch or so, and if you wish, you can also massage a little into your scalp by dipping just your fingertips lightly into the oil then doing a fingertip massage of the scalp, but do not saturate your hair. And *do not put oil on the soles of your feet* or they'll be too slippery when you're stepping into and out of the tub.

7. When the tub is full, and with the oil now spread over your body, **get into the tub and soak in the hot water**. Be careful getting into the tub as you will be quite slippery! Once in, try to lie back so that everything but your face is under water. If necessary, turn over onto your stomach for five minutes, sticking your legs up out of the water to get the trunk of your body into the hot water. Sit up again once you start to sweat. Take a clock or wristwatch with you and **stay in the hot water for 15-25 minutes, or until you are sweating profusely.** If the water is shallow and starts to cool off, let a little bit of it out and put some fresh hot water in.

If you are really sick or weakened, it's a good idea to **have someone around to keep an eye and an ear out for you**. Ask them to come to the bathroom door once or twice during the soaking period to ask, "Are you doing okay in there?" If you need help, say so. If you live alone, ask a friend to come over and just read or have a cup of tea nearby while you're doing the sweat bath. If, by chance, you should become faint, or slip and fall, you'll have someone to help you.

If the water is nice and hot, you will usually start to be uncomfortably warm after about five minutes. The tendency is to hold your breath, but don't do this. Don't breathe in extra-deep gulps either. Breathe steadily, easily, and in a relaxed manner. You will feel most uncomfortable just before the body breaks into a full sweat. **Once you start to sweat, begin drinking water from the quart of purified R.O. water** you brought to the tub. Keep sipping at the water as you sweat. Drinking not only replaces the water you're losing through sweat, it gives you something to do when you're so hot, sweaty, and uncomfortable.

The hot bath allows the oils to penetrate to the deepest levels of the skin, and both the castor oil and the olive oil are nutrients as well as healers of skin and mucous membranes.

I usually tell people that, once I get in the tub, I stay until I get to the point that I think I'm going to melt or pass out, then stay for five minutes longer!

Once your heart is going at a very good clip in its efforts to cool down the body, you are ready to get out of the tub.

8. **When it is time to get out of the tub**, pull the plug to let the water out and climb out of the tub but *do not stand up straight. Stay bent at the waist to keep your head about level with your hips.* If you try to stand up straight, you may find you are too light-headed. Again, be careful getting out of the tub because you will be quite slippery. **You should also be sweating heavily, breathing fast, and have a pounding heart**. Take a towel, sit on the toilet seat cover or a nearby chair, and quickly dry yourself as much as possible, which will be difficult because of the continuous sweat.

9. In spite of the profuse sweating, **immediately put on the heavy socks, t-shirt, sweatshirt, and sweat pants. Wrap a towel around your head**.

10. **Get into your bed and cover up with two more towels, the top sheet, blanket, and at least two quilts**. Pull the covers right up to the bottom of your nose to keep you hot and sweating as long as possible. Stay under the covers for one hour. During this time you will feel like you have become one giant, beating heart, and you will sweat prodigiously. This sweating stimulates the release of poisons and toxic waste matter through your skin. It also has an extraordinary effect on the lungs, clearing them dramatically.

11. After about half an hour or so, you will notice that your heart is slower, you are cooling down a bit, and the sweating is beginning to slow up. If you are drowsy, drift off into a little nap. This will be wonderfully healing for you. **When an hour has gone by, or when you wake up, your heart should be quiet, your breath should be normal, and you, as well as everything around you, should be soaking wet.** At this point, the sweating portion is done.

12. **Get up, peel off the wet clothing (you *will* be soaked through), and go take a *warm* shower using an oatmeal or a glycerin soap,** both of which are gentle on skin. Do not use the commercial soaps you see advertised on television as they are often quite harsh and contain chemicals that are difficult for the skin to handle. Wash and condition your hair as usual. And be careful getting in and out of the shower if that shower is also the bathtub you were soaking in earlier. It will have a thin film of oil in it!

13. **When you get out of the shower, get a clean, dry towel and begin drying yourself off with a *slow*, pressured motion that removes dead skin. Sometimes the dead skin on your arms and legs comes off in thousands of tiny rolls**. Continue removing dead skin until the new skin underneath is bright pink, soft, and glowing. If an area of skin dries before you have a chance to rub it with the towel, dampen the skin with warm water for a few minutes or so, then continue rubbing with the slow, pressured movement.

14. When you are done rubbing dead skin from every area of your body you can reach, **get dressed in clean, preferably cotton clothing. Do not put any creams, oils, or lotions on your skin for 24 hours**. Leave it clean and clear to breathe easily, without the impediment of lotions and potions.

15. **Strip the bed of its wet sheets. Throw these into the washer and then the dryer, along with your wet clothes and towels**, and you are finished.

❖

When you have completed the entire sweat bath routine, you will notice a distinct difference in the depth, clarity, and ease of your breathing. Not only does it feel like you are breathing easily all the way through your chest, this feeling extends down into the abdomen! It's almost as if every organ and system in the trunk of the body has been turned into a set of lungs. It can also feel as if you are breathing through your skin, and there is an unusual sense of being alive that has to be experienced in order to be understood.

After 24 hours, you may take a *warm* shower using a washcloth or back brush to rub the body briskly but without soap. Let the water run over your skin as long as you can. Afterward, massage in a thin coating of a good, herbal oil or moisturizing lotion. You will be surprised at how beautiful, flexible, and healthy your skin looks, even after 24 hours with no lotions! You will realize that your skin becomes old-looking, dry, wrinkled, and sallow because you haven't bothered to clean it well and a thick layer of dead cells has built up on the surface. This is the layer that cracks and wrinkles, making you look years older than you are.

The castor oil/olive oil sweat bath is one of the most valuable of the detox routines and is a potent restorative. This is especially true for someone who has cancer, lung disease, asthma, or one of the forms of arthritis. As a side note…if you have cancer, don't be surprised if the water in the tub turns brownish or blackish after you've been sweating a bit. This just means you are getting rid of a lot of toxins.

In a full detox program the **castor oil/olive oil sweat bath should be done once a week for 12 weeks** in the first three months of the program. After that they can be discontinued until the following year when they should be repeated.

I live in Michigan and have found that it is best to do the sweat bath series each year from mid-December through mid-March. This is the coldest time of the year and the sweat baths are a wonderful way to ward off lung congestion, head colds, sinus infections, and the stiffness that generally accompanies cold weather. You can certainly start them at any other time of the year if you have contracted a catastrophic illness and need to implement a full detox program, but for annual maintenance the winter months are a great time to do them.

Don't hesitate to do a sweat bath if you should get the flu, catch a cold, or develop any other temporary problem. It is wonderful for healing almost everything. ❖

23
The Coffee Enema

THE COFFEE ENEMA HAS BEEN USED FOR OVER 100 years as a generalized detox procedure and was formerly listed in the Merck Manual as a powerful detoxifying and healing practice. Despite rumors to the contrary, coffee enemas are perfectly safe when you follow the guidelines. Coffee enemas stimulate the liver and gallbladder to release stored toxins and wastes, and this improves and enhances liver function. When Dr. Nicholas Gonzales inquired as to why coffee enemas were removed from the Merck Manual, he was told that it was considered "too old-fashioned."

To do a Coffee Enema you will need:

A stainless steel or glass coffee maker, drip style is fine.

1 QT plus ¼ cup of distilled, or R.O. water, or spring water

2-3 TBSP of organic coffee (no decaf)

1 disposable enema bag (can be re-used many times)

KY jelly (or wheat germ oil, olive oil, Vitamin E oil)

A hook on the wall to hang the bag from, or a hanger to hang the enema bag from the shower curtain rod.

1 rubber colon tube (optional)

1 TBSP unsulfured blackstrap molasses (optional)

A nearby chair, bed, or a chaise lounge chair

1. To make the coffee, use a regular, automatic drip coffeemaker just as if you were making coffee to drink, although this coffee will be weak compared to what you drink. **Put 2-3 TBSP of organic coffee in the**

filter basket. Pour 1 quart plus ¼ cup of distilled or R.O. water into the coffeemaker and turn it on to make the coffee. Do not use city tap water, as it is full of chemicals and other less-than-helpful substances. Do not use an aluminum coffee pot either, because aluminum is a toxic metal and can leach into the coffee while perking.

2. Once the coffee has been made, you should have about 1 quart of coffee, the extra ¼ cup having been absorbed into the coffee grounds. At this point, you may wish to **add 1 TBSP of unsulfured blackstrap molasses to the entire quart while the coffee is hot and stir it in**. The molasses aids in retaining the enema and increases the efficiency of the detox effect.

3. **Let the coffee cool to body temperature**. It is acceptable to make the coffee the night before and then warm it a bit before using.

4. **Get your disposable enema bag, make sure the *tube* on the bag is closed using the stopper or clamp, then pour the quart of coffee into the bag.**

5. **If the coffee is quite cold, run some hot water into the sink and set the bag in it for a few minutes**. This will warm it slightly to body temperature. If the coffee is still hot, run cold water into the sink and cool it. Then hang it on a hook above the bathroom sink, or put it on a hanger and hang it from the shower curtain rod. In our healing rooms here at the farm, we have attached a flower-pot holder to the wall above the sink in each bathroom. The flower pot holder swings out to hold an enema bag nicely, then swings back to lie flat against the wall when not in use.

5. **Put some K-Y jelly, Vit. E oil, or Vaseline on the end of the tube,** release the stopper or clamp just long enough to allow coffee to fill the tube, then re-clamp. If you leave the tube filled with air, you will end up pushing this air into your colon when you start the enema and that may make it more difficult to retain the coffee for the full 10 minutes.

6. Then **bend forward slightly while in a standing position near the sink or the toilet and gently insert the tube into the rectum about 5-6 inches**. Release the stopper or clamp and allow half, about 1½ - 2 cups of coffee to flow slowly into the rectum.

7. Pull the tube out and set it carefully in the sink or a container (bowl, can, etc.) or in the tub or shower, and **move slowly and gently to a**

chair, a bed, or bathroom bench and sit quietly for 10 minutes, then go to the toilet and expel the coffee. At first it may be difficult to retain the enema, but with experience you will be able to hold it with considerable ease.

8. **After expelling the coffee into the toilet, repeat Steps 5-7, using the remaining two cups of coffee, holding for ten minutes, then expelling.**

10. When you are finished with the second pint of coffee, **rinse out the bag, washing the end of the tube with warm, soapy water. Hang the bag to dry** on a clothes hanger or hook in open air in an inconspicuous place.

11. **Wash your bottom, and wipe off the underside of the toilet seat, and you are finished.**

The reason for doing a coffee enema is that there is a sympathetic resonance between the liver and the colon. Putting weak coffee into the rectum induces the liver to dump its wastes into the colon, which then expels them into the toilet. "Doing a coffee," as I refer to it, has a powerful effect on the liver. If you do not remember anything else about coffee enemas, remember this: *you do not do a coffee to clean out your colon. You do a coffee because it detoxifies the liver.* When the coffee enters the rectal opening and comes in contact with mucosal membranes, it immediately causes the liver to start a series of gentle contractions that dump toxins and metabolic waste, gradually promoting better liver function.

This information is especially important for people who are going through chemotherapy. The liver is greatly stressed by the load of dead tumor tissue and chemicals that must be filtered from the body immediately after a chemo treatment. If the liver becomes overwhelmed, it will shut down. This is what people mean when they say, "The chemo killed him." What actually happens is that the liver stops working and death follows quickly. A coffee enema is a godsend in that it supports the liver and prevents the shutdown during periods of intense toxicity caused by tumor die-off. Dr. Gonzales recommended that during these periods, the patient do a set of 2 coffee enemas every four hours until the nausea disappeared and the individual was restored to feeling normal again.

The coffee enema is one of our most useful tools for healing. When I first started my own detox program, I did NOT want to do coffee enemas. It was not until that first Liver Flush that I discovered the magic of a coffee enema and its nearly miraculous relief from the intense nausea, headache, vomiting, and night sweat caused by the build up of a lot of toxic waste in my liver. It is my perspective now that you should not attempt to do a detox program, a serious exercise program, or a weight loss program without doing a set of coffee enemas daily. You will just be too miserable, and that misery is what causes 90% of people to quit the program. The coffees can be done in the morning, mid-afternoon, or early evening after work.

During a full detox program in which there is not a life-threatening situation, the usual recommendation is to do two sets of coffee enemas every day for the full length of the repair and rebuild program. The coffees can be done in the morning, the late afternoon, or early evening.

Once you are past a crisis or have completed your rebuilding program, there are various ways of maintaining yourself and a healthy, functioning liver. Many people continue to do coffee enemas daily, some every 3-4 days, some only on the weekend, and others only when they have a cold, flu, or headache. Still others only do the coffees during their monthly detox procedure as they rotate through the year. Those with a poorly functioning liver or who have a tendency toward gallstones and gall bladder trouble may do a coffee every day because it greatly reduces the difficulties caused by liver-gall bladder sluggishness. Then there are those who have a tight, demanding, stressful schedule who do not have time to listen to their body or to go to the bathroom several times a day. They do a set of coffees daily simply because it keeps the liver at a peak of function and their energy stays high.

Coffees are meant to be used to provide support for the body and relief from a host of things that make us feel bad...things like the flu, a fever, colds, sinus problems, headaches, hot flashes, PMS, nausea, many kinds of illness, during the early stages of a new exercise program, or any kind of difficulty that leaves you feeling achey, pained, or fatigued.

One of the fears you may hear about doing enemas over a long period of time is that you will become dependent on them and won't be able to have a bowel movement without an enema. While this may be true for taking laxatives, I have found that it is not true with coffee enemas. The diet of whole foods that are required for you to heal contains large amounts of fiber and fat, and this guarantees that your bowels will continue to work without problems. Even after very long periods of coffee enemas, the most sluggish of bowels takes only a day or two to work on its own. For many people on a real food diet with its very high amounts of fiber, it is not uncommon to have a bowel movement on their own on days when they also do a coffee enema. Each of us is different, and thus each will use the coffee enema a little differently. Regardless of how and when it is used, the great value of a coffee enema is its ability to detox and clear the liver, which boosts the liver's filtering action and keeps you healthy and energized.

Here are some practical closing thoughts regarding coffee enemas. I would highly recommend that you invest in a rubber colon tube. It is not absolutely necessary, and you can use the enema bag as is. However, some chemotherapy treatments for cancer create conditions that require up to six sets of coffee enemas a day for a couple days. Since the tube on the plastic enema bag is a rather hard plastic, there is a possibility of irritating or scratching the delicate membranes inside the anal opening. The rubber colon tube is much softer and gentler on these tender tissues.

If you decide to use the rubber colon tube, you have to attach it to the plastic tube on the bag. To do so, look at the end of the plastic tube on the enema bag. You will see two holes…one in the *end* of the plastic tube and a second hole on the *side* of the plastic tube about an inch from the end. Cut off 1 inch from the end of the plastic tube about where the small side hole is. Slide the rubber colon tube onto the cut-off end of the plastic tube, pushing the rubber as far onto it as possible, and you're ready to start.

If you are using a rubber colon tube, you should not use vaseline or any kind of oil. Use KY jelly instead. If you use oil on the rubber tube, it will not last very long. The oil will gradually affect the rubber until it is soft, sticky, loses its shape, and disintegrates. Since rubber colon tubes are relatively expensive (about $45.00) compared to the enema bag (about $6.00) taking steps to make it last is a good idea.

If you have had a colostomy, you can still do a coffee enema although it might be necessary to lie down on your side instead of standing up. Insert the tube from the enema bag into the colostomy opening about 6 inches, and *very slowly* release only ½ to 1 cup of coffee into the colon. Some people have worked their way up to two cups, but even one cup will do the job. My experience with colostomies is that people who have them very quickly train their colon to empty at the same time every day in order to make clean-up easier. Thus, you can train yourself to hold onto a coffee for ten minutes. During these ten minutes, replace the colostomy bag, and then release the coffee into the colostomy bag. Your liver will respond just as well as if you were introducing coffee into the rectum. Empty the colostomy bag, rinse it, and reuse it for the second coffee enema in the set. It's a little more work than doing a coffee without a colostomy, and you will use more colostomy bags, but the health benefits are well worth it.

The best place to go while you're holding the coffee is a nearby chair that is fairly close to the toilet or right outside the bathroom door if your bathroom is too small to put a chair in it. Read a book, watch a video, do some email, or just doze and rest.

A few people who have never been coffee drinkers may feel slightly jittery at first, but this passes and most people quickly find the enemas very relaxing. If the jitteriness continues, try adding the molasses to it, which adds minerals, aids retention, and usually leaves you calm. If you are still jittery afterwards, you are making the coffee too strong. Visually, the coffee should look like light brown water and works very well at this strength.

I have read a variety of instructions for making the coffee to be used in a coffee enema and was quite surprised to find that some instructions said to put one quart of water in a pan with a cup of ground coffee and let it boil!! My personal opinion is that this is much too strong. The body is not a stupid or unresponsive organism. It will respond in just minutes to the *energy* of even homeopathic-strength coffee introduced rectally. ❖

*Part 4*_____

Supplements for Building the Body

24
Enzymes and Glandulars

ONCE UPON A TIME NOT SO VERY LONG AGO, a young man named Ed Howell graduated from college and went out in the world to work. He didn't get very far with his career, however, because he was so tired, so fatigued, and so sick that he couldn't get himself out of bed in the morning. He did everything he knew to heal himself and get going with his life, but nothing worked. He went to one doctor after another, but no one was able to help him. As a last resort, he checked into a place he had heard of in Illinois, a place where only "health nuts" and the desperate went. It was a place where the emphasis was on diets using raw foods and other nutritional therapies.

To his surprise, Ed began to feel better. When he asked the head of the institution what secret they were using to create such miraculous results, the doctor said, "Enzymes." It was the direction Ed Howell was to pursue for the rest of his life.[73] He obtained a degree in medicine, joined the staff of the Lindlahr Sanitarium, and later started the Food Enzyme Research Foundation. Over his life, he designed and carried out a number of powerful research projects which showed conclusively that enzymes, especially pancreas enzymes, were largely responsible for continuously rebuilding and repairing the body, and that many, if not all, degenerative diseases that humans suffer and die from are caused by the body's slowing production of pancreatic enzymes. Every living thing, be it plant, animal,

---

73 Dr. Nicholas Gonzales MD, from a lecture given at Boulder Colorado Medical Center, Boulder, CO, March, 1992.

or human, is alive because of enzymes. *Enzymes are life energy,* and scientists have been unable to synthesize them. Without enzymes you would die quickly.

"Enzymes are the substances that make life possible. They are needed for every chemical reaction that takes place in the human body. No mineral, vitamin, or hormone can do any work without enzymes. Our bodies, all of our organs, tissues, and cells, are run by metabolic enzymes. They are the manual workers that build our body from proteins, carbohydrates, and fats, just as construction workers build our homes. You may have all the raw materials with which to build, but without the workers (enzymes) you cannot even begin." [74]

Says Stephan Blauer, "Without the life energy of enzymes, we would be nothing more than a pile of lifeless chemical substances—vitamins, minerals, water, and proteins." [75]

Everything we do...working, sleeping, breathing, healing, and more, depends on our ability to produce enzymes, and in this effort the pancreas is the key producer. "Indeed, each of us could be regarded as an orderly, integrated succession of enzyme reactions." [76]

In his small but spectacular book, *Enzyme Nutrition*, Howell wrote:

"The living body is under a great daily burden to produce the volume of enzymes necessary to run efficiently... (and) enzymes are continually being used and eliminated in the urine, feces, and sweat. The laboratory in every hospital can find them there. They are needed in digesting food; running the heart, kidneys, liver, and lungs; and even in thinking.

"Life could not exist without enzymes. Enzymes convert the food we eat into chemical structures that can pass through the cell membranes of the cells lining the digestive tract and into the bloodstream." [77]

---

74 Edward Howell, *Enzyme Nutrition* (Wayne, NJ: Avery Publishing Group, 1985) p. 33.

75 Howell, p. ix.

76 Howell, p. 33.

77 Howell, p. 33.

There are basically three kinds of enzymes…

1. Metabolic Enzymes are used to rebuild and repair the human body, as well as run many of the ongoing reactions that take place within us. At present, science estimates that there are at least 6,000 metabolic enzyme systems in the body, and perhaps as many as 10,000. I call these *pancreas enzymes* or *R&R enzymes* because they are essential for the constant *repair and rebuilding* that goes on.

2. Digestive Enzymes are those produced by the body specifically to help digest food that we eat. I separate digestive enzymes into two broad categories: stomach enzymes and intestinal enzymes. The most widely known digestive enzymes are protease, amylase, lipase, and cellulase, all of which are also known as *stomach enzymes* because they break down foods in the stomach. Protease is used to digest protein, amylase digests carbohydrates, lipase is for digesting fats, and cellulase digests cellulose, part of the structure of green plants.

3. Food Enzymes are enzymes that exist naturally in whole foods before they are cooked, baked, fried, or otherwise processed. All fresh foods contain complete sets of highly specialized enzymes designed to help the body digest that particular food so its nutrients and nutritional co-factors will be made available to the body. These enzymes are provided by nature to assist in the digestion of that food so the body does not have to spend its precious life energy producing digestive enzymes and can be free to concentrate on the continuous work of repair and rebuilding. For instance, raw milk has the enzymes lactase, catalase, galactase, amylase, oleinase, peroxidase, dehydrogenase, and phosphatase, among others, all designed to help you digest the milk once you drink it. [78]

Enzymes are very sensitive to heat and begin to die when the temperature of the food goes above 117° F. [79] You can hold your hand in water at temperatures below 117° F, but when the water goes above that, it begins to sting and become quite uncomfortable. This is a convenient test for whether or not something is hot enough to destroy enzymes. [80]

---

78 Howell, p. 36.

79 Howell, p. 72.

80 Howell, p. 5

The enzymes in fruits, vegetables, grains, and meats don't stand a chance in our highly industrialized food processing industries. And as if that weren't enough, cooking and baking temperatures in the modern kitchen are very high, and the result is complete destruction of the enzymes in anything that is cooked. Most food enzymes are destroyed by the time the food reaches 140° F, and the destruction of any remaining life energy is complete by 180° F.

When we eat cooked foods, there are no living enzymes left in it to help the digestion process. From this, it should be clear that if your pancreas has to stop producing repair and rebuild enzymes in order to start producing digestive enzymes, then the body has to suspend or at least cut back its repair and rebuilding processes. In short, the body's continuous healing program slows drastically, and may even come to a halt whenever we eat cooked or processed food.

If eating were a temporary and occasional interruption, we might overlook it. But think about what happens for millions of us every day. It takes anywhere from one to six hours to digest cooked or processed food. During this time, the body's effort to repair and rebuild itself is seriously compromised, if not halted. If you are one of the many people who snack endlessly throughout the day, sometimes right up to the time you go to bed at night, your body will be too busy trying to deal with what you are putting in your mouth to focus on the structures and processes it needs to repair. You then have the foundation for a slow-but-sure degeneration of the body, just like an old house that no one bothers to take care of any more.

If you are interested in serious healing, adding digestive enzymes to your daily diet is very important. Doing so helps the healing process immeasurably by reducing the body's need to produce digestive enzymes. When it can do this, the body is free to focus on the metabolic enzymes that keep everything healthy and running smoothly.

To help your body do its best, you should know that some digestive enzymes work in the acid environment of the stomach, and others work in the alkaline environment of the intestine, and you will probably need both. Of course, the enzymes that come in raw food are perfectly created by nature to do an excellent job no matter what area of the gastrointestinal system the food is in, but most of us don't eat much raw food. If you eat a lot of cooked food, adding enzymes to your diet is essential.

You can easily buy capsules containing protease, amylase, and lipase to take with your meals. These *digestive* enzymes will sometimes have additional things like papain, bromelain, betaine, beet root, ox bile extract, ginger, or peppermint in it. These substances all help make the process of digestion easier and more complete so you get the full benefit of whatever nutrients are in the food without exhausting the pancreas.

You can also buy *metabolic* or *pancreas* enzymes that do the work of both digestion and repair or rebuilding. Pancreas enzymes greatly improve your ability to absorb nutrients in the small intestine. After doing so much work to prepare the food for digestion, pancreas enzymes are a godsend in terms of their ability to help the body absorb whatever nutrition it offers.

If you have active stomach ulcers, be careful with enzymes. You may have to do a long juice fast in which you drink mainly carrot and cabbage juice in order to allow the stomach to heal before you start taking enzyme supplements. You might also avoid stomach (digestive) enzymes at first and try starting with pancreas (metabolic) enzymes for a couple of months, until your ulcers have become less troublesome and your stomach walls have repaired themselves somewhat. Chewing your food extra well will also help make up for the lack of stomach enzymes.

When you put food in your stomach, it goes into the upper area of the stomach known as the "cardiac portion" where it sits quietly for a while. During its time in the cardiac area, the food enzymes in the food (if any) continue the all-important process of predigestion, which actually begins in the mouth when you chew the food and douse it with saliva. Fruits stay in the cardiac portion for 15 to 20 minutes if they are raw, longer if canned or cooked. Vegetables like peas, broccoli, lettuces, and tomatoes stay in the stomach for up to an hour if raw, up to two hours if cooked. Carbohydrates like bread, cereal, and pasta stay in the stomach for two to three hours, while meats, cheeses, other dairy products, and nuts stay in the stomach for three to six hours.

As the enzymes in the food – plus any stomach enzymes you've taken – successfully predigest the chewed food, known at this point as "chyme," some of the food begins to sink into the lower portion of the stomach where it soaks in the stomach acid known as hydrochloric acid

(HCL) and where the peristaltic churning of the lower stomach continues to prepare the food for the remaining journey through the gastrointestinal system.

The importance of enzymes cannot be overstated. If everything you eat comes out of a box, bag, can, or jar, you are, in effect, levying a heavy enzyme tax on your body because the body must produce extra enzymes to make up for what is missing in the food. [81] You might consider this to be a 50% tax since the effect on the body is to shorten life by half. Since the body is designed to easily last ten times your age at puberty, most of us should be living to at least 120 years of age.

Obviously this is not the case. Many of us are dead and buried by the age of 75. This is why our governments and institutions have no wisdom and no long-term perspective in them. We die too early and never live to see the long-term effects of our decisions, processes, and creations. We are gone before we have a chance to learn anything.

I see lives in terms of "thirds." We spend the first third of our lives gathering information and learning how this reality we were born into actually works. Around age 40, we move into the second third of life. Just as we should be reaping some of the benefits of our long tutelage…just as we step into our power and should begin applying what we have learned… we start falling apart with fatigue, high blood pressure, diabetes, cancers, heart disease, arthritis, and other physical nightmares.

Of course, the last third, which begins around the age of 70, doesn't have a chance! We are gone without ever having time to evaluate or assess whether what we created is working without disastrous long-term effects. Time for reflection is gone. We settle for short-term effects because the term of our life is so short. Too often, we look at something that has been working for a relatively short time and decide it is good. We then assume it will work forever. It is always convenient to make a decision once and not have to pay attention to it after that, but this is a poor strategy for surviving and thriving. If all our attention is caught up in coping with a body that is falling apart, we have no time or energy for changes within the larger system that require more time and energy.

---

81 Howell, p. 81.

Your body has an endocrine system of strategically placed glands whose job it is to manufacture the various chemicals that will then trigger specific activities and reactions in the body. The main glands in this system are the pituitary, hypothalamus, thyroid, parathyroids, thymus, pancreas, liver/gall bladder, adrenals, ovaries, and testicles. The pituitary is the master gland that often sends commands to the other glands in the endocrine system.

The pituitary and hypothalamus are structures in the brain that are responsible for managing some of the most basic balance points, such as the body's need for oxygen and water, our fight-or-flight response, and the hormones that create many emotional and perceptual states.

The thyroid is heavily involved in digestion and absorption processes, as it helps maintain steady energy, body temperature, and a host of general body operations from the sex drive to attitude to sleep.

The parathyroid glands are responsible for the metabolism of calcium in the body, which affects all muscle movement, including the heart muscle.

The thymus is a major player in the immune system and its many functions, whereas the pancreas is the main center for production of thousands of enzymes and their work in the body.

The adrenals not only regulate many heart activities, they produce the chemicals that allow us to cope with stress. And the ovaries and testicles are key players in our ability to reproduce.

In addition to the glandular substances produced by the endocrine system, your organs also create chemical instructions (hormones) for each other and for all of the systems of the body, especially the brain, heart, kidneys, liver, spleen, lungs, and reproductive organs. These chemical messengers not only carry out the functions of the body, they also help create the emotional states and feelings that accompany or trigger the actions themselves.

For instance, when estrogen levels are high, a woman will feel much more romantically inclined. When thyroxine levels are high, she will have enough energy to go to work all day and clean closets all night, even if her family complains that she is disturbing them.

Sometimes aging will slow the activity of glands, and sometimes a disease process interferes with their work, but in today's world of toxic materials, oxygen-deprived air, poisoned water, dead soil, and foods empty of any nutrition, the most common causes of poor glandular activity are interference from heavy metals and an absence of nutritional factors that would allow ongoing repair and rebuilding of the glands. Once your glands begin to falter, the production of hormones, neurochemicals, and enzymes that run your body begins to slip. The result is that your organs begin to malfunction. When an organ begins to malfunction, all sorts of diseases can manifest, and life can become both painful and difficult.

Taking glandulars allows the entire body to carry on with the chemical reactions that must occur to stay alive. Glandulars support both the glands themselves and the processes that the glands are responsible for inside the body. They also reduce the stress on organs by allowing many chemical sequences to continue, which keeps the body functioning while repair and rebuilding goes on. The effect is to reduce or eliminate the tendency for diseases to become an entire string of difficulties, each one triggering the next in a sequence of breakdowns.

When designing a program to heal yourself, you may have to include several glandular supplements to support certain functions until health and balance can be re-established and the gland can take over again.

For example, if you have asthma, you would likely want to include raw lung glandulars, as well as liver and pancreas glandulars in your healing program. One lung glandular capsule each breakfast, lunch, and dinner directly supports lung function, as does the liver glandular if taken with each meal. When the liver gets sluggish or is chronically overloaded, the lungs often back up with fluids or are over-sensitive and can spasm, which leaves you coughing. Taking two to four pancreas glandular capsules with each meal supports *all* enzyme systems within the body and helps you absorb nutrients from your food, thus these three glandulars would prove to be very powerful assistants toward healing.

In another example, if you have heart trouble, you may want to add raw heart glandular, maybe parathyroid glandular, as well as liver, adrenal, and pancreas glandulars. The liver and pancreas would be taken for the same reasons given above, whereas the heart, parathyroid, and adrenal glandulars would support normal heart function.

If you have cysts on your ovary, a healing program might include iodine as well as ovary, pancreas, and liver glandulars.

If you have osteoporosis, you might want to include pituitary, pancreas, and liver glandulars on your supplement list. If the osteoporosis is severe, you might want to get injections of Human Growth Hormone (HGH), a powerful glandular that increases bone density and muscle mass, while greatly improving lung function and health in general. [82] Since bone density will also increase greatly in response to exercise, the HGH glandular plus a regular exercise program will do wonders for the problem of bones that break any time sudden pressure is applied to them.

In the case of arthritis, you might want to begin taking thyroid and parathyroid glandulars to support metabolism and the body's use of calcium, which is managed by the parathyroid glands. In addition, liver glandular supports the liver, which is a critical organ, and when combined with pancreas enzymes, will reduce the pain and inflammation of arthritis.

As you may have noticed above, in almost every case of serious illness, the liver and pancreas need support, and thus liver glandulars and pancreas enzymes are frequently included in a good healing program. This is especially true of cancers, since the *pancreatic enzymes trypsin and chymotrypsin will directly dissolve the fibrin covering that shields tumors and cancers from the immune system,* allowing your own killer cells to get at the cancerous growth and destroy it.

Dr. William Kelley's healing program suggests that people with cancer get up at 2:30 am to take up to a dozen pancreas enzyme capsules because the pancreas itself is very active at that time of the day. The combined effect of what the pancreas puts out, plus the dozen pancreas capsules, overwhelms cancers and tumors, killing them outright and breaking them down. The liver then filters the dead tumor tissue out of the blood so it can be excreted. Generally speaking, in cases of cancer, you might take an entire complex of glandulars plus extra amounts of thymus and spleen glandulars in order to break down tumors, support the immune

82   James F. Balch MD and Phyllis A. Balch CNC, *Prescriptions for Natural Healing* (Garden City Park, NY: Avery Publishing Group, 1997) p. 552-553.

system, assist the body's ability to make new blood, and to repair itself perfectly.[83]

It is highly recommended that you do not take pancreas glandulars and enzymes to dissolve a cancer unless you also embark on a full detox program. I would like to emphasize again that dead, dissolving tumor tissue is *extremely* poisonous and will quickly overwhelm the liver. If the liver gets plugged, you will be very ill. If it shuts down and you don't get it functioning again, you can die quickly. Constantly detoxifying the liver and lymph system becomes a steady challenge and requires daily coffee enemas plus a continuous rotation through the major detox routines of Liver Flush, Colon Sweep, and Purge on a monthly basis until the cancer is gone.

As mentioned earlier, we have all heard of people who started a chemotherapy program for cancer and then died from the effects of the chemo. Now you know why! The chemo kills the cancer, along with a lot of other living tissue in the body. Both the dead cancer tissue and the chemicals used in chemotherapy are highly poisonous substances in themselves. The liver is seldom given the support it needs to handle the onslaught of dead and toxic material that accumulates in the body during chemotherapy treatments. The result is that the entire body/mind system weakens terribly and sometimes gives up. Much of this can be avoided with the practice of detox and a good supplement program consisting of: 1. Amino acids (for rebuilding), 2. Minerals (for rebuilding), 3. Vitamins (for function), 4. Enzymes (for repair and reduction of inflammation), and 5. Glandulars (for temporary support). Together, these constitute key parts in getting well again naturally. So, let's do a quick review of what the amino acids, minerals, and vitamins actually do. ❖

---

83 Teaching of Dr. Nicholas Gonzales MD.

25
Amino Acids, Minerals, and Vitamins

IT HAS BEEN KNOWN FOR A VERY LONG TIME that any group of people who wish to survive must eat a combination of foods that will supply all of the amino acids that the body uses to create the entire array of proteins needed for the body to survive. There are usually key foods in any given culture that become staples simply because they provide a combination of essential amino acids that are not found elsewhere.[84] For the Japanese, it is rice and fish. For Mexicans, it is beans and corn. For Americans, it is meat, milk, and potatoes.

If you want your body to be able to produce enzymes and glandulars, you have to get enough amino acids and minerals in your diet. In fact, in the hierarchy of supplements, these two are at the top of the list.

Minerals, which are needed to build…

Amino acids, which are needed to utilize…

Vitamins, all of which are needed to produce…

Enzymes, which run the body and are necessary for making…

Glandulars (aka hormones), major players in your endocrine system that act as chemical on-off switches!

---

84 The key word here is *essential*, which means the body cannot make these amino acids for itself and they must be supplied from the diet. Since not every food contains these essential amino acids, certain foods become critical because they supply the missing aminos, without which, civilization would die out.

In fact, all of these elements are intimately interconnected. You can't build perfectly working amino acid chains without minerals, and you can't utilize minerals without the correct amino acids. You cannot use vitamins well without all the necessary minerals, and you will have great difficulty producing the enzymes and glandulars that run the body without a proper supply of well-built and well-functioning amino acids, plenty of minerals, plus a steady supply of vitamins. All of these are needed to run the body smoothly and maintain physical, mental, emotional, and spiritual health.

As we have already seen, amino acids are the critical building blocks used to make a human body. Aminos are the pieces and parts used to create proteins in their thousands of forms. Hair and toenails are protein, muscles and tendons are protein, your organs and glands are made of protein, your blood is protein, and so are many of the tissues and fluids that make up your body.

When you eat food with proteins in it, your body breaks down the proteins that once formed the body of the plant or animal you are eating, turning it into its original molecular form of vitamin, mineral, and amino acid components. It then recycles these components to build its own highly specialized proteins, each of which has unique uses and applications.

Amino acids can run short in your body if you are under stress, are suffering from a trauma or infection of any kind. This is also true if you are getting older, have impaired absorption of nutrients, take drugs – including over-the-counter and prescription drugs, or have a poor diet characterized by too much sugar, too little fiber, and too few nutrients.

The body can produce about 80% of the amino acids it needs, but the rest must come from your diet. Without the needed types or sufficient amounts of amino acids, you can easily fall prey to illness and disease. If you don't pay attention to the warnings of nutrient deficiency, you are liable to develop an entire cascade of problems, each one feeding on the one before it, complicating the situation immensely.

When you buy amino acids, look for the words *free-form amino acids* on the label, which means that the aminos do not have to be digested or worked on by the body and are ready for absorption directly into your bloodstream. You can also look for a statement that says the aminos came from organic sources and are *L-form* aminos, which has a left-hand molecular spin, (as opposed to D-form, which have a right-hand spin) so that they are more usable by your body. And make sure that the full set of aminos is included in the capsule or powder you buy. There are nine essential aminos, which your body cannot make and must get from food or supplements.

These nine essential aminos that you must supply are:

Histidine improves digestion, increases interest in sexual activity, is used in growth and repair of tissues, helps remove heavy metals and protects from radiation.

Methionine helps prevent fat build-up in arteries and the liver, is a potent antioxidant and detox agent, helps excrete excess estrogen, is important in cell building and maintaining muscle strength, assists in reducing allergic reactions and preventing osteoporosis, and increases the energy of cell metabolism.

Isoleucine maintains energy and endurance, is used in making new tissues including hemoglobin. It also stabilizes blood sugar.

Leucine promotes healing of bones, skin, and tissues; is used to produce Growth Hormone; and provides energy for the body's use.

Phenylalanine is used by the body to synthesize neurotransmitters, which are utilized by the brain. It helps with alertness, memory, and learning; keeps appetite down and spirits up; helps with everything from PMS to Parkinson's disease; and even works to control pain.

Lysine is used to improve and manage calcium absorption; fights cold sores and herpes outbreaks; assists the immune system in building antibodies; aids tissue repair, collagen formation, and muscle formation; lowers triglycerides; helps the body build enzymes; prevents hair loss and irritability; keeps energy up; maintains reproductive ability; and prevents anemia.

Threonine assists liver function, prevents fatty deposits, keeps proteins in balance, forms collagen, and is used in a number of key organs like the heart and brain.

Tryptophan is used by the body to synthesize serotonin, stabilize moods, relieve migraines, reduce appetite, fight insomnia and depression, reduce stress, manage hyperactivity in children, and maintain correct coronary artery tension.

Valine is used as an energy source, maintains nitrogen balance in the body thus improving cell construction, and helps with tissue repair.

The remaining amino acids:

Alanine is used to metabolize glucose in the body.

Arginine is important for tumor control, muscle metabolism, and production of pancreatic enzymes. It builds bones, tissue, muscle, and collagen; triggers sexual maturity; enhances immune function; and helps produce a variety of hormones and enzymes.

Asparagine helps create balance in the nervous system and in transforming other amino acids into useful forms.

Aspartic acid enhances immune function, removes toxins from the blood, assists DNA and RNA functions, prevents disorder in the brain and central nervous system, and reduces fatigue.

Citrulline is a detoxifying agent and helps release energy in the body. It supports arginine's efforts to retard tumors and cancers, and is an overall stimulant to the immune system.

Cysteine & Cystine are two closely related and very important aminos in terms of their detox effects. They are needed for healthy skin, hair, eyes, collagen, and digestive enzymes; help fight cancers and arthritis; promote healing; burn fats; and relieve respiratory problems.

Gamma-aminobutyric acid is known as GABA. This amino relaxes nerve activity in the body and, thus, helps with conditions like epilepsy, ADD, hypertension, anxiety, and some neuralgia.

Glutamic acid is used as a neurotransmitter and is important in the metabolism of carbohydrates and fats. It also transports potassium, can serve as fuel for the brain, and improves nerve action and reaction.

Glutamine is a key amino needed for brain function and good mental activity. It helps detoxify the brain; builds good muscle and connective tissue; is essential for maintaining DNA, the digestive tract, and acid/alkaline balance in the body. Glutamine reduces cravings for sugar, and is useful for treating everything from alcoholism and arthritis to ulcers, MS, impotence, and senility.

Glycine helps the body synthesize other amino acids; builds muscle tissue; maintains DNA and RNA; and promotes conditions like a healthy prostate, good digestion, and fast repair of injured tissues.

Ornithine promotes production of growth hormone, aids in detoxification of the liver, and supports the synthesis of other amino acids in the body.

Proline helps create a strong heart, good connective tissues and tendons, healthy joint capsules, and good skin.

Serine is used in the body's metabolism of fats and as a major support for the immune system.

Taurine, another key amino in the body, promotes utilization of the six major minerals: calcium, magnesium, sodium, potassium, zinc, and iron, as well as trace minerals. It helps produce bile, which allows digestion of fats, which in turn allow absorption of fat-soluble vitamins. This amino also supports everything from a steady, even heartbeat, good eyesight, and healthy cholesterol levels to healthy blood, muscles, and brain function.

Tyrosine aids in raising your mood and keeping depression at bay while suppressing your appetite and burning fat. It assists the thyroid, reduces fatigue, eases chronic headaches, Parkinson's disease, and allergies.

For a more complete discussion of amino acids, read the section on Amino Acids in *Prescription For Nutritional Healing* by Phyllis Balch, CNC, and her husband James F. Balch, MD. This is a reference that every home should have. In addition to having excellent information about supplements, it is overflowing with suggestions for a wide variety of problems and illnesses that we humans run into. Their suggestions include what to take, how much of it, and what each supplement does, all in order of importance. And one of the nice things about this reference is that they update it with new information regularly.

Minerals – The Six Majors

In order for your body to carry on the basic processes of metabolism and the constant replenishment of basic supplies and structures, you need minerals. The basic six minerals, sometimes referred to as the *six majors*, that you absolutely must have on a steady basis in order to stay alive are:

Calcium is essential for good bones and teeth, keeping blood pressure down, maintaining a healthy heartbeat, lowering cholesterol, eliminating depression, and relieving literally dozens of other difficulties and conditions.

Magnesium assists the body in utilizing calcium and potassium. It's also needed for a smoothly working nervous system; to provide support for enzyme systems; and help prevent osteoporosis, PMS, and depression as well as many other irritating conditions.

Sodium supports the work of the stomach, nerves, and muscles; maintains proper blood pressure; keeps the liver and kidneys healthy while helping to prevent a wide variety of symptoms such as depression, confusion, poor memory, gas, headache, loss of coordination, infections, and lack of energy.

Potassium is a co-worker of sodium that aids nerve and muscle function, especially the heart. It keeps blood pressure steady, helps keep the heartbeat even, maintains water balance in the body, aids respiration, keeps cells functioning normally, prevents salt retention, and assists with many of the same difficulties that sodium prevents.

Iron is necessary for high energy and a well-functioning immune system as well as for producing red blood cells and many enzymes. It helps create healthy hair, skin, and nails; prevents digestive upsets; reduces overweight and nervous irritability.

Zinc keeps the immune system healthy; promotes healing at all levels; is an ingredient in many enzyme systems; counters fatigue and lethargy; helps keep vision, hearing, taste, and smell in good working order; and is necessary to prevent infertility and impotence.

Additional Key Minerals

Your body uses over 90 other minerals to maintain good function. Although you can buy a good book that focuses on mineral supplements in great detail, I have listed a few here that are critical but get little attention.

Iodine is necessary to keep your thyroid gland healthy and working properly. It is needed for development and maintenance of your entire physical, mental, and emotional self. The body needs iodine in order to utilize the fats that construct both cell membranes and nerve sheathing. It also prevents fatigue and weight gain.

Dr. David Brownstein wrote a critical book titled *Iodine: Why You Need it, Why You Can't Live Without It*. I cannot say enough about this book. If you get a chance, read it. If you're trying to heal, read it. For no reason at all, read it. We have an iodine deficiency epidemic in the U.S. and yet we hardly ever hear about iodine. If you have any form of cancer, catch every kind of cold and flu, are struggling with depression, have constant fatigue, low sex drive, pain, ADD/ADHD, ovarian cysts, Fibrocystic breasts, cysts in your thyroid or anywhere in the body, hemorrhoids, headaches and migraines, high blood pressure, hardening of the arteries, prostate disorders, macular degeneration, Parkinson's, goiter or other thyroid dysfunctions, wounds that don't heal correctly and end up with excess scar tissues, yeast infections, swelling in your feet or legs because of poor kidney function, acne, erectile dysfunctions, liver diseases, stones in the gall bladder, kidney, or parotid ducts, lupus, proteinuria, high cholesterol, or extremely low pH, any form of tumor or cancer, especially breast cancer, you probably have serious deficiency of iodine.

The Recommended Daily Allowance (RDA) of iodine set forth by the FDA is 125 *micrograms*. Brownstein points out that the thyroid alone uses 12-13 *milligrams* of iodine daily. A milligram is 1,000 times more than a microgram. In addition to what the thyroid uses, the rest of the body needs another 10-12 mg per day, and sometimes as much as 50 mg daily during times of stress, which is when your body often uses nutrients four times faster than normal. Iodine is needed in every single cell of your body, and is especially concentrated in the glandular system.

Without enough iodine, the thyroid slows down and a host of troubles that seem unrelated and intractable will appear. The most common of these are depression, thinning hair, always being chilly even on warm summer days, lack of interest in sex or physical exercise, dull skin, fading eyesight, failing ears, as well as major problems like autoimmune disorders and cancers, especially breast cancer.

Everyone needs differing amounts of iodine depending on how deficient you are in the first place and how efficient your body is at utilizing it. Here is a key factor in taking iodine. When you have enough in your system, you will begin to have little heart palpitations. This is the body signaling to you that you can cut your dosage back and maintain at a lower level. Okay, enough about iodine! Let's return to other key minerals.

Sulfur is a basic ingredient of the major amino acids and, thus, is a requirement for building every cell in your body. It is also a powerful disinfectant, acts as an anti-aging substance by keeping cell walls flexible, improves digestion and elimination, builds collagen, and protects us from radiation. Recent research indicates that sulfur is a key in keeping your electrical system working smoothly and well!

Phosphorus is a necessary co-factor for many of the vitamins and provides a great deal of the *oompah!* in the hundreds of chemical transactions that go on in the body. It works closely with calcium and magnesium to continuously form and maintain bones and teeth. It is important for normal breathing and a steady heartbeat, for healthy, functioning kidneys and the ability to use vitamins.

Copper is necessary for your body's ability to create its cells and enzymes. It also helps keep energy and strength high, assists in all healing processes, helps maintain normal levels of triglycerides, keeps your hair from turning gray prematurely, and is necessary for zinc to do its work.

Chromium is essential in assisting your body to utilize insulin and keep blood sugar normal. It helps you metabolize amino acids, lower your cholesterol, keep weight down, and avoid osteoporosis.

Manganese is a trace mineral used to build bones and keep joint capsules in good working order. It also metabolizes fats and proteins, produces important enzymes, maintains normal blood sugar, and keeps the immune system healthy.

Selenium is a powerful anti-oxidant that protects the immune system, heart, and liver; supports the pancreas; maintains fertility; and helps prevent cancer, heart disease, and liver disease.

Boron is a bone and brain enhancer that promotes the absorption of calcium thus helping you avoid osteoporosis and stay mentally sharp.

It is also a co-factor in being able to keep and use other minerals within the body.

Germanium improves oxygen levels in your cells thus leading to better resistance to infection and disease. This mineral also supports the immune system while acting as a detox agent in the body.

Silica works with calcium to form bones and is a key mineral in the formation of collagen and connective tissues, and in reducing arthritis and osteoporosis. It keeps you flexible and young; is necessary for healthy hair, skin, fingernails, and arteries; helps your body get rid of aluminum toxicity; and helps prevent Alzheimer's.

Molybdenum is essential for normalizing cell operations and keeping the tissues in your mouth and gums healthy. Molybdenum is important for good bones, your liver, and teeth, and helps keep male sexual potency alive and well.

Vanadium, like molybdenum, is necessary for normal cell function and for the processes that form good bones and teeth. It is also needed for reproduction, a healthy cardiovascular system, and good kidneys.

Gold is seldom thought of as a necessary mineral, but when taken as a trace element, it stabilizes mental and emotional balance while promoting a sense of well-being. It is also used as a pain-killer for burns and arthritis, to ease the difficulties of menopause, and lift the spirits of those who suffer from Seasonal Affective Disorder (SAD).

Silver is a powerful supporter of the immune system. It is effective in keeping your body clear of hundreds of viruses, fungi, and bacteria thus helping prevent inflammation and clearing internal and external infections. Like gold, it is used as a pain-killer for burns and arthritis

Vitamins

Once you have the amino acids, six major minerals, and other key minerals in place in your diet, it is time to think about vitamins. Most people think of vitamins first and give little thought to minerals, although you must have minerals in your system before you can properly utilize vitamins.

The major oil-soluble vitamins include:

Vitamin A is known as "the healing vitamin" because without it you cannot heal, no matter what else you take or don't take. Its presence is necessary for your body to utilize protein. Since amino acids, fats, and many of the body tissues are forms of protein, Vitamin A is critical. It is essential for bone and teeth formation, protection of the major organs, good eyesight, healthy skin, and clear mucus membranes, especially those involved in asthma, as well as protection from cancer.

Vitamin D is known as "the sunshine vitamin" because your body will convert cholesterol substances in your skin to Vitamin D precursors if you expose your skin to the sun for about 20 minutes three times a week. Vitamin D is necessary if you want to utilize the calcium you take in! It is essential for bone growth, the immune system, normal thyroid function, good eyesight, normal weight, strong muscles, and regular heartbeat.

Vitamin E is known for its protection against heart attacks and cardiovascular disease. Vitamin E not only improves your general circulation, it lowers blood pressure, promotes normal blood clotting, and repairs capillary walls. As an anti-oxidant, it preserves Vitamins A and D from attack by free radicals, preserves fertility, helps to maintain vision, hearing, and prevent cancers.

Vitamin K is the last of the oil-soluble vitamins (that we know of) and is required for the formation of bone and its repair. It is closely involved in the production of your body's chemical factors that maintain blood clotting ability and resistance to infections, especially ear, nose, and throat infections. It is necessary for healthy liver function, normal blood sugar, for anti-aging protection, and in preventing cancers, especially of the organs.

The major water-soluble vitamins include:

Vitamin B-Complex is a star player in the body. The B's, known as B1 (thiamin), B2 (riboflavin), B3 (niacin), B6 (pyridoxine), and B12 (cyanocobalamin) are involved in an extremely wide variety of functions. Usually taken together so that they are taken in the correct ratios, each is highly unique. A very partial list of their activities includes circulation, blood-building, cell building and longevity, protection of nerve sheathing, good digestion, brain function, learning capacity, good memory, good muscle tone, anti-oxidant abilities, regular heartbeat, pain reduction, good vision, healthy skin and eye tissue, normal growth rate, fertility, preventing birth defects, clear skin, stimulation of bile, production of adrenal and sex hormones, utilizing other vitamins, boosting stamina, preventing neuropathy, maintaining mental health, cancer immunity, and the production of DNA and RNA. Of them all, B-6 is a necessary ingredient in more bodily processes that any other vitamin, and without it, you will quickly go downhill.

Vitamin C is a major anti-oxidant as well as promoter of tissue repair. It also stimulates immune function and boosts iron absorption. It works as an anti-bacterial and antibiotic agent; protects against blood clotting; lowers cholesterol and blood pressure; strengthens arteries, veins, and capillary walls; and supports the immune system against infections and cancers.

Folic Acid is actually part of the B-family of water-soluble vitamins. It is critical for being able to produce and maintain healthy blood, preventing birth defects, keeping the processes of protein metabolism healthy, and in helping prevent the breakdown of DNA, thus guarding against cancer, TB, and other serious diseases.

Co-Q 10 is a powerful companion worker with Vitamin C in keeping the immune system in good working order. It helps cells to generate the energy necessary to do their work, keeps us from aging too soon, increases circulation, and is especially good for heart function.

Conditional Vitamins include:

Conditional vitamins are those that your body will manufacture under normal circumstances if deficiencies are not present. Without the necessary amino acids, minerals, and major vitamins as building material, the body may fail to make them and problems can result.

Biotin is needed for metabolism of all major nutrients: fats and oils, carbohydrates, and proteins. It is also a key player in preventing anemia, depression, hair loss, dry or flaky skin, and pain.

Choline is another key raw ingredient in building a healthy physical body. It is used in a large number of bodily processes, especially those of the brain and nervous system, the gall bladder, and liver. It is needed for smooth, coordinated movement, for carrying fats through the blood so all cells that are in the process of rebuilding their cell membranes (which are made of a double layer of both saturated and super-unsaturated fats) will have access to these fats. Choline also helps prevent the deposit of fat in the organs of the body. It is an assistant in avoiding angina and other heart problems, ulcers, and high blood pressure.

Pantothenic Acid (B-5) is another member of the B-family. Like choline, it transports necessary fats to and from cells. It is important in the production of hormones, reducing triglycerides and cholesterol, easing stress, the development and maintenance of cartilage, and producing other important substances in the body, including antibodies, neurotransmitters, and those enzymes that manage glucose in the blood, thus assisting with prevention of diabetes.

Inositol and its total role are not yet well understood, but it is found in every single cell of the body. It is especially abundant in the heart, brain, and skeletal muscles and serves to lower cholesterol, prevent arteriosclerosis, relieve constipation, irritability, and mood swings. It also keeps fatty deposits from forming in the liver, keeps eyes healthy, helps prevent hair loss, and helps with recovery after illness.

PABA, also known as para-aminobenzoic acid, is actually a component of folic acid. Similar to the other conditional vitamins, it is essential in the metabolism of proteins. Other effects include maintaining hair color, maintaining healthy intestinal bacteria, creating normal, healthy blood cells, and preventing sunburn and skin cancer.

You have now been introduced to the most basic and most familiar amino acids, minerals, and vitamins. This is not an exhaustive list by any means, it is just some of what we know so far. Mineral deficiencies affect your moods, perceptions, and feelings. The chart below lays out some of what we know.

Deficiency of	Effect on Perception, Mood, & Feeling
Calcium	Gives up easily; no persistence or patience; confusion, anxiety; immature attitude; weakness, lethargy, unable to establish a routine or sense of regularity in life.
Magnesium	Doesn't want to be touched; short attention span; poor sleep; muscle cramps; cravings; tendency toward hysteria and being over-dramatic; selfishness; lowered ability to maintain individuality in presence of others.
Potassium	Paranoia; difficulty keeping perception focused in this dimension; perception wanders into other dimension; picks up frequency sets that are generally ignored by the majority; tendency to see and hear things others do not see or hear, combativeness.
Sodium	Sleepiness; fatigue; a feeling of being heavy or overweight even when not; poor sense of self.
Zinc	Inability to smell or taste; alternating moods of near-suicidal depression followed by moods of unrealistic invincibility and adventurousness.
Iron	Doesn't want to interact; sluggish; unwilling to physically get up and move; unable to swallow properly.
Copper	Anger; irritability, sometimes explosive
Iodine	Feels achy; pain with no specific source; crabby; persistent depression; lowered ability to differentiate between Self and others; no interest in sex or intimacy; difficulty seeing oneself as you really are.
Vitamin A	Lack of interest in sex; jumpiness; inability to cry; tendency to hold one's breath; inability to forgive; poor self-image.
Vitamin B-1	Easily confused; panic attacks.
Vitamin B-2	Headaches; tiredness.
Vitamin B-3	Unwilling to think for one's self; agitation, anxiety, depression, psychosis.
Vitamin B-5	Guilt; irritability; impatience; burning hands & feet; insomnia; difficulty falling asleep and staying asleep; sense of weakness in muscles; poor coordination.

Deficiency of	Effect on Perception, Mood, & Feeling
Vitamin B-6	Feeling of constant stress; irritability; dizziness; depression.
B-12	Anxiety; feeling weak and fatigued; afraid that you might fall or tip over; tearful and weepy; mental fog; unstable perception shading into a catatonic-like absence of perception altogether; sleep disorders; depression; dementia; rapid heartbeat; light-headed or fainting spells; vision problems; tendency to want vegan diets because other foods disturb them; numbness and loss of sensation in skin; feeling like you can't take a deep breath; intermittent fever without accompanying conditions or symptoms.
Vitamin C	Unable to see the big picture in situations; tendency to focus on details that are meaningless; loss of will power.
Vitamin D	Sadness; poor attention to everyday reality; feeling of impending death or disaster; moodiness; schizophrenia; feeling of claustrophobia.
Vitamin E	Unable to see or grasp the meaning in words or events; unable to care or love; vague feeling of confusion.
Vitamin F (Omega 3, 6, 9)	Loss of creativity; lack of stamina and unwillingness to finish things; low interest in life.
Vitamin K	Feeling disorganized; unable to structure perception or activities; easily distracted
Folate	Procrastinates and puts things off indefinitely; lack of interest in everyday living; tendency toward drama

There are at least 75 additional trace minerals used by the body in its many and varied processes. If you eat at least some of your food as *real food* that has been grown in a healthy manner, you should be able to get many of these other trace minerals into your system.

One of the key goals of this chapter is to help you grasp the fact that your body is a self-healing system that depends on you to supply it with raw materials for repair and maintenance. These vitamins, minerals, and amino acids are another set of tools for healing.

This is also an opportune moment to warn you against something that happens all too often. Some people are perfect examples of the old belief that "if some is good, more is better." This is not always the case.

Let's say you read or hear about something that might help you with a problem you've been having, so you run out and buy that supplement and start taking it without doing your homework. Your homework is to find out how much you actually need, and what *supporting* supplements might be needed to make the new supplement work, and more importantly, what the cautions and contraindications might be.

For example, many of the amino acids need Vitamin B-6 to work properly. So you buy a bottle of B-Complex capsules with 100 mg of each B-vitamin and start taking it three times a day. But be aware! Sometimes Vitamin B-6 in excess can conflict with medication taken for Parkinson's, making the medicine ineffective. This may not happen in your case, but you at least need to be aware of the possibility. All things have a *relationship* to one another! Get on the web and do a little checking. Go to the bookstore and search out a good, complete reference on vitamins and minerals, then buy it. Or go to the library and do a search there. Gradually you will learn the nature of the relationships between these substances and come to honor them.

Read, ask questions, and then experiment with the new supplement for a few weeks. If all goes well, extend the experiment for a month or two or three, *always* paying attention to what you experience and how you feel. If something comes up, read or search for answers until you find them. If all is well, keep going, but keep your eyes open. After three weeks to three months – sometimes only three days – you should notice signs of improvement. If nothing happens after two or three months, your healing program needs further tweaking.

Often, vitamins do not work as well as they should because the body is so clogged with wastes. Worse, when you start taking a full complement of amino acids, minerals, and vitamins, your body enthusiastically goes to work breaking down old, poorly built material. This adds to the waste and congestion problem! Dr. Gonzales recommended frequently that people not even start a supplement program until they had completed one round of detox procedures first.

Since research is ongoing and our base of information is ever-changing, this introduction to aminos, minerals and vitamins will certainly be deficient before it ever goes to press, but you have to start somewhere.

There are many other books that go more deeply into the intricacies of amino acids, minerals, and vitamin effects within the body, and if you are going to be your own healer, or be one of the healers in your family, you should have one or two of these references in your home library (see suggested references in the Appendix). Get one, read it, and work at understanding yourself as a body/mind system that functions as an integrated ecological system with many needs, checks and balances. ❖

*Part 5*_____

Lifestyles and Stress

26

Foods, Moods, and Stress

IN EARLIER DAYS OF HUMANITY'S EXPERIENCE on planet Earth, our bodies developed an elaborate response to danger that was designed to help us survive. Today, our lifestyles run counter to the ways that we were designed and built to live, and this is very stressful to us. Lots of people think stress is just another vague mood, but it's not. Stress is a series of biochemical and physiological changes in the body. These changes are disastrous over time.

Imagine you are walking through the jungle and a tiger starts to chase you. This threat to your life sets in motion a chain of events called the General Adaptation Syndrome, known popularly as *stress*. The minute you recognize that you are in danger, your brain immediately downshifts from the higher brain functions found in the cortex to the mid-brain functions of the limbic system.[85] When a tiger is chasing you, you don't need to be figuring out which species of big cat you are dealing with or calculating the tiger's rate of approach. These are analytical activities made possible by the cortex. You *do* need to fight or run for your life, and these kinds of responses are handled in the limbic area of the brain.

Stage 1 of the stress response is alarm and begins as soon as the threat is perceived. Instantly your adrenal glands go into high gear, dumping adrenocorticotropic hormone (ACTH), cortisone, and cortisol into your

---

85 Leslie Hart, *Human Brain, Human Learning* (New Rochelle, NY: Brain Age Publishers, 1983) p.108.

bloodstream. This ACTH brings quick energy, heavy breathing, and a fast heartbeat within 30 seconds. You are immediately ready to fight or run for your life. Your blood pressure rises, and sugar pours into the bloodstream, giving quick energy to muscles and brain. Digestive processes shut down so the energy normally used to digest food can be used for defense. Red blood cells flood the arteries to take in more oxygen and dispose of carbon dioxide, while clotting factors pour into the blood to clot quickly in case the tiger bites or scratches you. Blood is withdrawn from your extremities and moved into the deep interior of the body to protect and feed vital organs and big muscle systems, and within two minutes of the start of the stress response, endorphins (brain-generated opiates) pour into the blood stream to dull perception and ease pain in case the tiger gets hold of you. The endorphins also "loosen" attention from your usual points of interest and habitual behaviors so you can move into survival mode and do whatever is required of you. The cortisone and cortisol loosen up joints and relieve stiffness, allowing you to run like a gazelle or fight with gusto.

Stage 2 of the stress response is resistance in which the fight or flight is on. During resistance, more and more of the above chemicals are released, and your body will rally intensely to defend you against the threat.

Stage 3 of the stress response is exhaustion in which your physical resources are used up, the defense and immune system wear down, and without immediate relief and attention to healing, your body gives up and dies. [86]

From this, you should be able to see that stress is not just a convenient psychological excuse for changing your life – stress is a killer. The wonderful thing about the stress response is that, if a tiger really is chasing you, it gives you the energy to run without pain (the work of the endorphins) or even a thought about being tired. If the tiger gets you (or your boss verbally blasts you), you will be so drugged by your own opiates that you may not suffer as much as usual. The bad thing about the stress response is that it is triggered whether the threat is a tiger, an angry spouse, a final exam, a rough business meeting, a screaming two-year-old, or anything else you find difficult to deal with.

---

[86] *Stress* by Walter McQuade and Ann Aikman, Bantam Books, 1975. p. 7-9.

If you spend any amount of time in stress, not only will you exhaust your endocrine system and your immune system, you will suffer nutritionally simply because the processes of digestion shut down during stress (note *Stage 1* above). All of the nutrients you put into yourself are wasted because they are not absorbed, the body has no supplies for repair and rebuilding, the immune system is disabled, and serious degeneration sets in. This is why so many people come down with cancers, high blood pressure, diabetes, heart attacks, or other serious diseases about 1½-2 years after a period of great physical or emotional difficulty. They were caught in the stress response, and their entire body was degenerating at an extremely rapid rate. This is why you need four times the ordinary level of nutrition when you are ill or in a state of stress. The illness itself causes stress and very little nutrition is absorbed. Worse, you are using up the nutritional supplies on hand at a tremendous rate.

You should also be able to see why more heart attacks happen on Monday mornings than any other time of the week. High-pressured executives going back to work get caught in the stress response, and the clotting factors released into the blood make it easy for clots to form in veins and arteries that are already narrowed or full of plaque and other obstructions.

During periods of stress it is difficult to sleep because your endocrine system is too exhausted to produce serotonin to keep you calm or melatonin to help you sleep. Your creative abilities suffer because the downshifting of the brain from cortical to limbic functions leaves you without access to the great creative abilities of the frontal lobes of the cortex. This leaves you dull, foggy and fatigued, and interferes with your ability to see clearly what is happening around you. Thus, intelligence, decision-making, and energetic action remain just out of reach.

When Weston Price was traveling the world back in the 1930s, he found that people who were getting high levels of nutrition did not experience the bad moods, petty jealousies, periods of depression, damaging competition, juvenile delinquency, or high crime that were prevalent elsewhere in society at that time and are even more so in our time. People were healthy, relaxed, creative, and cooperative. They loved the everyday processes of growing, collecting, or hunting their food. They enjoyed the personal involvement needed to gather fiber for clothing, to tan hides for pouches (purses), jackets, and other everyday items. There was no separation between art and the making of dishes, tools, blankets, rugs, or other household items needed for everyday living. A spirit of joy in their oneness with each other was expressed easily and naturally in the music, dance, and rituals that connected them to their intuition, healing abilities, wisdom of their ancestors, or the great Source that lies at the heart of everything.

Today, millions live in constant stress. Sometimes war is the cause, other times sickness or financial need is at the root of our difficulties. In many places around the globe, we are slaves to our economic system and a great deal of effort goes into making sure that the system stays in place.

Many people have accepted the routine of just going to work, staying in their cubicle or rut, and repeating the one set of behaviors they were hired to do over and over and over. Yet in order to accept this kind of confinement, we must set aside, or at least seriously compromise, our need for a secure and trusting connection to Mother Nature. This compromise makes us uneasy in our soul. Worse, we are naturally creative beings, and the effort to find outlets for our creativity causes considerable stress because artificial outlets demand extra money, time, and energy. When creativity is divorced from the routines that bring us food, water, shelter, and tools, then a creative life begins to seem like a luxury instead of the necessity it really is.

The demand that we be at the office or in the factory for set, specific hours so many days in a row interferes with our freedom to travel when and where we need or want to go. The expectation that we will show up at an office or factory at the same time every day, day after day, also disrupts our natural sleep rhythms, which tend to rotate through a variety of cycles.

Sedentary lifestyles interfere with our need for full physical activity that uses the body the way it was designed to move. All of the expectations and habits of contemporary life stress the body/mind system terribly and cause us to get old before our time. When you add the fact that the nutrition we're getting is totally inadequate, you begin to see why the outcome is widespread degeneration and depression that has become epidemic. We are stressed, irritable, and impatient on a regular basis.

Back in the days when we were trading tools, furs, metals, fabric, and a few specialty items directly with one another, we were somewhat on the safe side. The biggest danger was in the travel. The moment we began marketing an entire array of manufactured and artificial foods, we started down a destructive and dangerous path that is quickly leading to the collapse of our entire civilization.

No group of people has ever survived, thrived, and maintained their power on foods that do not contain the high-level nutrition required by the body. This has been the lesson for every group from the Mayans to the Romans to the Persians to the Sumerians. As I have already pointed out, get too far away from Mother Nature's soil, and you will either collapse from illness and fatigue, or someone will invade and you'll be too weak to care and too tired to defend yourself properly.

When I first started studying the mind, it led me back to the body again and again. I ignored these early observations and conclusions because I was caught up in the New Age idea that the body was just an incidental thing, completely subject to the mind. It was a long time before I realized that the mind is also subject to the body it is conjoined with. *It is a body/mind system.*

I have come to recognize that, contrary to the idea of the body as a messy, embarrassing incidental in this life, we all come here precisely to experience the great joy and sensuousness that a body offers, to create with love and enthusiasm, and to evolve that body toward full enlightenment.

Our lives are filled to the brim with the textures, tastes, sounds, feelings, sights, movements, and expressions of the body – but we are too tired and stressed to enjoy them. Yet, we are all deeply affected by what goes on around, in, and with the body. Our participation here in this reality is completely dependent on having a body to experience it with, and one of the most overlooked factors of that body is how it affects the mind.

Although most people separate physical feelings such as the pain of a stubbed toe from emotional feelings such as worry about money, the truth is that all feelings and emotions are the result of our thoughts. When we have a thought, the body then uses neurochemicals and hormones to produce feelings that match our thinking.

Although it is true that much of what you spend your life thinking about is the result of the way you've been taught to think and feel about reality, the fact still remains that what you feel at any given moment depends on whether or not your endocrine systems and brain can produce the chemistry that will create the feelings you would like to have, for these are the drivers that push behavior.

If your body does not have enough aminos, minerals, and vitamins with which to produce the neurochemicals that make you feel happy, sad, curious, compassionate, guilty, rushed, or any of the other emotions that are part of life, you will not be able to experience appropriate feelings or share the wholeness and richness of life. With a limited range of feelings, you end up caught in the same few emotions over and over. When this happens you become bored, angry, listless, and can behave inappropriately in situations that require a new set of feeling responses. Do this often enough as a child and you will be diagnosed as emotionally disabled, a condition that often accompanies learning disabilities. If these disabilities continue into adulthood and you never to develop the capacity to produce the chemicals that create a wide range of sensitivity and caring, you may be labeled everything from depressed, to incompetent, to a sociopath.

You may try to develop yourself to a more expansive consciousness or advanced level of spirituality, but the body may not be able to respond to your intention to remain calm and loving because it does not have the supplies it needs to produce the neurochemicals that maintain a positive attitude of calm clarity, patient compassion, or loving kindness. Your moods are directly dependent on the level of nutrition you give yourself, the amount of exercise you do, and the amount of sleep you get.

If you are depressed, feel generally anxious, or have a constant sense of restlessness or irritation, it is time to survey your life and begin making changes. Although many people blame outer circumstances for their depression, if you are not superbly healthy in the first place or have high levels of inflammation, you will not have the energy to make needed changes in your life whether they are physical, mental, emotional, or spiritual. People who aren't healthy can't deal with the fallout resulting from inner or outer change, so they refrain from making changes at all.

To relieve stress and create or maintain a sense of emotional well-being and balance, all of the things we have talked about in this book are critically important. This includes changing your diet to real foods, detoxing your body regularly, balancing your amino acid, mineral, and vitamin intake, avoiding foods that you are allergic to, making sure you are *absorbing* the nutrition you're taking in, and getting enough general exercise as well as aerobic exercise.

Be sure you are getting enough of the right fats – saturated and superunsaturated – because you need these to utilize the major, oil-soluble vitamins. Avoid eating a low-fat diet because this quickly causes depression, irritability, unsocial behavior, fatigue, and a host of conditions characterized by mental or emotional degeneration.

If you live a highly stressed life, you may be deficient in amino acids, magnesium, calcium, Vitamin B-6, and the entire Vitamin B-Complex, as well as the essential fats Omega 3 and 6.

It is important to avoid all white sugar/white flour products, and at least one meal a day should consist of raw foods. Either eat fruit all morning, or have a very large salad with lots of vegetables in it for lunch or dinner. Extra tyrosine, glutamine, tryptophan, phenylalanine, or methionine (see amino acids, Ch. 25) may also be needed, depending on the specific and individual symptoms that result from the stress. Dr. David Brownstein MD recommends iodine plus ATP Co-Factors to end depression. SAM-e plus B6 also work very well with a very nice side effects of stopping arthritis pain!

Even mild but continuous stress can result in depression and we just feel irritable and dissatisfied all the time. In his book, *Nutrition and The Mind*, Gary Null quotes Dr. Lendon Smith as saying…

"What we've found is that if their level of GGT (a liver and gallbladder enzyme called gamma glutamil transpeptidase) is below 20, they're more likely to have some of these magnesium deficiency symptoms – short attention span, trouble relaxing or sleeping, little muscle cramps in the feet and legs, a craving for chocolate. Most of these people don't like to be touched. They may be a little crabby. (All of these) symptoms go with low magnesium… which is one of the first minerals to disappear from food when it's been processed. Magnesium is also one of the first minerals to leave the body when there is stress, which accounts for how so many women behave a day or two before their periods. They feel stressed because they're losing their magnesium."[87]

Good nutrition is a non-negotiable factor in your life as well as a miracle worker. Even the more challenging mental problems such as bipolar disorder, schizophrenia, alcoholism, ADHD, autism, chronic fatigue syndrome, premenstrual syndrome, aggressive behavior, Alzheimer's, anorexia, and bulimia respond well and sometimes disappear with high-density nutrition, a good diet, and exercise.

If you are constantly fatigued more so than depressed, you're probably deficient in light exercise, amino acids, magnesium, calcium, the entire Vitamin B-Complex, iron, and potassium. You may need DMPS chelation and might also benefit from any therapy that increases oxygen, such as 2 droppersful of Oxy Life Force and a gingko biloba supplement, which improves circulation and increases delivery of nutrients to the tissues.

One caution – I do not take iron and Oxy Life Force together as they cancel and complicate one another. Since I need booth, I take the iron first thing in the morning, and the Oxy Life Force after supper. This helps build reserves of energy and makes oxygen available without the complications. And sometimes, the iron does the entire task if you also exercise enough to do some heavy breathing.

Manic depression, known today as bipolar disorder, is often the result of the body's inability to metabolize zinc properly. Often, there is a need for the natural mineral lithium, extra Vitamin B-Complex, the right combination of fats, and the complete set of amino acids.

Schizophrenia responds slowly but well to a full detox program, complete elimination of sugar, elimination of all foods that the body is allergic to, Vitamin B-12, Vitamin B-3, Vitamin C, the entire Vitamin B-Complex, calcium, magnesium, zinc, manganese, chromium, selenium, amino acids, acidophilus, pancreas enzymes, raw butterfat (from milk or

---

87 Null, p. 42.

butter), and Omega 3 and 6 fats.[88] Drinking distilled water regularly and taking 1-4 droppersful of Oxy Life Force is also very helpful. Adding C60 in Coconut Oil, plus regular exercise, is even more beneficial.

It would also help if the extraordinary abilities that schizophrenic people have for dipping into other dimensions of reality could be shaped, channeled, or put to good use rather than dismissing this skill as craziness. Schizophrenia is a problem in bio-chemistry that interferes with the ability to filter out other realities while in this reality. The result is a garbled reality here, coupled with a tendency to visit other realities, some of which have very different basic assumptions and laws of perception. We could learn much about consciousness if we could get past our diagnostic prejudices.

Alcoholism is usually an addiction to sugar and thus, it is absolutely necessary to eliminate sugar as well as many carbohydrates. Supplements include a good amino acid capsule containing the full set of aminos, the B-vitamins, especially Vitamin B-3 in the niacinamide form, a good multiple-vitamin/multiple-mineral capsule, extra zinc, Vitamins A and C, chromium to help regulate blood sugar, manganese, milk thistle to repair the liver, and flaxseed oil or hempseed oil to supply Omega 3 and 6. The Liver Flush is very important here, as is walking and stretching on a regular basis.

As children, many alcoholics and drug addicts made very poor decisions about themselves and life. Often, these old decisions have not been examined, updated, or re-decided in the light of adult perspective and consciousness. Specific forms of guided imagery have proven to be startlingly powerful in healing the emotional pain of alcoholics and can result in an 80% rate of rescission among alcoholics, something almost unheard of in most drug and alcohol counseling centers. [89]

Aggressive, autistic, or ADHD children almost always have calcium and magnesium deficits, are low in Vitamin B-6, and have heavy metals in their brain and blood, and thus, suffer from neurotoxicity. A number are

---

88 Read *Nutrition and Mental Illness* by Carl Pfeiffer PhD, MD, Healing Arts Press, Rochester, VT, 1987, for an eye-opening look at nutrition and its effect on mental illness.

89 Michael Hutchinson, *Megabrain Report* (Sausalito, CA: Megabrain Inc, Vol. 1, Number 3 and 4).

also allergic to the food in their diet – especially sugar. Neither are they getting enough of the necessary fats. Often, they have a sluggish liver and colon, and are not getting the full range of vitamins and minerals they need because of poor absorption. Through chelation, plenty of outdoor play and exercise, whole foods, a good supply of the saturated and superunsaturated fats, as well as a steady supply of nutrient-dense foods, supplements, and enzymes, even cases of autism are being reversed completely. [90]

Exercise

Notice that all of the above healing programs utilize exercise and/ or active physical play. Physical movement in the form of exercise is essential to the success of any healing program. I recommend getting a copy of the book *The Ancient Secret of The Fountain of Youth* and doing the five exercises described in it on a regular basis.[91] These exercises are basic to a healing program. I have been doing them for 20 years and have found them to be invaluable because they help keep the endocrine system in good working order, which is needed to run the body smoothly and well and to slow down the aging process.

I love these five exercises because they take only 15 minutes to do, and they are extremely powerful. They keep the core muscles of the body in good shape, keep the body flexible, eliminate fatigue, and produce a huge amount of energy, which lasts for approximately 60 hours – over two days! They also eliminate cellulite from thighs and arms, tighten sagging jowls, keep the bladder from leaking, clear sinus passages, reduce headaches, keep the neck flexible, and restore strength to the upper body in the shoulders, arms, wrists, and hands.

It is a good idea to get a few weights and lift weights a couple of times a week because weight-bearing exercise keeps your bones strong. You don't have to bench-press 200 lbs.! Just lift 5 lbs. with each arm or leg a dozen times or so and that is enough.

---

90 "A Guiding Light in Nutritional Intervention" in *The PPNF Journal*, Price-Pottenger Nutrition Foundation, LaMesa, CA, Spring 2000, Vol. 24, No. 1.

91 Peter Kelder, *The Ancient Secret of the Fountain of Youth* (New York, NY: Doubleday, 1998).

A wonderful tool for maintaining good health is a rebounder, which is something like a small trampoline. You stand on it and bounce lightly up and down, which helps drain tissues and clear the lymph system.

I recommend getting at least one exercise video, perhaps a beginning yoga routine, then using it at least once or twice a week as an alternate set of movements. And walk. Go outside and walk briskly, swinging your arms and taking big strides. Jog a little now and then. Run a little if you feel like it. Breathe deeply. Allow yourself to sweat. Above all, try to reclaim some of the huge range of movement and motion you enjoyed as a child.

Inner Work to Change Yourself

Excellent nutrition goes a very long way toward creating a balanced mind that matures beautifully into a wise, tolerant, peaceful personality. Yet it cannot make up entirely for poor child-raising practices, education that teaches competition rather than cooperation, or a socio-cultural system that promotes victimhood and the "every man for himself" approach to living.

Be aware that every behavior is accompanied by a feeling to which we have assigned a specific meaning. Many of these assigned meanings are contradictory from family to family or culture to culture. This results in a great deal of confusion and miscommunication. Some well-known examples of this are that in some cultures (American), you are taught to feel good if people respect your personal space "bubble" and stay an arm's length away when talking. In other cultures (Middle Eastern), you are taught to feel insulted if someone remains an arm's length away. In some cultures (American), you are taught that it is okay to clean your teeth with a toothpick after meals and it is not okay to pick your nose. In other cultures (Thailand), people are taught that it is the grossest of habits to pick one's teeth, yet it is perfectly acceptable to pick your nose in public. In some families, it is acceptable to openly discuss one's finances or one's age, whereas in others it is considered the height of rudeness to bring up such subjects. In some families, it is okay to use sarcasm as humor, to stand up to others to the point of bullying them, or to use alcohol freely. In other families, sarcasm is considered a slap in the face, pushing one's own ideas forward is considered argumentative, and alcohol is an escape.

In addition to the stress that results from learned prejudices and biases, there are dozens of conditions in the body that result in bad moods, poor attitude, slow cognition, or mental and emotional fatigue. Some of the more common are PMS, low thyroid function, chronic fatigue syndrome, heavy metal toxicity, and disruption of the endocrine system by exposure to fungicides, pesticides, or other chemicals. Although these moods and attitudes are a problem for some, the bigger problem is that too many people are not self-aware and do not realize they don't have to feel the way they do.

When you are faced with the need to heal yourself, spend time examining *why* you think and feel the way you do. Get support from a counselor, coach, or therapist who will help you change habitual patterns of thinking and responses that have proven to be destructive or that no longer work for you.

With good nutrition, some detox, a bit of exercise, less stress, more rest, time for oneself, a little support, and some common sense therapy, life can be much sweeter and more peaceful.

High-nutrition foods are necessary if you want to maintain a life of restfulness, calm insight, dynamic creativity, and a peaceful demeanor. When the diet is nutrient-poor, you will not be able to produce the internal biochemistry and neurotransmitters that allow you to experience good moods while handling stress and avoiding perceptual confusion, mental difficulties, and depression. ❖

27
Thinking Ourselves Well...

FEW THINGS ARE MORE IMPORTANT TO YOU and your quality of life than high-nutrition food on a consistent basis. Few things are more detrimental to you than manufactured food filled with sugars and chemicals and lacking in nutrition.

A decade ago when I was working as an educational consultant, a couple of men came to visit me one day. One was head of a learning program for gifted and talented children in Warren, Michigan. The other was the principal of a Lansing-area school. As we talked, I discovered that the principal's wife had cancer and was struggling terribly with the disease.

Knowing that I was into New Age thinking and believed in alternative health, the principal asked me if there was anything I knew of that might help his wife. Not really knowing what to say, I handed him a popular platitude of the times, "Well...you know, she must want that experience, and you should ask her why she created that disease for herself..." The implication being that she could just think otherwise and she would be well again.

Almost explosively he interrupted me. "Oh god! Don't ever say that to her. She's heard that over and over, and her response is, 'I don't *want* this damned disease, I *never* wanted this damned disease, and don't try to tell me that I did! No one ever wants cancer, and no one in their right mind would ever create such a nightmare for themselves, so don't tell me I created it! That's bull----!'"

After he left, I thought deeply about what had been said. I had to agree with his wife. No one in their right mind ever wants cancer, even unconsciously. I wouldn't want it, and I could see how his wife would feel outraged when offered such a cheap answer. She was beyond the shallow excuses of most New Age thinking and needed something real, something she could trust to guide her toward healing. This was life and death for her.

I loved the whole New Age movement because it was a refreshing change of pace that made room for more of my humanity. Yet in that moment, it came up woefully short. The whole movement looked like the emperor without any clothes, and it was at this moment that I discovered the difference between *believing* in something and the *knowing* that comes from real experience with something. Fluffy-sounding, sophisticated platitudes were useless. The woman was dealing with cancer. Her life was on the line. Where was the core of information and solid experience that would lead to something constructive, in this case, health and life?

This little episode made a big impression on me, one I've never forgotten. However, it was years before I could address the implication that we could just think ourselves well. After wrestling with the whole thing for a very long time, one day the question I had posed to the principal revised itself from, "W*hy* did she want to create that disease for herself?" to the question "H*ow* did she create that disease?"

Suddenly, there was the answer. *Of course* she didn't want the disease! She wanted to be healthy. But perhaps she also wanted to eat a lot of sweets…maybe she was too busy and on the run to find and prepare excellent meals…maybe she hated to deal with food at all…maybe she didn't like taking supplements or couldn't afford them…maybe she was being swept up in the pressures and politics of her husband's school district and had been living in a state of stress for years…perhaps she was struggling with a child or aging parent and didn't realize that time for herself was critically necessary… maybe she didn't realize the importance of avoiding pesticides, heavy metals, and all the other toxins that were being sprayed on our foods…maybe she never learned how to feed herself correctly and take care of her body in a way that would result in good health. Wanting all of these things and wanting good health amounted to a situation that was overflowing with contradictions. If so, she would not be able to regain good health unless and until the contradictions were resolved.

If we *think* we can eat foods with no nutrition in them...if we *think* we can get away with spraying pesticides and other extremely poisonous chemicals on our foods...if we *think* we can manufacture food instead of eating the foods Mother Nature has produced for us to eat...if we *think* we can lead lives of great stress and dismiss that stress as a necessity of modern life or as a mere emotional figment that we just need to get through...if we *think* we can cover up the early warning signs of physical degeneration with drugs...then we are going to end up creating nightmarish diseases that we will have to deal with or die. It is in this way that we can think ourselves ill or think ourselves well. We do create our reality with our choices, and the body reacts accordingly.

The principal's wife may have been caught in the gap created by wanting contradictory things not recognizing this or knowing any better. All too often, we live an unexamined life dictated by forces outside ourselves.

Life in America seems to be organized around the concepts of "grow up, get an education, get a job, get married, buy the best and biggest house you can afford, establish a nuclear family, work hard to make as much money as possible, collect as many symbols of the good life as you can, retire, and travel before you die."

What I am suggesting in this book is that we must begin to organize ourselves around a different set of concepts.[92] They are similar, yet powerfully different. They are: grow to full maturity, commit to personal growth and the development of your natural potentials, learn to feed yourself, learn to educate yourself, learn to heal yourself, find work you like and be disciplined enough to figure out how to live on the money that work will make, organize your work and home life to maintain balance and health, marry if you can find someone who is as committed to your own development as to their own, find a group of people you can live and work with and invest there to create a family of small businesses that all complement one another, think twice – no, three times – before having a child, work in such a way that you contribute to, support, and are celebrated by the entire family of people and businesses you are part of, learn to enjoy your work as much as possible (even the parts you do not

---

92 See my book, *Robes: A Book Of Coming Changes,* for views of the future that may inspire you.

care for as much), age wisely allowing your work to change as you change and age, give up the idea of death, travel only when absolutely necessary, and communicate with people and the world on an ongoing basis.

It has been my experience that *if you really want to heal yourself, you have to heal your whole life*. You can do some of this healing yourself, and some can be done by others who help you. The most important factor in whether you get well or not is whether you *begin* a healing program or not.

Thousands of people don't feel good on a regular basis, but the doctor cannot find anything wrong with them. This does not mean they are healthy. You should be aware that by law, an allopathic doctor cannot treat you for anything until something is clearly and obviously wrong. The rules of current medicine require the doctor to send you home and wait until a condition develops to the stage where he or she can diagnose it with current medical tests, then treat it with common drugs or surgical procedures. This is tragic because things should not have to get critically bad in the body before you do something. However, for a doctor to do otherwise is to open himself and his practice to being disciplined by the hospital he is connected to or being rejected by the insurance company because the treatments don't arise from a clearly defined and delimited diagnostic procedure. By delaying diagnosis and action, the doctor satisfies the requirements of the medical world he works in, yet opens himself to being sued for not taking action much earlier. The problem is not with the doctor, it is with a system that demands a clearly defined disease to which a host of standard medical procedures can be applied.

It is too bad that our current medical system evolved into such a rigid creature because it truly hogties our physicians. They are not encouraged to learn about nutrition, herbs, detox, or natural therapies, many of which allow for full healing in very early stages of disease or illness. Instead, they are forced to wait until there is a disaster or an emergency. I know that things are changing, but it's oh so slowly.

In the meantime, make your health a high priority and take the steps you can to keep yourself in good health. When you have to see a medical doctor, choose one with the idea that you are selecting a partner who must work *with* you, not *on* you. Find one who is aware of the power of nutrition, detox, herbs, and exercise. For most of us, it is not a choice of either/or…either allopathic medicine or alternative and holistic medicine. Think in terms of sustainable, complementary medicine. Sustainable medicine does not do as much or more damage than it does healing. And complementary medicine requires deciding what you need from all sides of the various healing traditions – allopathic included – then knowing how to mix and match or blend drugs, herbs, foods, surgeries, exercise, and the many healing practices that are our heritage at this point in time.

While you are healing the body and changing your physical routines to those that support and nurture life, consider healing your heart, your mind, your house, your clothing, your room arrangements, your relationships, your perceptions, your work, and the earth. Start now with something small. Continue each day with another step. In time, you will be healed. When you are, it will feel like the world is a wonderful, beautiful place. It is…and that is how it should be. ❖

Part 6

Healing Techniques and Programs

28
Tools and Techniques Used in Natural Healing

IF THERE IS ANYTHING TO BE AWARE OF as you look through this section of the book, it is that all of the procedures described here call for you to not only be involved in your own healing processes, but to also give yourself permission to take the time you need for yourself and your healing.

For you to get sick, it takes time and a willingness to ignore the signs and symptoms of approaching disease. For you to heal, it takes time and the willingness to learn, to become more aware, to pay attention to what you are doing to yourself, and to do the things that support and nurture the body. If your ill health has become a way of life for you, then returning to good health requires that you develop an entirely new way of living. This is a tall order, but well worth the effort. The suggestions in this chapter are certainly not all that can be done, but they will get you started.

Start With A Blood Test

One of the best ways to start your healing is to have your blood tested for its pH balance (its acid/alkaline balance). If you have had some recent blood work done, ask for a copy of the report. If you haven't had anything recent, ask for a *comprehensive* blood test, sometimes called a *full chemical scan* or a *CMP*, and get a copy of the test results. You can also arrange for a hair test, and this test often tells you which heavy metals are in your system as well as how much of them you have ingested.

Blood pH should be somewhere between 6.8 and 7.2. Rarely is it 7.0 because this is neutral and not helpful in terms of chemical reactions! If you're 7.1 or 7.2, you're in a reasonable state. If you're more than 5 points above or below the ideal, you should start making changes in your diet. If you are too acid, begin eating large amounts of raw vegetables and fruits, and drink a cup of hot water with the juice of one lemon in it once or twice a day. If you are too alkaline, change your diet to include red meat, cheese, and dairy products every day until your system is back in balance. Have your acid/alkaline balance tested every three months to see where you are at so you can eat accordingly.

As pointed out earlier in the book, if you are too acid, your cell membranes will close up tightly and nothing will be able to get in or out of your cells. Even if you are eating the best foods and taking supplements, you will not be getting the benefit of this good nutrition because the cells cannot open up enough to allow the available nutrients in. Acid conditions in the body create *sclerosis,* or hardening of tissues, and being too acid is a slow, painful route to malnutrition and degeneration.

If you are too alkaline, the cell membranes will be too loose and open. Not only will the hundreds of toxins from our world get into the cell interior to do serious damage to mitochondria and other internal cellular structures, they will derange cellular function. Your efforts to supply the cell with needed nutrients for repair and rebuilding will be thwarted because the nutrients will flow in and flow right out again due to the extreme permeability of the cell wall. Overly alkaline conditions in the body not only cause a too-drastic softening of tissues to the point they begin to break down, but this opens you to attack by every virus and toxin out there.

Correcting your pH is necessary for healing, balance within the body, and support of your immune system. It is also critical for optimal absorption, retention, and use of minerals and vitamins. It can take some time to change your pH permanently; often at least six months, and sometimes a year or two is necessary to shift the acid/alkaline balance and stabilize it at the new position. Once you know your starting point, begin your healing program. The following are many additional tools and techniques you can use to feel better and get well again naturally.

Castor Oil Pack

For many problems, it's hard to beat the pain-relieving and restorative power of a castor oil pack. This is an old Edgar Cayce remedy that is worth its weight in gold. It can be used regularly for every kind of healing from asthma, arthritis, and PMS to colds, cancers, infections, and ulcers. Not only does it help draw toxins from the body, the oil itself contains nutrients that nourish tissues and structures.

To make a castor oil pack you will need:

About ¼ yard of wool flannel or cotton flannel fabric

16 oz of cold-pressed castor oil (Home Health is the Edgar Cayce brand)

A piece of plastic about 12" by 15"

A bath towel and a hand towel

A heating pad

8 oz of water and a good book

1. To get the many benefits of a castor oil pack, you will need to use the pack **2 hours a day for 5 days in a row, then take 3 days off, then use it again, 2 hours a day for 5 more days in a row.**

2. To make the pack, fold and trim the flannel so that you have a rectangle of fabric that is big enough to cover the area you want to heal. I usually use sizes that range from 4" x 6" to 9" x 12". Fold the fabric so it is **2-4 layers of fabric thick**. Cayce recommended wool flannel but I use cotton flannel because I am so allergic to wool.

3. Next, get a plastic bag, piece of plastic wrap, or old shower curtain and **cut off a piece that is about 12" by 15"**. It should be larger than the flannel piece by at least 2 inches on all sides, and if you're a squirmy, wiggly kind of person who has difficulty sitting still, the piece of plastic should be even bigger in case it shifts and gets out of place. Of course, if you're truly resting, the plastic should stay in place easily!

4. Lay the folded flannel on the plastic. **Open the castor oil and drizzle it in a thin stream back and forth over the flannel**. Let that soak in for a few minutes, then add more castor oil and let that soak in. Continue this process until all layers of the flannel are saturated with castor oil. It

should be damp but *not* dripping, or later, you'll have oil everywhere once the oil warms up and gets runny. A 9" by 12" pack of cotton flannel will use about 8-10 oz of the castor oil. I'm not sure what amount the wool flannel would use, probably less. When the pack is saturated, fold both the flannel and the plastic in half, so that the flannel is inside the plastic. Your pack is now ready to heat briefly.

5. Pick a spot to sit or lay down, and **lay out the bath towel so that it will be under you to protect the chair or bed in case the oil runs.** Make sure you can also **plug in the heating pad** in that location. Once the heating pad is plugged in, turn it on "medium heat" and tuck the folded castor oil pack under it. Allow to warm for 3-5 minutes.

6. While the pack is warming, **get a hand towel, an 8 oz glass of water, a good book** or magazine (or the TV remote control) and put them within reach of the place where you will be sitting or laying down.

7. Meanwhile, **get undressed.** If you are going to put the pack on your chest (for colds, asthma, bronchitis, pneumonia, heart trouble, breast tumors, infection, injury, etc.), you need to undress from the waist up. If it is winter, wear a loose robe so that your arms and shoulders will stay warm once the pack is in place. If you are going to put it on your abdomen (for immune system stimulation, cramps, gastrointestinal difficulties, hip problems, PMS, tumors, surgical incisions, infection, or injury, etc.), you will have to undress from the waist down. Have a blanket or afghan available to put over your tummy and legs so you won't get chilled. You can also put the pack on a leg or foot, on your upper back and neck, on your lower back, your arm or hand, or wherever you have pain or difficulty.

8. When the pack is no longer chilly, get yourself comfortable, take the castor oil pack out from under the heating pad and **place the oil-saturated flannel against your chest** (or back, abdomen, leg, etc.). Then **place the piece of plastic over the flannel** to prevent oil from getting on other clothing or the heating pad. **Put a hand towel over the plastic** to absorb any oil that may seep out if the plastic and flannel get out of alignment.

9. **Put the heating pad over the hand towel.** You now have a stack of items that goes – from the bottom up – your skin, the oil-saturated flannel, the plastic protection, a hand towel, and the heating pad. Arrange

your robe or afghan over all this so you are warm and comfortable, then **sit and relax for two hours** while the castor oil soaks into you through the skin and goes to work. You can read, take a nap, watch television, knit or do other needlework, draw, write letters, or just think and daydream.

10. **Drink the water when you are half way through the time.** If you drink it too soon, you may end up having to get up and go to the bathroom, which can be a nuisance because you end up trying to hold the pack, the plastic, and the towel in place while moving about, getting to the toilet, etc.

11. **When the two hours are up, remove the pack from your skin,** folding it in half so that the oil-soaked flannel is inside the plastic.

12. Use a paper towel to blot up some of the oil on your skin, then **wash the remaining oil off with a warm, soapy washcloth,** rinse, and pat dry. This is to make sure that you don't develop any allergies to castor oil. It is a powerful healing agent and one that you want to be able to use whenever you need it. **After this, you are finished** and free to go on and do whatever you like with the rest of your day or evening.

Store the castor oil pack in the refrigerator or a cool, dark, dry place. Depending on where you keep it and how often you use it, it should keep well for several months and can be used again and again during that time. You may have to add a bit more oil if you use it a lot over a period of time and your skin has sucked most of the oil out of the pack.

If you live in a warm, moist climate, be sure to store the pack in the refrigerator or it will get moldy. I store mine in the refrigerator as a general practice in all seasons. Each person should have their own pack and use it for several months before getting new flannel and making a new pack. Depending on what you're trying to heal, you may have to make a new pack every month or perhaps only once a year.

I have seen some wonderful improvements using the castor oil pack. Some people notice a significant improvement in just the first one or two days. If this happens for you, don't stop using the pack until the entire thirteen days (5+3+5 days) is up. All kinds of secondary benefits and strengthening of the immune system take place during that time.

Mustard/Cayenne Foot Soak

Sometimes called the "mustard foot soak," this particular detox procedure is very helpful for headaches, the muscle aches and pains of colds and flu, water retention in the ankles or other parts of the body due to arthritis, diabetes, gout, poor circulation, and heart trouble, or the overall "blahs and goopiness" that accompany fasting, dieting, infections, and cancers or their treatments – chemotherapy, surgery, or antibiotics.

Your feet are a major outlet for toxic waste and since many people have such poor circulation in their legs, the feet become a storage site for waste instead of an outlet. The combination of warm water plus the healing properties of mustard and cayenne serve to both increase circulation and draw toxic waste right out through the feet.

To do this simple but powerful procedure...

1. You will need **a towel** and **a dishpan** or **basin of very warm water.** One of those foot-soaking appliances sold at the drug store works very nicely as well. The water should be deep enough to cover your feet without overflowing the pan when you put your feet in.

2. Add one tablespoon **(1 TBSP) of powdered dry mustard** and one teaspoon **(1 tsp) of cayenne pepper** to the water. Stir briefly just to distribute these two herbs.

3. Sit in a comfortable chair and **soak your feet in the basin for 30-40 minutes**. When finished, dry your feet with the towel and dump out the water, since it should not be re-used. **And that's it, you're done**.

The mustard soaks can be repeated 2-3 times a day and should be continued at least daily during periods of intense toxicity when the body is getting rid of a lot of waste, old cells, and metabolic structures that the body is breaking down because they are diseased or of poor quality construction. As you soak your feet, you will feel the intense heat of the mustard and cayenne working on your feet and legs. Even if the water cools off a bit, you will still feel the heat of these two herbs, and you will continue to feel them for several hours after you are finished with the soak.

Many people have thick, crusty skin on their feet or a variety of corns and calluses. These are the result of poor circulation and lack of care of the feet. In addition to the poor circulation mentioned above, there can be poor bone and tendon construction that started right from birth or as the result of bad or absent nutrition, badly fitting shoes, poor choice of shoes, being on one's feet for long hours every day, broken toes or injuries that didn't heal correctly, and many other difficulties. If you begin doing mustard/cayenne foot soaks, you have an opportunity to soak and scrape away much of this thickened skin, which interferes with your ability to eliminate toxins through your feet.

I often encourage people to take a very dull knife, one that is *not* serrated, and, using a flat, scraping motion, scrape the sides, heels, toes, tops, and bottoms of the feet to remove dead, thickened skin on the feet. You can also use a loofa sponge, a nylon "scrubbie," or a pumice stone, but they don't work as well as the knife. The loofa or scrubbie are fairly difficult to clean and can become so smelly after a few days that you won't want to touch them!

Even if you only do one mustard/cayenne foot soak, you will feel light on your feet afterwards. If you do them daily, there will be less pain in your feet and legs, less swelling, more healing of sores and tender spots, and even easier breathing and better clarity of mind, all because of the improved circulation and reduction of toxic waste inside the body.

I buy dry mustard and cayenne in bulk form, at least a pint of each at a time and sometimes more, from our local health food store. You can also get them from your regular grocery store, but they come in tiny amounts. You end up having to pay for all the little bottles or cans, which you then have to throw away. If you don't have a good natural food or health food store nearby, however, what's available at the grocery store will get you started.

The Salt and Soda Bath

A salt and soda bath can be used by almost anyone trying to recover from almost anything, and it is most powerful for those trying to heal the more challenging problems like cancer or tuberculosis, AIDS, MS, lupus, hepatitis, fibromyalgia, drug addiction, arthritis, or depression.

You should do a salt and soda bath when you are feeling your worst. It is during these periods of most intense toxicity that this bath shines! The baking soda and salt help to get toxins moving and released through the skin. This bath is especially helpful when you are nauseous, coughing, in pain, severely fatigued or unable to think and focus because of general irritability and restlessness. It is also very good for any sores on your skin.

To do a salt and soda bath...

1. **Run a bathtub full of very warm water.**

2. While the water is running **add one cup (1 c) of baking soda (sodium bicarbonate) and one cup (1 c) of salt** to the tub. The salt can be sea salt, real salt, natural salt, kosher salt, or if nothing else is available, regular table salt.

3. **Get in the tub and lie down** with as much of the body submerged as possible for at least **20 to 30 minutes,** although 45 minutes would be better. Add water if it gets too cool.

4. When finished, get up, **dry yourself by moving the towel slowly and with very firm pressure over your skin to remove as much dead skin as possible.** Then get dressed and **you're done**.

Do not put any lotions or oils on your skin for 24 hours, as these greatly reduce your body's ability to release toxic gases and wastes through the skin. It also interferes with the air available to skin cells, and if the lotion itself is full of toxins, it ends up putting back into the skin what you have just tried to remove.

If you are seriously ill, do a salt and soda bath every day until the nausea, weakness, fatigue, headaches, muscles aches, or other symptoms have diminished. The fact that your symptoms diminish usually does not mean that you are completely healed, however, it does mean that your immune system is coping with the problem much better than it was before. True healing usually has to be completed by detox and the top-quality nutrition that supplies the body with what it needs to repair and rebuild all of its structures.

When you are completely healed, fatigue disappears and you will have a steady supply of high energy, creativity, good spirits, curiosity, a desire to return to work or to find work you truly love, a sense of strength, and inner peace. You will sleep well, enjoy exercise, care about what you eat, and take an interest in your world. If you do not have the energy to do these things, then you are not well, even if there are no overt symptoms.

Fatigue, or lack of pep, is one of the earliest signs that your body is accumulating too much waste matter. To help draw toxins and waste out of the body, do a salt and soda bath regularly. This can be every day during a cold or flu or on the days you are doing one of the detox procedures. It can be once or twice a week for maintenance; right before, during, or just after menstruation; or any time that you are struggling with the symptoms generated by serious health problems.

Castor Oil, Aloe, and Honey Packs

If you have serious sores or ulcers on your skin, especially your feet, ankles, and legs, start your healing by drinking a gallon of water every day. Do the Colon Sweep for five days, followed by the salt and soda bath outlined above every day for one week. Then speed the healing of your skin using the following procedures.

1. On each of **the first two days of your salt and soda bath, rub castor oil on** *only the area of your skin that needs healing* after you have finished the bath. (It would actually work even better if you put castor oil on a compress and taped it over a sore or ulcerated area the day before you're going to take a salt and soda bath. Remove the compress just before the salt and soda bath next day, then put a new oil compress on after the bath that day.)

2. On **the next five days of your salt and soda bath, when you are finished with the bath, put a good amount of honey on a gauze compress and put the compress on the sore or ulcerated area** that needs healing. Change the compress daily.

3. If the sore or ulcer is not healed by this time, **return to using the castor oil** for one week after soaking the affected area in water for at least ½ hour each day.

4. If the sore is not healed by this time, **alternate back to using the honey** again, and continue the daily soaks.

5. Continue to **alternate between castor oil and honey, with daily soaks, until full healing is accomplished**. Take your aminos, vitamins, and minerals regularly. Consider doing a Liver Flush and Purge.

If You Have a Serious Burn

Begin with aloe vera for the first two days, or as soon as possible. Use *fresh* aloe vera, don't use something out of a bottle or jar.

1. Before you cut a piece from the aloe vera plant, take a minute to **touch the plant where you are going to make the cut and tell it you would like to use it to heal someone.** Then give the plant a few minutes to adjust itself. It will often mobilize its healing energies into the area you are going to cut so that the piece you cut off will do a good job for the person who needs healing. It also prepares itself to heal the wound that will be left behind once you remove a piece from the plant. While the plant is getting ready, get a sharp knife, a gauze compress, and some tape.

Step 1-2.   Step 3.

2. When you and the plant are both ready, **cut a piece from the plant** that is slightly longer than the burn or sore, if possible.

3. The next step is to **cut open the piece of aloe so that you can unfold it and make it lie flat against the skin.** To do this, take the knife

and carefully pierce the top layer of aloe skin (without cutting all the way through), and slice down the piece of aloe lengthwise. You now have a piece of aloe with a slice down the center and two flaps, one on each side.

4. Take the knife and slide it along under the left flap of the lengthwise cut you just made. Repeat this on the right side.

5. **Open up the piece of aloe, exposing the thick, meaty, juicy, gel-like interior and place this gel side directly on the burn**. If you need to cover a large area, cut two, three, or more pieces of aloe as described above and place them on the burn. If it is good aloe, you should be able to taste a slightly bitter taste in your mouth within five minutes of putting the aloe on your skin.

6. **Hold the aloe in place using a gauze compress** and tape. If the burn covers a very large area and the person is in bed, compresses and tape may not be practical. In this case, use something that is light in weight to hold it in place, like a folded towel. If the burn is on a leg or arm, use an ace bandage to hold the aloe pieces in place. **Leave the aloe in place for 12-24 hrs.**

7. **On day two**, (or after 12 hrs.), remove the compress, the weighted towel, or the ace bandage. Look at the aloe vera. All that should be left of the aloe vera will be a paper-thin piece of green plant skin lying on the burned area. **Remove this thin green skin carefully and replace with fresh aloe.** Cover or wrap as you did the day before, and **leave for another 12-24 hours**. Over these two days, your body absorbs all of the aloe vera's thick, meaty interior and uses it to stop the burn from going deeper, to alleviate its heat, and to limit its damage. If you are healing a third-degree burn, you may want to repeat using the aloe pieces for Day 3 and Day 4 or until the burning pain stops, then continue on with the rest of the steps in the healing

8. **On day three**, remove the compress, towel, or ace bandage and pick up the remains of the thin green aloe vera skin. If you had a first degree burn (reddened skin), it will probably be gone altogether. If you had a second-degree burn (blistered skin), the blisters will probably be gone, it will be much less red, perhaps smaller, and although it is seldom painful at this point, it will be tender, especially if it comes in contact with warm water. If you had a third degree burn (red, blistered, opened flesh),

the flesh will usually be smooth and closed, although it may still be bright red with no skin over it. If the third degree burn area is not smooth and red, you may want to use new aloe vera pieces for another day or two. In any case, after the skin is smooth and bright red, it is important to **begin using honey** to feed the newly forming cells that will take the place of those cells that were destroyed in the burn. Honey will provide such excellent nutrition for the burned skin that there will often be no scarring.

9. Spread honey – raw is best but not necessary – in a thick layer on a compress that is large enough to cover the entire burn. **Put the honey compress on the burn** so that the honey is directly in contact with the burned area. **Leave it on for 24 hrs.**

10. **The next day**, lift the honey compress off the burn and put new honey on the compress. Or simply **replace it with a clean honey compress.**

11. **Repeat steps 9 and 10 every day until the burn is completely healed**, which is about 2-4 days for a first-degree burn, 4-6 days for a second-degree burn, and 5-14 days for a third-degree burn.

Note: If the burn is a 4th degree burn and very serious (the flesh is blackened and shrunken), or if it covers a very large area of the body, using large quantities of fresh aloe vera for more than a week can cause stomach cramping. If this happens, stop using the aloe vera and switch to honey for a few days. If the burns are extensive and severe, return to using aloe vera after a 3-5 day break, then alternate between aloe vera and honey until the healing is complete.

This method of healing burns often leaves no scars or discoloration of the skin. Sometimes the healing is so perfect you cannot tell there was ever a burn there. The fresh aloe vera is a natural antibiotic, and the honey is an even more powerful antibiotic, since infection is the biggest problem with burns or any breach of the skin, the honey will prevent an infection. If an infection does get started, use The Purge to end it. Honey is so powerful an antibiotic that we use it for staph infections, including MRSA.

I keep a small jar of Manuga honey on hand as part of my medicine cabinet stock. At times I have used it even watered down for minor burns and infections. There is something very wonderful, almost magical about Manuga!

Skin Brushing

One excellent way of cleaning and stimulating your lymph system, while also detoxifying your skin, is skin brushing. Although it seems almost too simple, it feels very good and is a very effective healing technique.

To do skin brushing...

1. You will need **a long-handled brush with natural vegetable bristles**. Synthetic, plastic bristles are often rough and can make tiny cuts in your skin, so be choosy in selecting a brush. Except for an occasional wash and rinse, the brush should be kept dry and used dry.

2. A good time to do skin brushing is first thing in the morning when you get up, *before* you take a shower or get dressed. You can also do skin brushing at night, just before you go to bed.

3. Your body should be dry, and you should move the brush over the skin in long sweeping motions – no back-and-forth or scrubbing motions. Imagine you are brushing toward the heart...up the legs, up the arms, down the neck, and up the trunk. It is not necessary to brush the face, but I do so occasionally just because it feels so good.

4. Skin brushing can be done once a day for maintenance, twice a day if you are under the weather, and can be increased to four times a day in periods of intense toxicity when dealing with the effects of problems such as cancer, AIDS, TB, pneumonia, weight loss miseries, all kinds of infections, or anything that makes you feel awful.

It only takes a few extra minutes to brush your skin and is a startlingly wonderful way to begin the day simply because you will feel so alive all over. It is also a great way to end the day because it leaves you calm and relaxed.

Juicers and Juicing

When I first set out to heal myself, one of the prescriptions was a pint of carrot juice every day. The recommendation from Dr. Gonzales was to invest in a Champion juicer because it was, in his words, "a real workhorse, worth the money."

When I saw the price of the Champion, I balked. I did not want to put out $225 for a juicer. So I went to the store and came home with a nice looking juicer that cost $40. It lasted less than a week.

About that time, a friend offered to let me use his juicer – a $60 item – to do my juicing. That one lasted only two days, and I was back on the market looking for two juicers, one to replace his, and a good one with a decent motor for me.

An advertisement for a Vita Mix machine came in the mail just about then. After reading it carefully and swallowing hard at the $380 price, I sent for it because I wanted something that would do more than just juicing, and it had a sturdy motor. I was sure it would last more than a week even if used heavily. When it arrived, I plugged it in, put in my carrots, and ended up with carrot mush, a thick, mealy glob that was a long way from juice.

Hoping to salvage the situation, I got out some cheesecloth, thinking I would strain the juice out of the carrot cellulose and fiber. But the juice dripped out so slowly that, after half an hour, I only had half a cup of juice that was already turning bitter. My instructions from Dr. Gonzales were to make a pint of juice and drink it immediately, before it oxidized, so I was beginning to feel desperate.

In an effort to get the juice out of the carrot mush, I tied the four corners of the cheesecloth in a knot to form something akin to a bag. Slipping a broom handle through the knot, I laid one end of the broom on the cupboard, put the other end on the back of a chair, and hung the cheesecloth full of carrot mush over a large pot on the floor. Then I started turning the cheesecloth bag in an attempt to squeeze the carrot juice out of the mush and extract the required juice quickly.

However, as the pressure built up in the cheesecloth bag, the juice began squirting in every direction, sometimes three or four feet across the kitchen. I ended up with carrot juice all over myself and the kitchen, ruined a good shirt with stains that wouldn't come out, had a colossal mess to clean up, and got barely a lick of juice. I needed something that would actually produce juice and had easy clean-up.

After looking around for a while, I came across someone at a conference demonstrating the Omega Juicer. This looked like the answer to my prayer. It was only $180, had a good motor, produced a very high quality juice, and was very easy to clean up via a thin paper filter that prevented fiber from getting into the blades or screens. You just put the paper filter into the juicer, made your juice, pulled the paper filter out with all the pulp attached, rinsed the machine, and you were done. I bought it.

The Omega worked wonderfully for me. It was quick and simple and easy to use. But when my husband went on the same healing program I was on, I discovered that I couldn't make the required amounts of carrot juice without stopping the machine, taking it all apart, removing the filter paper and pulp, putting in another filter paper, re-assembling the entire thing, and continuing on with the juice-making.

When a third family member got interested in healing, I began to run out of filter papers, had to keep ordering, and was tired of stopping to take the machine apart several times just to change the filter. I needed a juicer that was designed for continuous feed operation.

In the end, I bought the Champion. It had the powerful motor I needed, made excellent juice, allowed for continuous feed operation, didn't require the purchase of filters, and was extremely easy to clean up.

I still use the VitaMix because it makes great whole-fruit smoothies, as well as excellent fresh tomato juice, and a variety of creamed soups. I bought a citrus attachment for the Omega and use it to juice the oranges, lemons, and grapefruit needed for the Purge, and it does an excellent job of making fresh citrus juice drinks for breakfast. For my everyday carrot juice or any type of vegetable/fruit juice (celery, beet, apple, broccoli, cabbage, spinach, etc.), I use the Champion. Each of these machines does an excellent job at one aspect of juicing. My daughter, who has access to each of my juicers, decided to try a Juiceman II for her own kitchen. She says the Juiceman also does a very good job with vegetables and fruits, although she, too, uses the Omega for citrus juicing.

My original wish to avoid spending $225 on a Champion ended up costing me over $900 by the time I was finished. The lessons were, "Don't try to skimp by buying cheap, poorly built equipment" and "Know what the equipment will really do." By ignoring these two rules, you could end up spending more in the long run, and if using the equipment is such a hassle that you avoid doing what must be done, your healing efforts will be delayed, and you will suffer longer.

All of this is just to make you aware that to take charge of your healing, you will have to make a few investments in your kitchen equipment. A good juicer is one of those investments. Remember, fruit juices tend to break up wastes in the body, and vegetable juices tend to rebuild the body.

The gift of healing that comes with juicing is that you get all of the vitamins and minerals in the fruit or vegetable, but the body doesn't have to put forth any effort to extract them. When you drink a freshly made juice, the vitamins and minerals go directly into your system. Much of the body's work of digesting and breaking down the component parts of a plant in order to extract useful nutrients is eliminated. The burden on the pancreas to drop repair and rebuilding efforts and switch to the task of digestion is also avoided, and the valuable pancreatic enzymes that consume cancers and infectious organisms are free to continue their work of healing. The pancreas does not get worn out, and you do not degenerate in the steady downhill manner that is so common today.

Drinking only fresh, raw fruit or vegetable juices is one very powerful way to heal and rebuild. When you are unable to digest foods or too weak to eat, you can slowly, gently nourish your body back to health with raw fruit and vegetable juices.

Mineral Broths

In addition to juicing, making broth is a fabulous way to restore health and get high-density nutrition. When broth is made properly, you use bones from beef, pork, chicken, lamb, or fish, and all of the minerals that were used to build those bones are extracted and end up in the broth, which you then drink or use to make soup. This kind of broth or soup is very healing and can be made in quantity then frozen to be used later.

To make a good broth, put the following into a large stock pot:

3-5 lbs of beef bones. These can be raw or leftovers from a roast. If making chicken broth I use chicken necks, backs, and wings

5-8 quarts of water

1 large potato

2 large carrots

1-2 large onions

3 TBSP dried parsley or ½ cup fresh parsley

¼ cup of vinegar or red wine to acidify the water, which makes
it possible to extract all the minerals from the bones

Simmer beef broth for 72 hours (3 days). Simmer chicken (or fish broth) for 36 hours. Strain everything out of the broth and do not re-use the vegetables. Add sea salt to taste, perhaps a little pepper, and it is ready to drink. If you are going to use some to make a soup, you may put cubed beef or chicken in the broth, add 1 TBSP of nutritional yeast, salt, fresh vegetables, and fresh or dried herbs such as 2-3 tsp of parsley, 1 tsp marjoram, basil or oregano. Simmer to cook vegetables, add ground pepper, and eat.

Raw Foods

There is nothing quite as drastic – or as powerful – as changing to a raw food diet for a while. Cooked foods take a heavy toll on your health…an extremely heavy toll, all because the natural enzymes in the raw food that would help with digestion and absorption of nutrients have been destroyed in the cooking process. Thus, I often tell people who need to do serious healing that raw foods are a major key to healing. Fruits, vegetables, grains, milk, eggs, butter, cheese, and even some organic meats can be eaten raw if you know how to prepare them.

Fruits and vegetables are easy – just wash and eat. Grains, as in 14-Grain Cereal, can be ground and soaked overnight. Raw milk may be illegal in your state, but can still be purchased if you can find a farm that sells shares of ownership in a cow. If you buy shares, then you have access to the raw milk, cream, and butter from that cow because it's your cow.

Raw eggs should be organic and can be eaten without cooking by adding one or two eggs to a smoothie, or by making an eggnog drink as follows: 1 cup milk

1 raw egg

1 TBSP honey

1 dash nutmeg and/or cinnamon

Put all ingredients in a blender and blend until frothy. Sprinkle a little more nutmeg on top and drink. It's delicious and so good for you. Sometimes I will add strawberries, blueberries, peaches, yogurt, or hempseed oil to increase nutrition and add variety.

Raw cheese can be purchased at any good health food store. And raw meat should be *organic* liver that is cut in ½" cubes and frozen individually. Then, you take out 1 or 2 frozen cubes, put it into a fruit smoothie, blend well, and drink immediately. I have seen this "smoothie-frozen liver" combination restore someone with fairly advanced multiple sclerosis to enough energy and health to set aside her wheelchair and heavy leg braces and return to walking.

I remember hearing long ago about people who were into raw foods, juicing, and a variety of other exotic practices like enemas, mineral baths, heavy exercise, and various forms of sweats. At the time, I thought they were just "health nuts" and wondered why anyone would bother with all that. Now I know…they were sick and had discovered the power of detox, raw foods, and the body's ability to heal itself if it was given complete support. In any healing program, raw foods, fresh vegetable and fruit juices, along with well-made mineral broths should be a mandatory part of your healing program.[93] [94]

If you're going to cook anything, make a good-quality broth. This, along with raw juices, brings healing and builds good, sturdy health.

At this point, several things bear repeating…If you are sick, change your diet. Start getting the high nutrition you need to rebuild. Exercise pushes nutrients into difficult-to-reach corners of the body; shoves waste materials out; promotes flexibility, strength, and energy; and allows organs to move around and stretch a bit within the tight confines of the body. Enemas, mineral baths, sweats, and specific detox procedures allow the body to return to youthful form and function, bring clarity, and zest for living.

---

93 To learn how to prepare excellent old-time foods, get *Nourishing Traditions* by Sally Fallon, ProMotion Publishing, San Diego, CA, 1995.

94 Another great book full of raw food recipes is *Living Cuisine: The Art and Spirit of Raw Foods* by Renee Loux Underkoffler. It was published by Avery Publishing in 2003.

Most people in first world countries are in terrible shape. Many are suffering from malnutrition. The first stage of malnutrition and starvation is a slightly swollen, puffy body. This puffiness then becomes a true overweight condition as people eat more than they should in an unconscious attempt to satisfy the body's need for nutrients. I hear people everywhere talking about trying to lose weight, or exhorting others to lose weight, or selling something to help people lose weight. You cannot be suffering from low-level malnutrition and attempt to cut back on eating without disastrous effects, the least of which are depression, fatigue, and irritability. You may look nice and trim for a while, but without the input of high nutrition, you will go downhill and may end up triggering one of your genetic weaknesses. At the very least, you will feel crabby and hungry, and you may return to gorging yourself because you're so miserable.

I would suggest that, instead of just talking about our health problems or engaging in less-than-helpful efforts, we educate ourselves well and learn to recognize where the source of the real problem lies, then make the necessary changes in our lifestyles, food systems, and the world.

Herbs

There are so many good books already written about herbs, what to use, how to use them, the standard dosages required for a therapeutic effect, and the contra-indications to be aware of that I will not duplicate those efforts here. But I do have several things to say about the use of herbs.

The first is that herbs are powerful medicines. Everything you eat affects the body immediately. And anything that you take in a consistent manner – three times a day for more than two days in a row – is going to shift your biochemistry seriously, for better or for worse. Therefore, do not take herbs recklessly or without knowing their effects.

The second is that herbs you use should be grown here in the U.S. on an organic farm, or wildcrafted, otherwise you have no way of knowing whether pesticides like DDT or fungicides – banned here in the U.S. but still legal in foreign countries – have been used on them. Also, many imported herbs are irradiated before they are allowed into the U.S., and that destroys both the medicinal potency and leaves you taking in a substance whose energy fields have been seriously deranged.

The third is that, too often people take herbs in doses that are much too low because their potency has not been determined. Or the herbs they take are old, irradiated, or were poorly grown.

Many people try a few herbs and when nothing spectacular happens within a few days, they try something different. When you decide to take an herb, you must commit to taking it for at least three months as they work slowly and very gently. It won't usually take that long for you to notice improvements, but it might be helpful for you to understand that herbs work in terms of "getting to the source" of the problem. They start by correcting imbalances in the body and, like antibiotics, need to be taken for a certain period of time in order to do the whole job. They do not usually have unpleasant side effects, so at first you may not notice them working – but they are!

Often you should take an herb for three months and then stop for a couple of weeks, then resume for another three months. If you have a chronic problem, an herbal program can be repeated every year at the same time, as this allows the body to cope with the problem better.

Herbs are a perfect accompaniment to the exercise, detox, high nutrition diet, and supplement approach to healing. If herbs aren't working for you, it may be because you have too much waste matter in your body and you're too plugged up to absorb anything, or your circulation is so poor that nothing is reaching its destination, or your nutrition is so wretched that the effects of the herbs are overpowered. Clean yourself out, change your diet, and herbs will have a quick, powerful impact.

Clay Packs

I first heard about clay in the book *Secrets Of The Soil* by Peter Tompkins and Christopher Bird. The book noted that trees, plants, and animals whose water contained traces of montmorillonite clay had extraordinarily fine health, resistance to disease, and all sorts of other beneficial effects. Since I was aware that what is good for plants and trees is often good for humans, I immediately made note of the power of clay. [95]

Shortly after that, I read somewhere that the Indians of South America made small clay balls, dried them, and kept them in their pocket to swallow now and then, keeping their gastrointestinal tracts free of parasites, worms, and harmful bacteria.

When I came across a book called *Our Earth, Our Cure* by Frenchman Dr. Raymond Dextreit, [96] I started exploring the uses of clay in all sorts of situations in which people and animals required healing.

I put clay in the water our chickens drank, and they grew thick, shiny feathers while producing eggs with thick shells and bright orange yolks. I put clay in the cow's water and got rich, creamy, delicious milk and butter. I put clay in the dog's water and achieved some relief of her arthritis and a clearing up of her "dog breath." I put clay in the greenhouse beds and got healthy greens all winter, greens that froze again and again but then thawed out and kept growing, refusing to die. They eventually went to seed the following summer. Finally, I started taking a tablespoon of clay in a liquid suspension every morning and discovered that my hair and fingernails improved, I had less gas and bad breath, and enjoyed a general improvement in health overall.

When clay turned up as part of the Liver Flush in the detox program that was outlined by Dr. William Kelley and Dr. Nicholas Gonzales, the whole family adopted it.

Now I use clay for lots of things...on bee stings or bug bites; for small burns; for sores, acne, and ulcers – both internal and external; to stop bleeding; for nausea, diarrhea, or constipation; as a poultice to draw poisons and toxins out of the body; to reduce fevers and pain; help bring organs back to healthy functioning; to restore beauty, color, and texture to facial skin; and a host of other applications.

There are two kinds of clay you might come across. One is Montmorillonite clay, the other is Bentonite clay. For all practical purposes,

---

95 Peter Tompkins and Christopher Bird, *Secrets of the Soil* (New York, NY: Harper & Row Publishers, 1989) p. 213-225.

96 See Appendix B for a list of suggested references every home should have.

they are the same as long as they are both food-grade clay, not the kind used to line the bottom of a pond so it will hold water. I don't know who came up with the name Montmorillonite or when they came up with it, but the Montmorillonite moniker was fairly well-known and had been used for some time when another fellow named Benton came along, discovered a clay deposit, started mining it, and named his brand Bentonite.

When it comes to application, I pay more attention to the color than the name. Green clay is the most potent, so I try to get green clay first. If I can't find green, I go for red clay. Other colors (gray, yellow, white, pink, brown, etc.) are also useful, but not quite as potent as green or red.

It is usually easy to find green or red clay in a small tube containing a few ounces of moist clay at your local health food store for around $8 per tube, but this is really expensive. I buy a 25 lb. bag of powdered clay for about $20 from a local supplier and use it all year on people, plants, and animals.

To prepare the clay, put 2 cups of the dry clay in a glass or ceramic pot that has a cover. A covered casserole dish is a good "clay pot." So are the old-fashioned baked bean pots you can sometimes find at flea markets. Do **NOT** use plastic or metal to hold the clay, as clay will react with both of these materials, either turning the plastic to mush or absorbing some of the metal. Next, add clean water (distilled or reverse osmosis) that has not been boiled or treated in any way. Do not stir!

Let the clay sit without touching it until the water has been absorbed into the clay evenly. If necessary, add more water a little at a time. If it is too thin, add a little more dry clay to thicken it. Again, do not stir. When all the water has been absorbed and it looks as though it has a paste-like texture, put the cover on and leave it in a sunny place if possible. After a day, it is ready to use. To keep it from drying out and cracking, add a little water every week or so and let the water soak in slowly. It will keep for months.

For reasons that are not well understood, clay has the ability to draw toxins from everywhere in the body to the site where the clay poultice is sitting. Thus, if you have a leg ulcer due to diabetes, and you decide to use clay to heal the ulcer, it will pull all the toxins in your body to the area of the ulcer. This means the ulcer will get worse before it gets better. To avoid frightening yourself into thinking that you are getting worse or creating a more monstrous problem, it is helpful to eat only fresh fruits and salads for several days and take 1 TBSP of clay orally in the morning and in the evening before you begin applying a series of clay poultices.

My grandson is very allergic to mosquito and spider bites and any bite site tends to swell and become very red, sometimes reaching a diameter of two inches of angry, red skin that burns and itches for days, while he scratches and makes it all worse. One day, he had a particularly nasty bite, so we decided to apply clay to reduce the inflammation. Because he was only seven years old and fairly free of toxins – or so we thought – we didn't think fasting or a few days of oral clay was necessary, so we put the thick, clay poultice on his thigh, put a folded paper towel over it, wrapped the whole area with an ace bandage, and left it overnight.

The next day his entire leg was swollen and red! The day after that it was worse, taking on a dark red color. The clay had drawn all the toxins from his entire body into his thigh. It took nearly a week of clay poultices, warm baths, drinking lemon water (to fluidify the blood for better circulation), treatments with hot and cold water, and careful eating to bring the leg back to a normal state. A side benefit of using the clay was that, for a while, he was much less reactive to mosquito and spider bites because the clay had removed some of the toxic load his body had to deal with, leaving his immune system more able to deal with the small poisons deposited by mosquitoes and spiders when they bit him.

Getting Rid of Parasites - See Chapter 17 where getting rid of parasites is covered in detail.

Using a Rife or Other Frequency Generator

A frequency generator is an important and useful tool that helps maintain good health and freedom from debilitating as well as nuisance problems in the body by canceling the frequencies of various bacteria, viruses, parasites, and degenerative conditions. There are a number of manufacturers making these amazing tools in spite of efforts to obscure their effectiveness. They cost anywhere from $500 to $40,000 and the cost seems to be related to how many frequencies they will generate, how difficult the machine is to put together and use, and how much research the manufacturer has done to catalog the frequencies of various critters, conditions, and diseases.

I started out in love with the Spooky frequency generator at $500 because the cost was low and a good friend of mine was able to eliminate his bipolar disorder with it.

The Spooky II came out next, and another friend bought that version. However, he was overwhelmed by the complexity of putting all the pieces together and getting it to work correctly. He eventually gave up when someone he knew gave him a BCX frequency generator. The BCX was compact, portable, didn't require any assembly, had a good list of conditions and their frequencies, and was easy to use. If he'd had to buy it, the cost would have been around $2500. Eventually, he ended up with two or three BCX machines and had a steady stream of people coming to see him to ask if they could use the generator for one thing or another.

Next, someone I was working with to help reverse Parkinson's disease bought a VieLight frequency generator. These generators have been specifically designed for healing and regenerating the brain. Although they have a few inexpensive models that are available on Amazon, the ones that address the more complex regeneration needs of the brain run from about $1,800-$2,400. They produce both alpha and gamma frequencies and the improvement in the man who was using the VieLight was quite remarkable after only 3 days.

Then there is the Bicam, a German-made machine that is very versatile. It will erase unwanted frequencies, tell you what frequencies you are missing, and send you the frequencies you need, including the frequencies of various fruits and vegetables. I don't know what the cost is, but it is not prohibitive.

There are other frequency generators out there, some of them able to do amazing things. A few people have worried that using a frequency generator is not very natural, but drugs and surgeries are even less natural. As mentioned earlier, why should we have to deal with the destructive side effects of drugs and surgeries when problems can be addressed at their core causation level, that of frequencies that are either out of tune or shouldn't be there at all?

I think it is important to note here that frequency generators are amazingly effective, however, the experience that several of us have had with them is that the condition will return if you do not change your basic lifestyle in order to maintain the healed condition. In other words, your food, water, exercise, supplements, and sleep are still critical. The BCX or other frequency generator will give you a leg up to get on that horse and ride into good health, but you have to do the follow-up work to keep going forward, keep living.

From my point of view, these machines are here to stay and are a taste of the "energy medicine" of the future. I can foresee whole research efforts to map the body and develop a set of basic frequency blueprints of the human being, and use those to regenerate us in ways we never dreamed possible.

Using Natural Products

If you are like I used to be, you probably don't give much thought to use of fancy flavored, and perfumed items like toothpaste, deodorant, lotion, soap, or detergents. If you haven't given much thought to your toothpaste and toilet cleaner, it's quite likely you haven't even considered the sorts of things that are spread, dumped, or sprayed around your kitchen or onto your lawn. Perhaps you wouldn't think your house was clean if you didn't use powerful chemicals designed to kill everything on contact. And maybe you think your lawn would die or be ugly if you weren't spraying serious toxins and fertilizers on it.

You can't change your whole life, your mind, your habits, and perceptions overnight, but while I have your ear, I want to mention that once you get serious about healing and have gone through a detox program designed to remove toxins, you are going to begin noticing what you put in, on, or around your body. It's a slow-dawning awareness, but once begun, it continues. The most important thing for you to grasp at this point is that there are good, non-toxic substitutes for every commercial substance you currently use and a variety of alternate procedures for every process you are in the habit of performing. Our ancestors were not ignorant, suffering savages. In my opinion, they were practical, creative, observant, and even brilliant. They came up with a wide variety of solutions for every problem.

Today, we are too dull and stressed to do this. We gape around for a one-size-fits-all, manufactured solution that we think we can afford.

To get beyond this, make yourself aware of "spincasting!" This is the ability of governments, corporations, and Madison Avenue to:

1. Spin a web of perception designed to make you believe what they want you to believe so you will either acquiesce to something, ignore something, or buy something. Some people call this propaganda. I call it outright deception.

2. Slant the facts just enough to create an attractive – but unbalanced and therefore unhealthy – view of someone, something, or some event.

3. Distract you with something interesting but irrelevant so that you will ignore the truth or fail to ask the really important questions.

The truth is that commercial toothpastes do not prevent cavities. The only thing that prevents cavities is a high nutrition diet. Toothpastes only cover the bad breath that often results from eating foods containing sugar. Rinsing the mouth with water or brushing with a dry toothbrush has as much power to deter cavities as brushing with toothpaste.

Most toothpastes have fluoride and sodium laureth sulfate in them, neither of which is good for you. In spite of the widespread effort to make us believe that fluoride prevents cavities, the only thing that fluoride prevents is the uptake of iodine in the thyroid, and this creates a witch's brew of conditions – from depression, weight gain, and falling hair to cysts, cancers, and death.

In the 1940s the government produced a lot of fluoride for the atomic bomb project. The fluorine gases emitted from these factories killed plants, trees, and sickened people and animals along the East Coast.

New Jersey area farmers who lost crops, cows, horses, and some family members sued. The government lost their case and eventually paid the survivors a very small sum of money (about $200) while hushing up the case. Looking for the perfect way to cover their need to continue producing fluoride for the Manhattan Project, the government suddenly declared that not only was fluoride harmless, it was good for you! In a perfect example of spincasting, they announced a decision to do "further research" because a few studies on fluoride indicated that "it strengthened bones and teeth."

This was simply not true. In fact, the exact opposite was true. However, the research project gave the government an excuse to experiment and added an aura of legitimacy to fluoride use. It also allowed them to see how bad things could get when fluoride was introduced into the general population. They published a study that said fluoride was *not* harmful, and the men who worked in fluoride factories had fewer cavities. The actual truth was that most of these men had no teeth left because their teeth had been disintegrated by the fluoride fumes in the workplace! There was no mention either of the rubber boots the men had to wear because the nails in their leather boots kept disintegrating. [97]

Since the 1940s, other research has indicated that fluoride disrupts endocrine function, especially thyroid function. Fluoride in the water supply has been seriously implicated in Alzheimer's, Down's syndrome, autism, hip disorders, brittle bones, thyroid cancers, stiffness in joints, central nervous system effects, and a general drop in overall health and mental brightness, as well as mental and emotional stability.[98]

Here at the farm, my daughter makes all kinds of soaps and lotions that are wonderful and do not have any toxic products in them. I have a friend down the road who makes a tooth powder from salt, soda, orange peel, and sage. I love it, and it cleans my teeth a hundred times better than any commercial toothpaste. People sometimes ask, "…but what does the tooth powder taste like?", and I tell them it tastes salty with just a touch of soda.

If you're into sweet stuff only, it may be a bit of an adjustment because homemade tooth powders are different from commercial toothpaste in that they are usually not sweet, and they certainly have a different texture, neither of which is disagreeable. It only took me a couple of days of using

---

97 "Fluoride, Teeth, and the Atomic Bomb," by Joel Griffiths and Chris Bryson; www.inter-view.net/~sherrell/bomb.htm, July, 1997. This page is no longer available on the Internet, but if you do a search for the authors' names, you will find other resources and information, including www.fluoridealert.org.

98 "The Greatest 'Scientific' Fraud Yet?" *Nexus New Times*, Jan-Feb 2001, pg. 14-15.

the tooth powder to get to the point of definitely preferring it to toothpaste. My teeth had never been so clean!

A good point to make here is that if you base every decision of what to eat or drink on whether something tastes good or not, you are using an immature system of judgment. This is like basing every decision on money. It simply doesn't work because the criterion is too narrow.

If your diet includes things like soda pop, candy, bottled or canned juice drinks, snacks, and processed foods containing sugars, you will be quite likely to reject anything that isn't based on sugar and doesn't taste sweet. This is disastrous for your body.

Changing your diet and eliminating sugar will allow your taste buds to normalize. If you do this for a few months, then go back to try your old diet for a day or two, you will be appalled at how thin and tasteless commercial foods are. You'll also be surprised at what a poor cleaning job regular toothpaste does. Then it will be easier to change to something that is good for you, including toothpaste.

As for deodorants, read the labels and you will find that a good many of them contain aluminum and aluminum compounds. Every time you put on deodorant in the morning, you are getting a dose of aluminum molecules. After a while, this can build up enough aluminum in your system to require chelation therapy. When added to the other heavy metals that you take in with your foods or in simply breathing, the effect on the body is deadly.

Do not use deodorants full of perfumes and chemicals or that are designed to inhibit wetness. There is nothing wrong with sweating; it is an important way of detoxing the body. Get a crystal stone from your health food store, wet it, and rub it over your armpits each morning. It prevents the growth of bacteria in your sweat and does not have harmful side effects. An added benefit is that you buy one stone for about $8, but it lasts two or three years, which is a tremendous savings. In addition, you are not buying the plastic cases or metal and plastic cans that many deodorants come packaged in, so you are reducing landfill wastes and ecological resources.

If you change your diet to whole food and eliminate white flour and white sugar, you will notice that your breath and sweat are much sweeter and your feet do not smell. Soon you'll become aware that many common products are designed and sold to cover up our poor physical condition. Most of them are marketed as if they will bring a sense of richness and luxury to your life, adding this illusion to the illusion of health and beauty.

Commercial shampoos are another illusion of luxury. They cost a fortune, yet most contain alcohol. Alcohol destroys hair follicles on your head and results in loss of hair. Many shampoos and bar soaps contain sodium laurel sulfate or sodium laureth sulfate, which create lots of foamy bubbles but are toxic.

When my daughter expressed an interest in making soaps and shampoos, I encouraged her. The soaps were wonderful but the shampoos left our hair with a thick, sticky build-up. To remove this build-up, we started rinsing our hair with vinegar until the hair squeaked. The results of using this odd combo were surprising. My hair, which is very fine and frizzy, had extraordinary body and still looked good after three or four days without shampooing. There was also much less hair loss on a daily basis. The norm for loss of hair is about 100 hairs per day. While I don't get down to counting actual hairs, I was surprised to notice that I was hardly losing any hair at all!

With commercial shampoos and conditioners, even the herbal kinds from health food stores, I had to wash my hair every other day or it looked flat and felt awful. Being able to stretch this to three days, or even four if I didn't have to go anywhere, and still look quite decent was a real bonus. Another benefit was less breakage and the disappearance of split ends. The bottom line for soaps and shampoos is to avoid commercial, synthetically perfumed products as much as possible. If you don't know someone who makes soap, get something as benign as possible from the health food store. After detox and a good supplement regimen, your itchy, scaly, patchy skin and scalp may clear up, and with natural products you may have far fewer allergies simply because you are not constantly exposing yourself to the chemicals used in so many common products.

There was a time when my cupboards were stocked with anti-bacterial soaps and detergents, bleaches, acids for dissolving limestone blotches around faucets, oven cleaners, spray polishes for furniture, cleaners and polishes for cooking pots, shower cleaners, floor disinfectants, water softeners, dryer sheets to prevent static cling, and a half-dozen other chemicalized items that I thought were necessary for any decently run home.

One day, I met a woman with breast cancer. She had come to visit the farm after reading one of my other books. For reasons I can't recall now, we ended up trading services, and to fulfill her part she wanted to do some housekeeping. I agreed, and we made the trade. When she went to work cleaning, she ignored all my expensive chemicals and asked if I had some vinegar, some baking soda, and a little dish soap for sensitive hands. I retrieved a bit of each requested substance from the kitchen, and she went to work, slowly and lovingly cleaning each guestroom.

I learned that day that my own cleaning style was crazy. I resembled a frenzied scrubwoman who spent most of the time holding her breath while running in and out of rooms so she wouldn't breathe in the chemicals she was spraying and splashing all over. I switched to simpler cleaning products and began to realize that the most powerful substance of all was just plain water.

Don't use powerful cleaning products that tell you right on their labels that you shouldn't get them on your skin or breathe in their vapors. They aren't necessary. How are you going to get anything done if you can't breathe? And when you think about it, it's a bit insane to use them in the first place. If the world were that dangerous and infectious a place, we would never have made it past caveman stage. As it is, half of us are suffering from the curse of Louie Pasteur who believed in the "war model" of bacteria-against-humans. The rest of us are suffering from the marketing myopia spread by those who specialize in advertising and marketing and who keep telling us what we need to buy/have/do.

The simplest products work merely by shifting the pH balance, thus making an inhospitable environment for bacteria. You don't have to kill bacteria, and in fact, you can't kill them. You only kill the weaker strains as well as the beneficial bacteria, leaving the more virulent strains to multiply without restraint or limits. When the beneficial bacteria and weaker strains are left in place, they compete with the more virulent strains for nutrients and space, thus providing an effective means of controlling these more vicious forms. And with a healthy immune system, bacteria are not a threat. After all, we survived very well without commercial chemical products – whether for cleaning, antibiotics, or personal hygiene – for thousands of years.

The simple cleaning products such as soap and water, baking soda, vinegar, and even hydrogen peroxide are easy on your body, your pocketbook, and the environment. Once you stop believing that the expensive Madison-Avenue chemicals are part of the American Way, or begin to discover how destructive the American Way is, you will begin to wonder how you ever got so paranoid about using certain products. ❖

29
Choosing a Healthy Way of Life

THIS CHAPTER IS NEW because I have refined my approach to staying healthy in order to make it more manageable on a daily basis. If you are going to take charge of your health and make it a way of life, it has to be do-able. It has to fit into a coherent daily routine as much as possible.

I am reminded of something Dr. Nicholas Gonzales said to me once, "I don't have time for people who want to peck at this or that pill with the attitude that they are looking for the magic bullet. I don't have time for people who aren't serious about healing. There are too many people who are desperate to live and will do everything they can to heal. Those are the people I want to serve."

This statement not only revealed his dedication to real healing, it exposes a truth that bedevils us. We often live hurried, pressured lives with no time for exercise, no time to find and prepare real food, not enough sleep, or not enough money to maintain a life that is healing and restorative. The result is rapidly accelerating degeneration, but we put off dealing with the little signs of a problem until a dysfunction or disease is no longer something we can ignore.

However, we then come to a bigger problem. If we didn't have the time, money, or bandwidth to take care of the body in the first place, does it make sense to set up a healing program that allows us to finally take care of the body...but doesn't allow us to take care of our career, pay our bills, maintain normal relationships, and enjoy life? We are just trading one unsustainable lifestyle for another. And why drop everything to run off and heal the body if you are going to go right back to the way of life that was causing the degeneration?

The deeper issues we have to face and the questions we will have to answer if we are going to be healthy include, but are not limited to, some of the following. Is the corporate lifestyle sustainable? Is our food system something we can live with – literally – or is it slowly killing us because it has little-to-no nutrient payload and a host of poisonous chemicals? Do we really understand how the body works and what we need to give it in order to remain vibrant and strong decade after decade? Are our electricity-based technologies compatible with our electricity-based bodies or are they canceling each other out? If the body needs healing, then our thinking, our feeling, and our spirit often need healing as well, yet where do we find support and help for the needed changes in these other aspects of self when such support is not part of the current medical system? If the priorities we always had are no longer relevant (priorities such as getting a college education, a high-paying job, a nice house, nice spouse, and a life that makes us feel good about who we are) because those priorities lead to disease and dysfunction, what other arrangements and goals for civilized life can we come up with? If we have lost much of our connection to Mother Nature and the survival options she offers, how do we reconnect? If the single survival option we now have is to get enough money to buy food, water, land, housing, and services in order to survive, why do we allow a tiny percent of the people (1%? less than 1%?) to hold and control all the money? And even deeper and more far-reaching...if other races of humanoid beings are living 600, 700, or 1,000 years, what are they doing and what do they know that we don't know and need to know? How have they structured their lives?

The truth about healing is that it requires an overhaul of our lives! Like remodeling the kitchen, it is messy for a while, but when you're done, it's beautiful, functions so much better, and is well worth it.

In trying to make my own healing more sustainable, I had to continuously research and revise what I was doing, see if it worked and how well it did so, then incorporate it into my program while phasing out some of the other less effective or more time-consuming pieces. The result is my discovery of something that isn't new or revolutionary at all. It is that the best way to get healthy again is attend to the basics without letting up! Yes, there can be an emergency situation that requires some temporary action or drastic step, but even as those are being utilized, it is necessary to begin putting together a plan that takes you back to basics.

The basics are what I listed in the beginning of this book. They are the tools in your toolbox. Your tools are: food, water, exercise, detox routines, supplements, and sleep. Some people think these are boring. They want some fiery, fast disappearance of the problem. There are some healing solutions that are pretty spectacular, but most are slow and require steady perseverance. Just start. If you fall off the wagon, get back on.

The suggestions and procedures described in the preceding chapter showed you some additional tools and techniques such as baths and soaks, various packs applied to the body, nutritionally potent foods you can prepare, herbs, juicing, frequency generators, and natural cleaning products. By combining these major cornerstones of all true healing, you can create a healing way of life for yourself or someone you love. Keep in mind as you read through these that every individual has to be considered through a unique lens. What heals one might be death for another. What one person tolerates easily, another is stressed beyond any useful point.

As you consider a way of life that is more healing, become aware of something called "healer's lag." This is a tendency to enter into a brief period of shock or delay in beginning a healing program. This lag often occurs because illness, even a slight fall-off in your health, affects perception immediately. You may not recognize the need to take action, or you may be unable to decide what to do. More often, people become frightened, which triggers the stress response, which then cuts off creativity and problem-solving abilities by blocking access to the frontal cortex of the brain. Others simply don't want to deal with the difficulty they are facing. Yet, true healing requires you to *think and act on your own behalf.* You must *do something different* today if you want to feel better tomorrow. You might also have to take time away from work in order to really heal. Oddly, many people want to be healthy, but they don't want to heal themselves. They want someone else to do it for them or at least to *make* them do it. This gives them the feeling that someone cares about them.

Over the last 30 years, Americans have gotten into the habit of ignoring how they feel until they collapse. They pop a few pills while continuing to run to work, to social events, and dozens of other places. In their mind, the pill is doing the healing and thus nothing more needs to be done. This is dangerous because the pills are merely covering up the body's warning signs, and if we are to become healthy, viable people once more, the idea of popping a few pills must be replaced with the truth: the *body* is doing the healing and must have widespread support for its efforts.

If you subscribe to the ways of modern chemical medicine and take a pill that only suppresses symptoms while allowing you to keep going at full speed without changing, you are going to get worse, not better. The little flags that the body raises must be taken seriously and corrections made, or there will be a serious disease, usually within a couple of months, sometimes a couple of years. Then, instead of a few alterations in day-to-day living, you may need major surgeries, extended time off work, expensive tests and medicines, and who knows what else.

If you are tired of your job, feel trapped in dull, dead relationships, or want to do something else with your life but are afraid to change, the thought of getting some time off because you've been diagnosed with a major disease may seem like it's not all bad. Perhaps going on permanent disability may seem like a viable escape at first because it allows you to do something different. However, playing the role of "sickie" ends up being a trap. If you get stuck in the limited incomes of those on disability, it will put a huge kink in your freedom to do anything new and interesting. It will also wreak havoc with your natural creativity, and it gets just as boring as the bad job or the dull spouse you were afraid to deal with in the first place.

Two other negative factors also work on people who manage to get a diagnosis of permanent disability. One is low-level fear based on the worry that if they heal up, they will have to go back to doing what they did before. If this was something they disliked, they have very little incentive to get well again.

The other negative factor is low-level guilt that they have succeeded in getting out of going to work. The burden of contributing to life has been put onto others. This half-unconscious guilt interferes with their freedom to do what they want to do each day. It prevents them from creating the life they might love to have because they must maintain the pretense of not being well. If they really *are* sick and disabled, the guilt is compounded with true anger, frustration, or sorrow that they cannot participate fully in what so many others do naturally and easily, and they cannot simply choose a different way of living.

The truth is that it is normal and natural to do what you want each day. It is not normal and natural to feel trapped by a corporate clock or an unnatural schedule. Neither is it normal or natural to do the same thing day after day for years on end, or to do work that is not what you love to do. If your dream is to become the CEO of a large organization, then pursue it. If your dream is to study art in Italy, become a surgeon, spend your days scuba diving among sunken ruins, dabble in real estate, or simply spend your days reading and reviewing books on Amazon – begin it. There is life in every decision that takes you in the direction of your dream. The universe will meet you half way!

Many people put off embarking on a healing program because they think they cannot take time off from work. When they are finally forced to do some serious healing, they discover that the world does not fall down if they do not show up at their office or their job. Sometimes this discovery is followed by a period of wild rebellion and a refusal to go to work at all. This is fueled by a deep recognition that the work schedule is a constant interference in life routines that would bring about full healing. This rebellion is healthy, truthful, and often temporary, especially if one's priorities include being healthy enough to stay alive and enjoy the life you want. Without exception, when people return to true health, there is an honest and excited desire to work at something that inspires and sustains them. If they are no longer interested in their former work, they have the clarity, energy, and creativity to create new work, jobs, or life situations for themselves. This is true healing, through and through!

Keeping a Record

It is a good idea to write down, or type and print whatever you do to heal yourself, making dated notes of what worked, how long it took, what you observed or experienced, what sequence of changes you went through, and what you might try next time. Keep these written or typed programs and notes in a notebook, or file them in a folder called "Family Healing Programs" or something similar.

Later, if the condition returns, you will avoid the anxiety and frustration of trying to remember what you did the first time you had to heal that problem. If it's all written down, it's right there. If there is a new intuitive flash or two, add that to the program. If something doesn't seem quite necessary from the old program, don't do it. As I have often said, healing is an *art* even more than a science. The science part is in knowing what kinds of effects a particular food, mineral, or procedure will have on *most* people. The art is in assembling the right pieces to support *your* body's healing work, and then adding or subtracting from the program based on your experience, intuitions, and current observations.

The body is a dynamic, living system. What is healing during one episode of illness may not necessarily work, or work as well, in the next episode. Many factors affect this – the nature of the illness, the conditions in the body, the seasons, the amount of stress going on at that period in life, things like age, sex, relationships, diet, physical activity, and the stage of the illness.

Quite often when you are trying to put together a healing program for yourself or a family member, something will come to you intuitively. You may not have any particular reason why you think such-and-such should be done, or avoided, or eaten, or practiced…but it keeps popping into your mind. This is often a key piece of the total healing program. Don't ignore it. Your intuition is a critical part of your healing program. Use it!

The Basic Healing & Maintenance Program for All Conditions

Over the years of working to stay healthy, it has become obvious to me that the most important thing to be done is to supply the basics and keep supplying them. Far too many people think they are doing okay because they don't have any obvious symptoms of a problem. When something does occur, they slap a few drugs or a few vitamins on the problem and hope the issue will go away. Sometimes this works for a while, but if you don't address the underlying conditions, the problem will return. Nothing is as powerful and long-lasting as rebuilding your entire system by maintaining a full-spectrum array of high-density nutrition, a varying exercise routine, a habit of doing some kind of detox every month, drinking excellent quality water, adding supplements to make up for what is missing in our food supply, taking time to relax a bit, and getting enough sleep. As mentioned earlier, it is very wise to start a 'get healthy again' program of rebuilding by the time you are reaching 50 years of age, unless you have developed a problem that demands an overhaul much earlier. There is nothing else that is as valuable as being healthy, feeling calm, having clarity of mind and the energy to do whatever you are interested in doing.

Food

One of the first things you have to do in order to heal is to give up your food biases. Some people insist that vegetarian diets are better for you. Others say a paleo diet of plenty of meat is the healthiest and most healing. Some pay no attention to what they are eating and eat whatever they can get their hands on. Others are religiously vegan and shun all animal products. Some lean heavily toward grains, some toward soy products, others toward fruit, and every one of these beliefs about food carries an attitude of moral superiority based on the belief that the way they eat makes them somehow better than others.

The truth is, none of them can claim a single ounce of moral superiority. Food is to be used to nurture good health, not an attitude of "I'm better than those others out there." If you've been vegetarian for years and suddenly come down with cancer or arthritis...if you've been scrupulously fat-free for years and suddenly show signs of dementia or leukemia...if you've been vegan and give birth to a child with spinal bifida...if you've been a big meat eater and begin having difficulty with asthma or kidney stones...the message is that your diet is deficient in some way and out of balance. At this point, moral superiority will not do you any good.

To heal, the vegetarian may have to eat meat, the meat eater may have to switch to vegetables and fruits for a while, the vegan may have to have dairy and eggs for a time, the soy products will have to be given up altogether, grains and fruit will have to be balanced with a much wider variety of foods, and the one who has not been paying attention at all will have to be much more conscious of what he or she is eating. *All diets are useful.* The goal is to learn how to use foods correctly to counterbalance the condition you are experiencing. You need to be open to all forms of food and be able to glide smoothly from one kind of diet to another as needed. Food biases will only dig your grave a little deeper.

Switch to organic foods as much as possible in order to reduce the amount of heavy metals and poisonous chemicals you take in. Many of these metals and chemicals seriously derange your endocrine system, and only a few molecules of a heavy metal are needed to create this havoc.

If you have been eating mainly processed foods with a lot of sugar in them, you will probably be quite acidic and have a very low pH. This means that there are hardly any chemical transactions going on in the body and healing will be very slow if it happens at all. To correct this, eat as much fresh, uncooked food as you can. This really amounts to salads, fresh vegetables, and fruits of every kind for almost every meal. Every day, eat a very large salad made from 30% dark greens and the rest chopped, raw vegetables. Put flaxseed or hempseed oil on it, then put your regular salad dressing on top of that to cover the taste. Some doctors and healers will tell you point blank, "Get used to having salad for breakfast."

Do not eat anything with white flour or white sugar in it, no boxed cereals, and *no* soy products. White flour products, cereals, and soy all prevent absorption of much-needed minerals that help repair and rebuild the body, and such products have little or no usable nutrition in them. According to Dr. Gonzales and research from the Price-Pottenger Foundation, soy products disrupt the endocrine system. Make or buy breads, rolls, and cereals with freshly ground, whole wheat flour in them. Choose old-fashioned pastas made with whole wheat, butter, and eggs.

Whatever you eat, food should be whole, not processed. A blood test is really the best way to determine what your pH is. If you've had one recently, ask for a copy of the report. If you're too alkaline, switch to meats, raw cheeses and unpasteurized dairy. Build your meals around meat, fish, eggs, cheese, milk, and grains.

Make 14-Grain Cereal and eat it 3-4 times a week. Use organic grape juice or apple juice to soak the grain overnight.

Make a very good beef or chicken broth regularly and either sip the broth as a drink, make homemade soup with it, or use it to make brown rice, which is delicious I might add.

Eat 10 raw almonds every day to help alkalinize the body if you are too acid. Eat cheese or yogurt snacks if you are too alkaline.

As much as possible, do not drink anything with caffeine or alcohol in it during the healing process. Caffeine pulls water out of your tissues, and this is something you cannot afford while healing. Once you are better, you will be able to return to a bit of coffee or tea.

Water

If you live in a city that serves up fluoridated water, call a water service like Culligan and have clean, purified, reverse osmosis (RO) water delivered every week. This is especially important if you have a cancer. Fluoride prevents the uptake of iodine, and iodine is necessary to prevent cancers and for your body to produce glutathione, a powerful anti-oxidant and defense against the spread of cancer.

When you need to heal, drink a minimum of 1/2 gallon of water (64 oz.) a day, preferably 10-12 glasses a day. If you are well and just maintaining, you can get away with 6-7 glasses of water a day. Yes, you will spend some time running to the bathroom. I do not like water, so to make it more attractive, I add 1 dropperful of ConcenTrace trace minerals and 1 drop of peppermint oil to every quart. The trace minerals are absolutely necessary for good health, whereas peppermint is refreshing and relaxing, keeps my breath fresh, and is known to promote mental clarity and focus.

Drinking plenty of water helps prevent aging. A great deal of aging is simply a physical system that has been allowed to dry out and stiffen. Water also conducts electricity through the body which helps prevent fatigue, provides oxygen, and prevents backaches caused by dried out spinal discs whose job it is to pad the spine, keep it flexible, and prevent pinched nerves. Water also adds a bit of hydraulic pressure that cells can use to clean themselves with and conduct chemical transactions. Water is one of those miracle substances that rarely gets the respect it deserves. I will say this, however, once you get used to the energy and magic that water affords, you will seldom have to be prompted to drink more.

Detox

When you need to heal yourself, the first thing you will probably think is, "What do I need to take to get better...what should I eat?" As mentioned earlier, rarely do people ask, "What do I need to get rid of... what kind of internal housekeeping needs to be done?"

The main detox procedures are the Parasite Cleanse, Liver Flush, Colon Sweep, Purge, Coffee Enemas, Castor Oil/Olive Oil Sweat Baths, and DMPS Chelation. These procedures have already been outlined in Chapters 15-22, however, the question remains, 'how to use them in the most effective manner?'

To begin renewing yourself and rebuilding your body, Dr. Gonzales and Dr. Kelley both recommended at least a year-long commitment to a regular detox schedule as follows:

1. Start with the Parasite Cleanse.

2. One week after finishing the Parasite Cleanse, start the Liver Flush, which takes 5 days.

3. Approximately one week after completing the Liver Flush, start the Colon Sweep, which takes 5 days to finish, and another five days of probiotics to begin replenishing your gut microbiome.

4. One week after finishing the Colon Sweep, do the Purge for two days, unless you have cancer, which then calls for a 3-day Purge.

5. One week after finishing the Purge, begin the series of Castor Oil-Olive Oil Sweat Baths, doing one bath each week for up to 12 weeks. While completing the Sweat Bath's, continue as follows...

6. One month after finishing the Purge, do another Liver Flush.

7. The following month, do another Colon Sweep.

8. The month after that, do another Purge.

9. The next month, return to the Liver Flush and complete this process for the third time.

10. Do the Colon Sweep again the next month.

11. Do the Purge the following month.

12. Finish out the year by repeating this cycle of one detox procedure per month.

13. Continue until you are completely healthy, and thereafter do steps 1 and 5 annually, or better yet semi-annually.

To carry out this program, you will need to put them on your calendar and not schedule anything else on those days. The detox program sounds like a lot – until you do it, and then you discover that they are really quite simple and they just involve being organized and ready. Although you may not experience any miracles the very first time you do these, if you keep it up, you will find that they have very powerful effects. As mentioned earlier, each year that you continue detox is a year that reverses your biological aging.

Restoring Your Microbiome and Immune System

As a minimum start, do a Colon Sweep to begin the process of repairing and rebuilding the microbiome in your gut. Although it often takes a year to completely restore the gut, you will begin to notice beneficial changes all the way through the process.

So many good things have been written over the past decade about the necessity of maintaining the correct balance of bacterial organisms in the gastrointestinal tract that it's difficult to cover it all. Some extraordinary research was done by a husband & wife team who were investigating what went on – or didn't go on but should have – in the digestive systems of children with autism. Dr. Marco Ruggiero MD and his wife, Dr. Stephanie Ruggiero, summed up their research as follows:

"In an ideal world a child is born naturally, and as it comes down the birth canal, a variety of bacteria and organisms that live naturally in the vaginal fluids are pushed up the child's nose and into the mouth where they are swallowed. Once swallowed, these fluids, which are loaded with a wide variety of beneficial bacteria, make their way to the gastrointestinal tract.

"Once the birth is completed, the mother begins to produce a substance called colostrum, which precedes her milk. As she nurses the child, it gets this colostrum for the first 3 days. The colostrum then combines with the natural bacteria and organisms ingested by the child on the way down the birth canal. The result is the genesis of a very wide spectrum of over 160 different and unique forms of probiotic bacteria that spread throughout the gut. These probiotics provide a high level of immune function, superior digestion and absorption of nutrients, and the kind of chemical balance that supports natural resistance to disease, excellent brain development, excellent emotional function, high intellectual function, and predisposes one to live a natural lifespan which is generally 125–160 years of age." (from *The Third Brain* by Greenlaw, Ruggiero, et al*)*

In our modern world, the ideal is rare. We do not often allow mothers to have babies naturally because doctors don't want to be bothered in the middle of the night to get up and go deliver a baby. They induce labor during business hours and then do a Cesarean section to get the process over quickly and efficiently. Mothers do not nurse babies so the child does not experience the magic that occurs when the vaginal bacteria and organisms combine with colostrum to produce very wide-spectrum probiotics in the child's gut.

Soy milk, another culprit, is often fed to babies, which further interferes with brain development and gut balance because it has no fat in it and the developing brain *needs* fat. This is followed by dozens of processed foods with almost no enzymes or nutrition in it. The result is a disaster for today's human who ends up with lower I.Q., poor health, a poorly built structure, serious anti-social tendencies, less resilience to environmental factors, and a lower immune response because so many factors and nutrients have been absent.

To restore your G.I. tract, high immunity, and ability to enjoy life, it is necessary to clean out the gut and restore as many healthy bacterial and probiotic agents as possible. I would do this with a Colon Sweep, followed by Bravo Yogurt, which was developed by the Ruggieros to replace what has been lost because of modern childbirth and child-rearing practices coupled with modern agriculture and food systems. I then go to this website to buy Bravo Yogurt:

https://www.bravo-probiotic-yogurt.com/.

It is expensive but well worth it. I would take it for a year because it takes that long to regenerate the microbiome, then maintain it with good quality probiotic capsules.

Once you have begun the process of restoring your microbiome, do a set of coffee enemas on a regular basis. This can be every day, perhaps twice a week, or at least every weekend. Do a set of "coffees" whenever you are not feeling well.

The bottom line is that, if you want to regenerate yourself, begin rotating through the entire set of detox procedures – Liver Flush, Colon Sweep, Purge, and Sweat Baths as soon as possible, and do the entire set at least once a year, twice a year would be better. Detox, combined with sufficient nutrition, is a miracle worker.

Exercise

I have already talked about the fact that exercise is non-negotiable (Chapter 7, p. 88) because it generates electricity in the body, so I won't say much more here other than to be blunt.

Walk at least 30 minutes EVERY day. Lift a couple of 5-8 lb. free weights a dozen times. Stretch frequently as if you were a cat, do the 5 Rites of the Fountain of Youth, do yoga for 15 minutes every day. There are plenty of good videos on YouTube that you could turn on to watch and let yourself be guided by.

Sleep

Get a full 8–9 hours of sleep every night or as often as you can. The body only heals when you sleep and your brainwave frequencies are allowed to slow down into the delta range of 0-4 hz. This is slow wave sleep and your need for it is cumulative, so there's no getting around it. Put yourself to bed and sleep every night for a minimum of 7 1/2 hours because it takes that long for the brain to finish detoxing and renewing itself every night. 8 1/2 hours of sleep is not a luxury, it provides enough healing to allow you to get ahead of whatever condition you are trying to correct.

About 40 years ago, I left the corporate world and decided I was never going to suffer the misery of alarm clocks again. I consciously decided that the one gift I would give myself for the rest of my life was the gift of enough sleep and waking naturally. I celebrate that gift regularly.

Supplements

As I worked to figure out the best way to heal myself and stay healed, I started with the program created for me by Dr. Nicholas Gonzales, which required that I take 156 capsules and/or tablets of various supplements every day. I did it because I was desperate to heal and regain full function again, but it was very expensive and the amount of gas created by such a large number of vitamins and minerals was enough to blow up an elephant. Originally, I was just doing what I was told was necessary. Gradually, I began to understand the what, why, and wherefore of what Gonzales had outlined. I then began to research and study for myself, experimenting as I went along.

You have probably heard me say that the human needs amino acids, minerals, vitamins, enzymes, and perhaps a few other things like glandulars, herbs, etc. in order to maintain great health.

Here is the list of what I eventually settled on for myself. Since I only eat 2 meals a day, getting some nutrition from supplements is essential for me. This is what I consider to be my minimum daily intake:

- *3 amino acid capsules*, spread out over the course of the day. Amino Blend is a good quality amino formula, available from www. ProgressiveLabs.com.
- *4 multiple mineral capsules* spread out over the day. (There are several good brands out there.)
- *1 capful of Source of Life Gold liquid vitamins* per day.
- *2 10 ml. doses of Floravital Iron liquid* formula.
- *12.5 mg. Iodine* in caplet form. Iodoral brand from www.optimox. com.
- *1 tablet of ATP Co-Factors*, from www.optimox.com. Take with the iodine tablet.
- *2 TBSP flaxseed oil or hempseed oil* on salads, in soups or smoothies. Do not substitute fish oils for flaxseed oil. If you can get it, take hempseed oil instead of flaxseed oil. As pointed out earlier in the book, hempseed oil contains both Omega 3 and 6 in the correct balance. The dose is the same, 2 TBSP/day on salads, in soups, or with steamed vegetables & butter. Don't hesitate to double your intake of Hempseed oil, as studies show that these essential fatty acids do an excellent job of destroying cancer. [99]
- *2-4 Probiotic capsules at bedtime*, on an empty stomach. The formula should have 30 million live cultures in it
- *1-4 pancreas enzymes with all meals*

---

99 Erasmus, p. 272.

In addition to the above, I may take the following extras a couple times a week or when I need to recover from an injury, a cold, or some other physical problem that demands a boost in nutrition. Remember, you need four times as much nutrition to heal as you do to maintain!

- 25,000 i.u. Vitamin A
- 1 capsule B-Complex 100s (100 mg. of each B vitamin)
- 1,000 – 2,000 mg. Vitamin C
- 2,000 i.u. Vitamin D drops, in divided doses
- 800 i.u. Vitamin E, in divided doses
- 45 mcg. (micrograms) Vitamin K-2 and K-3
- 1,000 mg. MSM (Methylsulfonylmethane), a nutritional sulfur
- 200 mcg. (micrograms) Selenium
- 50 mg. Zinc picolinate

The goal is to live in such a way that you never get sick or develop some disastrous disease. You have to get into the habit of living as if you matter. I spend roughly 2.5 to 3 hours on myself every day. I start my exercises before I even get out of bed. I have developed a set of small twist exercises that I do every morning while sitting up in bed. They generate a tremendous amount of electricity, and that electricity keeps me young and flexible. I swing my arms and stretch them over my head every time I walk through the house. I bend over from the hips to pick up things on the floor. I get on my treadmill and walk for 2 miles at a brisk pace at least two or three times each week, usually five or six times. I refuse to give up a single capacity for movement and motion. When I am not in bed sleeping, I am working, either on myself, in my garden, or one of my projects.

I attend online meetings or read email and respond to it while on the treadmill for a couple of miles. I return phone calls and watch or listen to informative videos while in the kitchen where I make various kinds of granola and large, elaborate salads. I work in my greenhouse to nurture a steady supply of fresh greens and vegetables and consider my refrigerator to be empty if I do not have fresh vegetables and fruits in it. I write, read extensively, or do research while in the bathroom doing my "coffees" or at my desk or while waiting for something to come out of the oven. I listen to podcasts while cleaning my house, not only getting good exercise but keeping up with the world around me. I put detox procedures on my calendar and consider them to be a firm date with myself. You can do similar things. You just have to give yourself permission to take care of yourself first, and then proceed to do so gently but firmly and consistently.

❖

30
Paths to Personal Healing

THIS CHAPTER PRESENTS A FEW IDEAS of how to put together healing programs for various health challenges. For purposes of legal safety, I have to say that these are only educational examples of what I would do if I were healing myself of various maladies and where I would look to find the healing agents. Each set of suggestions is meant to show you ways to use the tools in your toolbox that we have talked about in earlier pages. Again, your tools are: food, water, exercise, detox routines, supplements, and special procedures such as baths and soaks, Castor Oil Packs, or other techniques. By combining these major cornerstones of true healing in various ways, you can create a healing program for yourself or someone you love. Keep in mind as you read through these that every individual has to be considered through a unique lens. As I have already pointed out, what heals one might do nothing for another.

All of the sample programs that follow are based on the assumption that you have committed to the basic lifestyle outlined in the previous chapter that incorporates a diet change to real food, plenty of good water, daily exercise, regular detox procedures, enough sleep, and the full spectrum of necessary supplements. The healing programs outlined here are then *additional* things to boost your healing process. Keep in mind that you can't change your entire life overnight. Start doing whatever you can and just keep adding helpful things until you are superbly healthy.

There are many creative and useful ways to bring the body back to health and balance. Let me repeat...the art of healing is truly an art. Each person and the problems they present form a set of conditions. The true healer looks at all of those conditions and uses every tool at his or her disposal to bring the body back to health. All of the pieces presented earlier in this book are your tools. Use whatever tool you need to get the job done. Learning how to use these tools effectively will give you a feeling of security and confidence in your ability to take care of yourself and your family. This is sustainable medicine at its best. You might not use all of the suggestions in every case, but I list them because they are so powerful when used together.

In the programs listed here, you will find suggestions on what could be added to the basic tools of food, water, supplements, exercise, and detox. This may include other useful supplements, herbs, or practices. You might not use all of the suggestions in every case, but I list them because they are so powerful when used together.

Alzheimer's and Dementia

Start the Basic Program outlined in the last chapter (Ch. 29) slowly and gently, but begin immediately to make a breakfast of oatmeal or a smoothie to which you have added 1 TBSP of coconut oil. This can cause loose bowels at first, so don't overdo. Maybe start with a teaspoon.

After a few days, maybe even a week, if the bowels are stable, begin adding a second tablespoon of coconut oil. Put it in soup, on a salad, on vegetables, in a smoothie, or on meat. Again, watch for loose bowels. Have some Bentonite clay on hand to counter any diarrhea, if needed. You are now at 2 TBSP of coconut oil daily.

When bowels are stable, begin adding 1 dropperful of C60 in Coconut Oil daily. Time of day does not matter, but don't take it at the same time as the plain coconut oil. Working slowly, continue increasing the C60 in Coconut Oil 1 dropperful at a time until you are taking 4 dropdersful per day, spaced out over the day.

Work toward at least 4 dropperful of C60 in Coconut Oil and 4 TBSP of plain coconut oil daily. You should see signs of function and focus returning within a week or two, sometimes less. Keep going with the coconut oil and introduce coffee enemas and amino acid capsules. Consider adding the supplement "Cognitive Resilience" by Progressive Labs because it has both Lions Mane and Bacopa Monieri in it. Consider investing in a frequency generator like the VieLight that will help restore and regenerate the brain. Continue adding parts and pieces of the Basic Healing Program until you are doing it all.

Arthritis – Rheumatoid or Osteoarthritis

Arthritis, like cancer, diabetes, asthma and other serious challenges to your health can be healed but takes commitment and persistence. Start the Basic Healing Program immediately and don't hesitate. Arthritis can cause serious disfigurement and disability requiring expensive and painful surgeries. Dr. Gonzales once mentioned to me that at times he felt arthritis was more difficult to heal than cancer. He didn't say why he thought so, but I wondered if it was because people "fell off the wagon" (the food/ detox/supplement wagon) too easily because the threat of untimely death was not part of the disease.

Water is particularly important in arthritis. Drink 8-10 glasses of water, preferably purified R.O. (reverse osmosis) water every single day, no exceptions. Water alone can erase the pain of rheumatoid arthritis within a day because most rheumatoid arthritis is triggered by chronic dehydration in the body. Without enough water, the collagen tissues in joints shrink and dry out, leaving bones and tendons to grate, become inflamed, and swell painfully.

Detox should be started immediately as outlined in chapter 29 and continued for a minimum of one year, although three years is better. Following the initial set of Liver Flush, Colon Sweep, and Purge – procedures that are completed quite close together – begin rotating through them, doing one each month over the rest of the year.

Food – Arthritis is almost always the result of an extremely acidic state in the body. Get your blood tested to determine what your pH is. Begin changing your diet to a majority of fresh fruits and vegetables. Eat at least 30% raw food, which translates to at least one meal a day. In the case of severe alkalinity, begin adding more meat 3-4 x week, including beef, chicken, and fish, to bring your biochemistry into better balance.

Carrot/Garlic Juice – every day make 1 pint of carrot juice. Juice 1 large clove of garlic into the juice and drink immediately. You can add a couple stalks of celery, an apple, a beet, or other vegetable to the carrot juice for variety. If you are going to have surgery to repair a joint, ***stop taking garlic at least a week before the surgery***. Garlic makes the blood very fluid and reduces clotting, making excess bleeding a real problem during surgery.

*Supplements **in addition** to the Basic Program –*

- Source of Life Gold liquid vitamins, a second capful daily.

- 2-3 droppersful C60. C60 in Olive Oil is cheaper but tastes like gasoline (ugh!) However, if you are going to put it in a smoothie the taste won't matter and you can save a few bucks.

- Beta-carotene, 10,000 iu, 2 x daily, to allow your body to make more Vitamin A if it needs it.

- CBD oil, 2500 mg formula, 2 droppersful daily

- Vitamin B-Complex 100s 1 x day

- Vitamin C, another 1,000 mg, 1 x day, unless you have a history of kidney stones, in which case do not take any extra Vitamin C. Instead, take Glutathione, 500 mg, 4 x day.

- Co-enzyme Q-10, 30 mg, 1 x day, for its specific anti-oxidant properties and to enhance the activity of Vitamins C and E

- Magnesium, 250-300 mg, 2 x day. The magnesium will not only help alkalinize you, it will help you optimize the calcium you are taking.

- Zinc, 15 mg, 2 x day

- MSM (methylsufonylmethane) If you are in pain, you can take up to 3,000 mg/day in divided doses. MSM is nutritional sulfur and is used in every cell of the body to build the all-important cell membranes. MSM alkalinizes you but can cause diarrhea. If this occurs, reduce your dosage by one capsule at a time until the diarrhea stops.

- Rub castor oil or peanut oil into the inflamed joints daily.

- *Exercise* – Do not skip the exercises even if you are sore and stiff. At the very least, stretch gently and slowly. You will probably be surprised at how effective exercise is.

Asthma and Respiratory Issues

Asthma requires a long commitment to heal but it can be done if you start and keep going. You will literally rebuild your lungs.

- Start with the Parasite Cleanse by Dr. Hulda Clark and continue on through the entire set of detox procedures. Thereafter, rotate through the Liver Flush, Colon Sweep, and Purge, doing one of them each month for at least two years.

- Change your diet to one based as much as possible on fresh organic fruits and vegetables, a small amount of meat each week, whole grains, unpasteurized dairy, and good quality oils – olive, coconut, flaxseed, and hempseed. Do not eat too much at any one meal.

- Begin drinking a minimum of ½ gallon of good quality water each day.

- Begin taking ALL of the supplements in the Basic Healing Program in a 3 weeks on/1 week off pattern. Do your monthly detox procedure during the week you are not taking any supplements.

- At least once a week do a Castor Oil Pack for 2 hours on your chest.

- Order a supply of Oxy Life Force Elixir and OxyDHQ Elixir. Take 1 dropperful of Oxy Life Force and 1 dropperful of OxyDHQ together in a half glass of water or juice. Take 45 minutes before food and drink, or 2 hours after a meal, preferably before. Hold the elixirs in your mouth and let them slide under your tongue for 1 minute before swallowing. Do this twice a day.

- Do not start the Oxy Life Force or OxyDHQ before you do a round of detox procedures because they are powerful detoxifiers in themselves and you can end up going down with headaches, diarrhea, fatigue, congestion, and body aches and pains. If this happens, do a set of Coffee Enemas every day to help the liver stay clear and able to filter wastes out of your system well enough to keep up with what you are releasing.

- When you take the Oxy Life Force AND the OxyDHQ together, they produce 5 times more oxygen AND get it into your cells, also carrying amino acids, minerals, vitamins, and other nutritional elements into the cells. Consider taking these two elixirs for at least three months.

The combination of the two is usually recommended to prevent the spread of cancer, but it is a powerful combination for asthma, viruses, and bacterial infections.

Extra supplements in addition to the Basic Healing Program...

- 1000 mg. Vitamin C, 4 x per day, unless you have kidney stones or a tendency to develop kidney stones, in which case do not take extra Vitamin C at all, switch to Glutathione here below:

- 500 mg. of Glutathione, 2-3 x per day.

- 20,000- 25,000 i.u. of Vitamin A, 2 x per day

- 15 mg. zinc, 3 x per day

- Make it a regular practice to spend time before you go to sleep and when you wake up in the morning to do some breathwork. In a very slow and controlled way, allow your lungs to fill with air as if the air is just gliding in naturally in the form of a golden white light with pink edges. You may actually feel as if your entire body is filling with this golden light but stay focused on your lungs. When you are absolutely full and can't expand any further, breathe out completely by pushing the air out through pursed lips. Breathe naturally for a breath or two, then begin again with the slow, controlled intake. Do a dozen of these slow in-breaths then go to sleep if it is night, or get up and start your day if it is morning.

- Exercise lightly every day to increase the available electricity moving through your body, which helps rebuild and recondition your lungs. If possible, stretch, dance, do yoga, and walk briskly for 15 minutes each day, increasing as your lung capacity increases.

Comments on healing asthma...

The key thing to do in healing asthma is to stay with it. Even life-long sufferers of asthma have been able to heal and let go of their inhalers and puffers.

Be aware of the work of Dr. Harry Philibert and the thousands of people who suffered for decades with asthma then were cured – either completely and permanently or for years at a time – by a series of 2 or 3 injections of lidocaine, a local anesthetic, into the trigger point of the infraspinatus muscle. This muscle controls what Philibert called the Infrascapular Respiratory Reflex (IRR), and this is what cuts off the arterial blood supply to the lungs. I would imagine that Dr. Philibert has retired by now, but he trained many other doctors and with a little digging around, you may be able to find one. Dr. Joseph Mercola wrote about Philibert's work in his *Optimal Wellness News*, Issue 93, March 21, 1999. That was quite a while ago, but it may be another avenue of information.

Even just palpating the acupuncture point Small Intestine #11, which is in the infraspinatus muscle will bring quick relief in an acute asthma attack. Visit this link for diagrams of how to find the infraspinatus muscle: (http://www.newmediaexplorer.org/chris/2003/10/17/breathing_a_sigh_of_relief.htm)

Autism and Allergies

Many people are surprised that these two disorders are related, but they both stem from serious disruptions of the microbiome in the gastrointestinal tract that then lead to systemic inflammation of body and brain. I do not have enough experience with autism to say much, but I am quite familiar with allergies, and I do know that both can be reversed or at least greatly improved with even a few changes of diet that completely eliminate every kind of sugar, soy, and processed food.

- Begin with the entire Basic Healing Program as described earlier in *Chapter 29 - Choosing a Healthy Way of Life*, pages 302-311. Do not skip the pancreas enzymes!

- Next do the Colon Sweep to clean out the old bacteria from the gut and begin restoration of the microbiome using Bravo Yogurt. A greatly modified version of the Colon Sweep might be done for a child over the course of 30 days using ¼ to ½ tsp of Holistic Horizons Bulking Agent II in apple juice daily, or even in soup, to slowly remove as much of the gut bacteria and lining as possible. After the first week of this bulking agent in apple juice, begin introducing 1 TBSP of the Bravo yogurt daily. Once you are done with the first 30-day round of bulking agent, continue with the yogurt regularly for the next year. If adding the fiber of the bulking agent is too much because the child is too young, just start with the Bravo Yogurt, work up to ¼–½ cup per day, and keep going with the yogurt for at least a year.

- Start taking C60 in coconut oil, 1-2 droppersful daily, under the tongue if you have a cooperative child or adult. If not, put it in juice, a smoothie, on a salad, in soup, even in coffee if it's not too hot. C60 is a powerful regeneration for the brain, and the coconut oil adds medium chain fats that are also critical for brain health.

- For an adult, find a way to include 1-2 TBSP of flaxseed oil or hempseed oil in the diet daily. These are superunsaturated fats and are critical for brain health. The best way is a smoothie. For a child, 2 teaspoons is good.

- I would also make sure the child or the adult was getting the full range of aminos, minerals, and vitamins, especially plenty of Vitamin D along with CBD oil. You would have to experiment a little to find the best amounts for a child. I would recommend reading *Gut and Psychology Syndrome: Natural Treatments for Autism, Dyspraxia, ADD, Dyslexia, ADHD, Depression, and Schizophrenia* by Natasha Campbell-McBride. It is quite the eye-opener.

- For an adult, many allergies and food intolerances can be corrected by simply supplying the full range of aminos, minerals, and vitamins, the right oils, doing a Liver Flush and Colon Sweep at least twice a year, and restoring the microbiome to its natural, healthy state. The important thing to remember regardless of what you think is wrong is: Never give up on yourself...there is an answer somewhere.

Bee Stings and Bug Bites

The best thing for stings and bites is green clay. You can buy a tube of clay at most health food stores or find it online. We keep a bucket of green clay powder on hand and use if for stings, bites, and burns.

- Make a paste of 1 tsp. of green clay and water in a *glass* bowl. Do not use plastic or aluminum. Put a generous dollop of clay directly on the sting, bite, or burn and leave it to dry. The sting will stop stinging, the bite will stop itching, and the burn will stop burning.

- Over the next three hours, take a dose of the homeopathic remedy *Apis Mellifica 30x*, at a rate of one dose per hour. If the Apis is in the form of tablets, take 3 tablets per dose. If it is in the form of pellets, take 5 pellets per dose.

Burns – See pages 274-276 for how to handle a burn.

Candida

Candida is not just a nuisance that causes bloating, gas, burping, bad breath, indigestion and fatigue, it is a serious disruption of your gastrointestinal system as well as your immune functions.

- If you suspect you have Candida, do the Colon Sweep to clear all bacteria from the gut then follow with ½ cup of Bravo Yogurt every night at bedtime for 3 months. When you are done with the yogurt, take a high quality probiotic at bedtime for another 3 months.

- Change your diet to meat and vegetables and avoid sugar like the plague. Coffee, tea, and cream are okay, as are milk or eggs. Continue the diet change for 3-6 months.

- Take Caprylic Acid capsules, 4 capsules per day spread over the day. These are available from www.ProgressiveLabs.com.

- Do a Castor Oil Pack on the abdomen to stimulate the immune system, 2 hours each day for 5 days, then take 3 days off, use the pack again for 5 days, then 3 days off, and continue to rotate until the infection is cleared up.

Cancers and Tumors

This is a completely different approach to cancer than I would have originally taken. It is a little less complex and yet more powerful. The Basic Program of diet, detox, exercise, and supplement procedures are included as described in chapter 29, but the use of frequency elixirs has been added. Cancer demands that you do everything you can, and keep doing it.

Start with two decisions. One is a decision to continuously educate yourself about your own body. The education would come from reading, watching things on video & YouTube, trying things that appeal to you, paying attention to what works, and above all – making it an important goal to understand how the body works and then working WITH it, rather than against it. The other is the decision to take action that is comprehensive and ongoing.

I would take these actions steps and get organized as follows:

- Immediately begin a program to remove parasites. Hulda Clark has a parasite program that costs between $50-$60 and takes about 3 weeks to complete. Go to: www.DrClarkStore.com_-_https://drclarkstore.com/dr-clark-parasite-cleanse-w-freeze-dried-green-black-walnut-hull/ to get what you need to complete the program. NOTE: Just do Dr. Clark's Parasite Program and do NOT try to do her Intestinal Cleanse before or during the parasite program. It is often too much for the body to deal with at once. The Colon Sweep (below) will do this intestinal cleansing later.
- Know how to do a coffee enema before you start the removal of parasites because coffee enemas help avoid or quickly end a Herxheimer reaction, which occurs when the body is temporarily overwhelmed by dead parasite material. See the instructions in Chapter 21 on doing coffee enemas.
- Get a hair and blood test for heavy metals to determine if you need to do some chelation.
- Go to www.cancerfightingstrategies.com, download their 162-page book, and *read the entire thing*. Click on "Print version" in the upper right corner to get the book set out in an easy-to-read format.

Once you have read the book, I would go to www.gethealthyagain.biz and order the following 3 elixirs, which I will call **Elixir Cocktail #1**:
- *CMSD Elixir* – 3 bottles/month (blocks all pathways that cancer uses to feed itself)
- *Oxy Life Force Elixir* – 2-3 bottles/month (gets oxygen INTO cancerous cells to kill them, and into normal cells to prevent the spread of cancer)
- *Oxy DHQ* – 3-4 bottles/month (gets an amazing combination of minerals, enzymes, amino acids, oxygen, and hydrogen into cells, increases cell voltage, binds to toxins and helps detoxify)

As an alternative, I could order a different set of 4 elixirs, which I will call **Elixir Cocktail #2**:
- *CMSD Elixir* – 3 bottles/month (blocks all pathways that cancer uses to feed itself)
- *Oxy DHQ* (gets an amazing combination of minerals, enzymes, amino acids, oxygen, and hydrogen into cells, increases cell voltage, binds to toxins and helps detoxify)

- *Ronuv* – 3-4 bottles/month (enhanced frequency formula containing deuterium gets into cancer cells and reacts with water molecules to release oxygen that kills the cancer cell)
- BLA elixir, which dissolves tumors.

Once the elixirs have been chosen and ordered, I would go on to order the supplies to make Bravo Yogurt from https://www.bravo-probiotic-yogurt.com.

Detox
- While you wait for the elixirs and the yogurt supplies to arrive, begin your detox program with the Liver Flush.
- Two weeks from the start of the Liver Flush, make the Bravo Yogurt and start the Colon Sweep.
- Two weeks from the start of the Colon Sweep, begin The Purge. When finished, you will have completed one round of detox.
- When you are finished with the first round of detox, begin doing a set of coffee enemas daily.

When you have finished your first round of Detox...
- Start taking Elixir Cocktail #1 and the supplements from the Basic Healing Program with a few additions as listed here. All of These are non-negotiable. You will need them all to heal and stay healed. After 3 weeks, stop everything for 1 week.
- During this week off, do another one of the detox procedures.
- After finishing the detox procedure, start supplements again. If you have ordered both sets of elixirs, switch to Elixir Cocktail #2.

Supplements

To be successful with the complexity of a cancer supplement program, you will need to map out what to take each morning, each noon, each evening, and bedtime. It is also important to get a supply of small plastic bags and lay out a week's worth of capsules and tablets at a time, using four bags for each day and marking them appropriately as breakfast, lunch, dinner, and bedtime. Reuse the same bags again and again, keeping yourself and your program organized, and always taking them with food if possible. I would take the following *supplements **in addition** to the Basic Program*:

- Source of Life Gold liquid vitamins, a second capful daily.

- 2-4 droppersful C60. C60 in Olive Oil is cheaper but tastes like gasoline (ugh!) However, if you are going to put it in a smoothie the taste won't matter and you can save a few bucks.

- Beta-carotene, 10,000 iu, 2 x daily, to allow your body to make more Vitamin A if it needs it. You need the iodine to do this conversion.

- CBD oil, 2500 mg formula, 2 droppersful daily

- Vitamin C, another 1,000 mg, 1 x day, unless you have a history of kidney stones, in which case do not take any extra Vitamin C.

- Glutathione, 500 mg, 4 x day. This is an important antioxidant against cancer.

- Co-enzyme Q-10, 30 mg, 1 x day, for its specific anti-oxidant properties, to enhance the activity of Vitamins C and E, and to support your heart, especially if you have done chemo.

- Magnesium, 250-300 mg, 2 x day. The magnesium will not only help alkalinize you, it will help you optimize the calcium you are taking.

- Zinc, 15 mg, 2 x day

- MSM (methylsufonylmethane). You can take up to 3,000 mg/day in divided doses. MSM is nutritional sulfur and is used in every cell of the body to build the all-important cell membranes. MSM alkalinizes you but can cause diarrhea. If this occurs, reduce your dosage by one capsule at a time until the diarrhea stops.

- Plant-derived Multi-mineral Complex, 1-2 TBSP daily. Or other good quality, liquid trace minerals, ½ – 1 tsp. daily. Start slow or you'll have diarrhea. Put these minerals in juice or a smoothie. I add 15-20 drops in each quart or liter of water, add 1-2 drops of peppermint oil, and drink 3 quarts/liters of this water each day.

- Pancreas enzymes – Pancreas Pork or Pancreas Lamb Enzymes – 4/ meal and 4 at bedtime every night. These enzymes are made by A.R.G. (Allergy Research Group) and are available from www. willner.com. I would get the large bottle of Pancreas Pork, Catalog #29119. Alternatively, Pancreas Lamb only comes in small bottles, Cat. #10010. *Be certain that your pancreas enzymes contain trypsin and chymotrypsin because these proteolytic enzymes are the ones that actually do the work of dissolving cancers and tumors.* Once you begin taking these enzymes, it is essential for you to do the Coffee Enemas every day and rotate through the Liver Flush, Colon Sweep, and Purge, doing one each month in a continuously rotating order because these support the liver and other tissues by removing dead cancer tissue from the body.

- ½ cup of Bravo Yogurt every night at bedtime.

- 2 TBSP of coconut oil daily (this supplies you with medium chain triglycerides or MCTs. This, together with the flaxseed oil, is necessary to utilize the oil-soluble vitamins – A, D, E, and K. You can add oils to a smoothie, a salad, a soup, on cereal, etc.)

I would continue all supplements in a "3 weeks on, then 1 week off" manner. Ditto for the elixirs. If I had Elixir Cocktail #1 and Elixir Cocktail #2 on hand, I would alternate between them each time I started the "3 weeks on" portion of the supplement program.

Exercise, Water, and Juicing

- Do not skip the exercises even if you are sore and stiff. At the very least, stretch gently and slowly. You will probably be surprised at how effective exercise is. Commit to beginning and ending every single day with 10 minutes of stretching. This generates electricity in the body, which is essential for good use of nutrition and powering the healing transactions necessary. In the middle of the day, walk at a brisk pace for at least 30 minutes. Get some small hand weights – about 5 lbs. each – and do 10-12 curls every day (takes less than a minute). Be creative with your curls!

- Drink an absolute minimum of 64 oz of pure RO water per day, preferably 128 oz. if you can manage it. Do *not* drink tap water

- For lunch or supper make 1 pint of carrot juice and drink it immediately before it oxidizes. Juice 1 large clove of garlic into the juice for extra healing power. You can also add a couple stalks of celery, an apple, a slice or two of beet, or other vegetable for variety. If you are going to have surgery, *stop taking garlic at least 2 weeks before the surgery.* Garlic makes the blood very fluid and reduces clotting. You do not want your doctor to end up with a case of uncontrolled bleeding during your surgery.

- Eliminate smoking, caffeine. sugar, and alcohol except for red wine on occasion. As already noted, caffeine pulls water out of your tissues, and this is something you cannot afford while healing. Once you are better, you will be able to return to a bit of coffee or tea.

Comments on Healing Cancer:

If you are doing chemo or radiation, the number of Coffee Enemas can go up as the amount of dead cancer tissue circulating in your body goes up. The more of the tumor you kill, the worse you will feel because dead tumor tissue is very poisonous. The liver is responsible for keeping these poisons out of circulation, but it can be quickly overwhelmed, causing you to feel nauseous, full of aches, pain, fatigue, and fear. The Coffee Enema is an important and powerful tool for keeping the liver functioning and your spirits up.

With cancer, it's really a good idea to have your blood tested and to pay attention to your pH balance. A hair test is also a very good idea because this test often tells you which heavy metals are in your system, something that is important to deal with when you have cancer. You can find companies online that do hair tests if your doctor doesn't pay attention to the heavy metal load you are carrying. And consider doing DMPS chelation. It's very difficult to heal and stay healed if you're carrying an internal load of heavy metals.

One of the most powerful things you can do to help heal yourself is to "breathe into" the area of the tumor, envisioning that a beautiful golden-white light with pink edges is coming in directly through the skin right over the area of the tumor. Talk to the tumor, ask it to dissolve, and envision the light filling the tumor until it simply disappears. If I have a problem I'm working on and I wake up in the middle of the night and can't go back to sleep, I will "breathe into" some area of my body for as much as two hours. By then, I am quite tired from the intense breathwork and I fall asleep. Quite often, the problem is gone the next day.

If you have an estrogen-based cancer, take no more than 750 mg of calcium each day because an excess of calcium acts like the hormone estrogen and has estrogenic effects, which can complicate and worsen your condition. In addition, calcium acidifies the body and estrogens work best in an overly-acid environment. Therefore, you want to limit calcium, but you need at least some of this mineral to activate other enzymes in the body. It works best to take a small amount and take extra magnesium to make sure the calcium is utilized. The magnesium will alkalinize you and help you optimize the small amount of calcium you are taking. When dealing with an estrogen-based cancer, a good rule of thumb is to reverse the ratio and take 2 magnesium to 1 calcium. The suggested ratio, if you are too acid is 750 mg calcium to 1,500 mg magnesium. If you have an alkaline-based cancer, take 1500 mg of calcium and 750 mg. of magnesium daily.

Get a massage every two weeks to assist lymph system drainage. Between massages, brush your skin daily with a vegetable-bristle brush to increase lymph drainage.

Be aware that the most dangerous aspect of cancer is the fear that grips you and can even paralyze you from taking action. Fight this fear head-on. Use meditation, go for a long walk in a beautiful setting, and constantly re-affirm that you are alive, healthy, and loving. Find friends who will love and support the healing path you're on. Listen to positive, beautiful music.

As mentioned earlier, Dr. William Kelley also recommends getting up in the night at 2:30 am to take up to 12 pancreas glandular enzymes because the pancreas is quite active at that time of the day, and the intent is to support its work as fully as possible. He encouraged doing this at least once a week until the cancer is gone, but also notes that if you do, you can feel quite sick, nauseous, and have symptoms that indicate the pancreas enzymes are breaking up tumors and your liver is working overtime to remove toxic waste from your body. The same thing happens during chemotherapy, and detox is invaluable at this time as well. If you are focused on breaking down old tumor material, do an additional set of Coffee Enemas, or up to six sets on the days you are feeling awful.

You can also use the Salt and Soda bath, the Castor Oil/Olive Oil Sweat Bath, the Mustard & Cayenne Foot Soak, and the Castor Oil Pack regularly if you experience nausea, headache, fatigue, body aches similar to the flu, or a general sense of malaise. Not only do these procedures help detox your system so that you feel better, you have a sense of taking care of yourself.

Healing cancer takes time and energy, but once you have recovered, there is often a true feeling of power, humility, spirituality, and confidence that accompanies you wherever you go. You will have learned a lot about your body/mind system, much of it information that will be useful for your entire life.

Cataracts, Macular Degeneration, Glaucoma, and Eye Diseases

Cataracts, macular degeneration, and retina problems can often be stopped and even reversed if you embark on a healing program specifically designed to support your eyes. Although it may seem like a lot of work, your eyes are well worth it. The following is an example of a fairly complete program.

Start the Basic Healing Program outlined in the previous chapter (29), beginning with the Parasite Detox and continuing through the Liver Flush, Colon Sweep followed by Bravo yogurt, and Purge.

After the first round of detox procedures, begin the supplements being sure to include the amino acids, the minerals, the vitamins, and the following:

- Begin taking 3-4 droppersful of C60 in Coconut Oil daily. This alone will often improve the condition of your eyes and your vision.
- Glutathione, 500 mg, 2 x day
- Vitamin C, 3,000 mg in addition to the Vit. C in the Basic Program, unless you have a history of kidney stones, in which case do not take any extra Vitamin C. Instead, increase the Glutathione to 500 mg, 4 x day.
- Vitamin A, another 25,000 iu/day for 2 weeks, then stop for 1 week. Continue this rotation for 4-6 months.
- Vitamin E, an extra 400 i.u. daily
- 2 TBSP of Flaxseed oil or hempseed oil. Or Evening Primrose oil, 1000 mg, 3 x day
- Drink at least 8-10 glasses of R.O. water *every* day

Exercise is absolutely necessary when healing eyes.

- Every morning when you wake up and before you get out of bed, squeeze your eyes shut tightly, then open them as widely as possible, alternating these two eye movements 10 times. Then rotate your eyeballs in a circle, looking as far *up* as possible, then to the *left*, then *down* as far as possible, then to the *right* as far as possible, and back up. Rotate 25 times in one direction, then reverse and rotate 25 times in the opposite direction. Then close your eyes and relax them for a few minutes before getting out of bed.

- Sit facing the sun, with eyes closed, and very slowly move your head back and forth from left to right, for 15-20 minutes each day, allowing the sun to hit the closed eyes.

- Walk briskly for 30-40 minutes daily.

- *After you have been taking the Vitamin C* for the first two rotations of 3 weeks on/1 week off and are past the danger of rupture in small blood vessels and capillaries at the back of the eye, take up the following... do 10-15 minutes of stretching in the late afternoon, ending by bending forward from the waist, letting your arms dangle toward the floor (or resting on the floor if you're more flexible) and letting the blood flow into the head. Work at breathing as normally as possible while bent over, for at least 5 minutes, less when you first try this, longer as you get used to it. If you have high blood pressure, for the first two weeks lean forward from the waist, clasping your elbows, and resting both head and arms on a table, or a chair, letting blood flow toward your head and breathing deeply, exhaling completely.

Comments on healing your eyes...

Eat whole, natural foods as much as you can. Avoid sweets like the plague.

Get extra sleep for the first three months of healing your eyes, so say goodnight to everyone a couple hours earlier than usual and retire to your room. Even if you don't go to bed immediately, this should help lower stress and make it easier for you to go to bed at least one hour early. If you don't go to sleep right away, that's okay, too. Just lay there with your eyes closed and breathe deeply, as if breathing living light energy into your eyeballs. You can also daydream, think, plan, envision, or do a few more eye exercises. All of these are very healing for your eyes.

Do not overeat when you are trying to heal. You do not need to give up coffee or tea completely while healing your eyes, but it is good to cut back for a while because caffeine draws water out of your tissues, leaving them dry and unable to function properly. Also, avoid drinking a cup of coffee after you have just eaten. The caffeine interferes with the absorption of nutrients.

Colds, Sore Throat, or Ear Infection

Often, if the infection is minor, as in the case of a cold or sore throat, all you need to do is stop eating and start drinking water. In our experience, the cold or sore throat will disappear within 1-2 days. If you catch it early enough, it may never manifest at all, especially if you go to bed early and allow yourself extra sleep.

If you don't catch it early and it has a good hold on you, stop eating, drink 8-10 glasses of water over the day, and consider taking the homeopathic remedy *Mercurius Vivus 30x* or *200ck* at the rate of one dose each hour for 3 hours. If the homeopathic remedy is in tablet form, take 3 tablets as a dose. If it is in pellet form, take 5 pellets as a dose. Then, take a fourth dose of *Mercurius* 3 hours after your third dose, then a fifth dose three hours after that. The next day take 3 doses spread out over the day. I have also used *Hepar Sulphuricum* or *Kali Bichromicum* with good success in strep, sinus, and ear-nose-and-throat infections. See the appendix at the back of this book, *Personal Healing Checklist* for a short list of homeopathic remedies to keep on hand. If you want to learn to use homeopathic remedies, get the very excellent and user-friendly book *Everybody's Guide To Homeopathic Medicines* by Stephen Cummings, MD and Dana Ullman, MPH. See Appendix B, *Suggested Reading and References,* for more information about this book.

Continue fasting, take a long nap after midday, do a set of Coffee Enemas each day, soak in a warm tub of water with 1 cup of salt and 1 cup of baking soda in it, and go to bed early.

If you have a really sore throat, you can also gargle with salt water. Put ½–1 tsp salt in 6-8 oz of hot water. Stir to dissolve, then gargle with the salt water, using it all, mouthful by mouthful. Do this twice a day, morning and evening until the symptoms have cleared and you feel well again.

Typically, when someone is not feeling well, they are not very interested in food and thus it is relatively easy to stop eating and fast for a few days. If you get extremely hungry, eat an apple, or some celery, perhaps a banana or orange, nothing cooked. When your hunger returns full force, your body is telling you to put something nutritious in it. Start with uncooked food, and when you return to cooked food don't overdo.

Depression

If you are seriously depressed, all of the diet, exercise and supplement changes recommended throughout this book should help tremendously. Begin taking the supplements in the Basic Healing Program, especially the iodine and ATP Co-Factors.

Supplements

If you are too depressed to put together a healing program and get yourself started with it, then consider taking a specific form of amino acid called *S-adenosyl L-methionine E*, aka SAM-e, (pronounced săm-ēē'). This is a form of methionine that supports your mitochondria in their efforts to produce the adenosine triphosphate (ATP) that gives you the energy you need for living and enjoying life.

SAM-e must be taken with Vitamin B-6, Vitamin B-12, and Folic acid or it won't work, but many SAM-e tablets include these vitamins right in the tablet. If they are not included in the tablets you buy, then get a B-Complex 25 formula from your local health food store and take 1 capsule twice a day.

The usual way to take SAM-e is to start with what is known as a *loading dose* at first, then drop gradually until you get to the maintenance dose. For many people, this is:

1,000 mg/day, divided into 2-4 doses, for two weeks, then drop to

800 mg/day, in divided doses, for two weeks, then drop to

600 mg/day, in divided doses, for two weeks, then drop to

400 mg/day, in divided doses, for two weeks, then drop to

200 mg/day, in divided doses, and stay there for 3 months.

At the end of the 3 months, you might try dropping to 100 mg/day and see if you maintain your good energy and steady spirits. If not, go back up to the 200 mg/day and stay there for another 3 months. Do not take SAM-e for more than 6 months without a break. It is a wonderful supplement, and research has not been able to come up with any side effects, but you don't want to tempt fate. Take a 2-3 week break from it and rely on good nutrition to keep you out of the pits.

Food

Good food, plenty of water, steady exercise, and regular detox are critical in eliminating depression. Chronic depression is the result of a combination of poor nutrition, lack of enough electricity to drive the chemical transactions that should be going on, and a buildup of waste materials and toxins in the brain, the liver, and other organs, all of which results in inflammation throughout the body and especially in the brain.

Begin changing your diet to the best, whole, high-nutrition food you can get your hands on. Eat the entire spectrum of foods: meat, fish, eggs, cheese, butter, milk, whole grains, plenty of vegetables, and fresh fruits, avoiding only those things you know you're allergic to. Do NOT eat anything with sugar in it or you're likely to end up depressed again. Eliminate sugar, processed foods, and foods with little or no nutrition. These lead to serious depression over time, which is why half of our nation is suffering from depression. Learn to shop differently. Learn to prepare meals differently. Learn to snack differently.

Detox

Do the initial round of detox procedures and once completed, commit to doing a set of Coffee Enemas every evening to keep the liver clear, since a sluggish or plugged liver is a major factor in depression. Twice more over the year do the Colon Sweep. Make and eat Bravo yogurt for 3 months.

Exercise

Commit to walking daily and exercising at least 3-4 times a week to create the electricity you need to keep your spirits up . Exercise also forces the delivery of nutrients into the far corners of the body as well as through any resistant cell membranes simply because the heavier breathing you do during exercise helps alkalinize your body making cell walls more permeable. *The Fountain Of Youth Exercises* are particularly helpful here because they work on the endocrine system so effectively, which is implicated in depression. Walking, swimming, running, biking, dancing, and even gardening are very helpful in relieving depression.

Comments on healing depression...

For many people, depression is the result of malnutrition and exhaustion. Exhaustion can be caused by stress, poor relationships, and many other factors. Evaluate your job, your relationships, and your goals in life. Begin to live the life you are interested in. Don't ever shortchange yourself because you think you owe something to someone else! If your major relationship is not good, face this fact and be honest with yourself. There is no situation that cannot be handled well if you put a little mature thinking and compassion into how to do so. The stress of trying to lie to yourself or deny yourself drains the body and leaves it unable to produce the neurochemicals that allow you to maintain comfortable emotional and mental states. Poor nutrition, an over-loaded colon, and a poorly working liver then complicate this biochemical imbalance. The result is depression.

With the restoration of a steady supply of ATP, clearing the liver and colon, high-density nutrition, and a bit of exercise, the results can be magical in a really short time. As you slowly rebuild your body/mind system, you'll find you can maintain good energy and a sense of well-being without the SAM-e. The good thing about SAM-e is that it does not have any bad side effects and it is much cheaper than prescriptions. And it's even cheaper still to get the same effect from good food and a lifestyle that supports good health.

Diabetes

To heal diabetes, get the book *A Promise Made, A Promise Kept: One Son's Quest for the Cause and Cure of Diabetes* by Dr. James Chappell. It is excellent, and he outlines an 8-point program that is similar to the healing programs you see in this book – food, water intake, enzymes, detox, supplements, exercise, and a few other important things. You can heal diabetes!

Diarrhea

Diarrhea is very common, especially in children who are teething, in adults who ate something that didn't agree with them, after chemotherapy among whose side effects are the destruction of the critical bacteria that make up the microbiome in your gut. There are many other reasons for diarrhea, which often accompanies illnesses like the flu, irritable bowel syndrome, food poisoning, food allergies, taking too many laxatives, parasites, alcoholism, the need to take antibiotics, and many other conditions. The following are things that I would do. The first two help immediately. After that, you will have to rebuild your microbiome.

Clay – Bentonite clay not only stops diarrhea, it heals the intestinal tract, soaks up poisons, helps kill parasites, and does an amazing job overall. Usually one dose of clay is enough to stop the diarrhea. You can buy Bentonite Clay in a liquid suspension from Sonne's or Progressive Labs. Take 1 TBSP 1-3 times over the course of a day until the diarrhea subsides. You can also keep it on hand in powder form and mix 1 tsp in a half-glass of warm water and drink.

Charcoal – If the diarrhea is severe as sometimes happens after chemo, I would take 4 capsules of charcoal every hour until it stops, using only a small amount of water and *not* taking anything else by mouth, including food, medicine, or supplements. Charcoal tablets can be purchased at your local health food store. When the diarrhea has stopped and your gastrointestinal system is quiet, leave it that way for 24 hours, taking very small sips of water frequently, but not eating anything.

Foods – begin the following, eating tiny amounts – a mouthful at a time for the first day or two.

- 2 TBSP Bravo Yogurt once or twice a day.
- Ripe bananas in small doses.
- Peanutbutter (real, freshly ground is preferred, from a spoon, not on toast).
- One or two ounces of very well-chewed beef. Chew small pieces 30-40 times each.
- Mashed potatoes, no salt or pepper, no butter or margarine.
- Oatmeal or brown rice in small doses, 1-2 TBSP at a time.
- Foods to avoid would be beans of any kind, caffeine, fruit, (especially unripe fruit), any packaged or processed foods.

Comments on healing diarrhea...

Once the diarrhea has passed, it would be a very good idea to completely rebuild the microbiome in your gastrointestinal tract. This is a long process but it is simple. Start with a Colon Sweep, and then begin replenishing the bacteria needed in your gut with ½ cup of Bravo Yogurt every day, regular helpings of unpasteurized sauerkraut, and 2-4 capsules of a high quality probiotic every night at bedtime. Stay away from sugar because this will destroy your efforts to colonize your gut with the right bacteria.

Consider taking a year to commit to the Basic Healing Program including the detox and the supplements. When taking ANY vitamin or supplement program, don't forget, the rule is "3 weeks on, 1 week off." Do not take vitamins and minerals or other supplements continuously. They cause such a furious rate of repair, replacement, and rebuilding that the body can actually bog down in its rate of healing if you don't give it a brief rest from all supplements, and this is especially true if you don't do any detox. If you have had a serious operation or illness, get out a calendar and write on it what you need to be taking and when. Once that's done, just refer to the calendar, otherwise you'll forget, get confused, etc. It is well worth the effort to be organized in terms of your own healing programs.

Flu, including Coronavirus (Covid-19)

In December of 2019, my daughter who is a Registered Nurse, came home from work one day and left me with this warning, "There is a new kind of flu going around and it's dangerous. You think you're coming down with something for 3 or 4 days, and then it acts like it's going away and you're getting better. But a few days after you think you're getting better, it suddenly hits like a brick. You feel awful, your lungs start to fill up, and you end up in the hospital fighting for your life, so pay attention!"

Less than two months later, I came down with what I thought was a little touch of the flu. That was January 30th. It lingered for several days, but then I felt better and thought no more of it until 2:00 a.m. on February 6th. I couldn't sleep, couldn't get warm, had only a mild fever but was achy and uncomfortable. I also realized I was not breathing as easily as I always did. After tossing and turning for another hour, I suddenly sat up because I was having more difficulty breathing, and it seemed to be getting dramatically more difficult.

I remembered my daughter's warning and realized that I needed to do something immediately. I got up and took Oscillococcinum, Vitamin

B-6, Vitamin C, and Mercurius Vivus 30x. I immediately stopped getting worse, but my lungs were already full. It took me 4 weeks of coughing and rest to recover completely. If any flu, including coronavirus, were to happen again, I would revise what I took as follows:

- The minute you suspect you may have any kind of flu, stop eating and go to the health food store or drug store to get the homeopathic remedy called *Oscillococcinum*. If you feel too awful to go anywhere, call a friend or family member and ask them to pick it up for you. Inside the package, there will be 3 small vials containing tiny white beads of the remedy. Open 1 vial and pour the contents under your tongue, letting the beads dissolve. Do not eat or drink anything. Go to bed and stay there until it is time for the second dose, 6 hours later. After taking the second dose, return to bed until it is time for the third dose, 6 hours after that. This is absolutely the best flu medicine you will probably ever find. Even if you are already suffering, your flu will literally disappear within hours. If the flu hasn't quite got hold of you and you take *Oscillococcinum*, it will simply not materialize. Keep it on hand at all times.

- Vitamin B-6 – 200 mg. immediately, and another 200 mg. every hour for four hours. The B-6 helps keep the lungs from filling up with fluid and cutting off your oxygen.

- 2 droppersful of Oxy Life Force or Oxy DHQ, or 1 dropperful of each – available online from www.gethealthyagain.biz. These are oxygen and frequency elixirs that push oxygen into your cells, stopping the virus and countering the pneumonia. Continue taking 2 droppersful of the Oxy Life Force or OxyDHQ in the morning and evening until your lungs are clear. Keep one or both of these oxygen elixirs on hand at all times. They are part of your emergency healing kit.

- Glutathione, 500 mg. 2–3 x daily until completely recovered. If you do not have Glutathione on hand, take Vitamin C, 1,000 mg. 3-4 x daily unless you have a history of kidney stones, in which case, do not take more than 1,000 mg. of Vitamin C in divided doses daily.

- When you have finished the *Oscillococcinum*, begin a second homeopathic remedy called *Mercurius Vivus 30x* or *200ck*. If the Mercurius is in tablet form, take 3 tablets every hour for 4 hours, and thereafter 3 times daily for the next 2 days. If the *Mercurius* is in pellet form, take 5 pellets every hour for 4 hours, and thereafter 3 times daily for the next 2 days.

- When you feel well enough to get out of bed, do a Salt and Soda Bath, soaking yourself for at least half an hour.

- When you are sure the flu is gone and you are in recovery mode, eat lightly: fresh fruits, salads, beef broth with parsley and salt in it, homemade chicken vegetable soup, steamed vegetables, whole wheat rolls or biscuits, no sweets, for the duration of your healing. Remember, every time you eat, healing slows down!

- Do a Castor Oil Pack on your chest for 1-2 hrs. every day.

- Do a set of Coffee Enemas daily until recovered, which supports the liver, which in turn, greatly helps the lungs. When the liver plugs up or becomes sluggish, the lungs begin to struggle.

- Take M-S-M (methylsufonylmethane), 1,000 mg, 2-3 x day. This is nutritional sulfur and helps break up stringy mucous. You can also take the homeopathic *Kali Bichromicum 200ck* to help break up mucous.

- Once you are feeling better, exercise lightly but daily as this will help you break up the mucus in your lungs.

- Get a massage or some acupuncture to help clear the lungs.

Comments on healing the flu...

It would be very helpful to make Carrot/Garlic Juice regularly while you are in healing mode. Make 1 pint of (about 6-10 carrots, depending on size) and add 1 large clove of garlic to the juice. Drink immediately before it oxidizes.

Alternate between the Carrot/Garlic Juice and a Lemon/Honey/ Cayenne drink – Mix 2 TBSP of fresh lemon juice, 1 TBSP honey, 1/8 tsp of cayenne, and 2 cups of water in a quart pan. Heat until warm, but do not boil. Drink 1 cup in the morning and 1 cup in the afternoon. Do not warm in the microwave. In fact, do not use a microwave for anything.

Headaches and Sinus Problems

Nothing can make you as continuously miserable as headaches and sinus problems. Be sure to check the section on *Infections – Sinus* when dealing with sinus problems. Many sinus troubles come from allergies, air pollution, or are the result of a diet that does not agree with you. Be willing to at least change your diet!

Tension, Stress, or Allergy Headaches

- Start with a set of coffee enemas.

- Continue with a Mustard & Cayenne Foot Soak (p. 270) or a Salt and Soda Bath (p. 271).

- Take a homeopathic remedy – either Belladona, Pulsatilla, or Lycopodium. Take 3 doses 1 hour apart (3 tablets or 5 pellets per dose), then 3 hours later take a fourth dose. The next day, take 3 doses over the course of the day.

- Use a bit of acupressure by pushing up with your thumbs on the bone of your forehead at the edge of your eye sockets and right next to your nose. Keep up the pressure for at least 5 minutes. It helps to lay down to do this because your arms will get tired.

Sinus Headaches

- For quick relief of sinus *headache*, drink 4 cups of clear water, one right after another. Your sinuses will begin to drain almost immediately, and you may begin sneezing. Continue drinking, 1 cup of water every hour that you are awake.

- Do the 5 Rites from *The Ancient Secret of The Fountain of Youth* in the morning and the evening. These five exercises have an amazing ability to get the sinuses to start draining. You can do them 3 or 4 times a day if necessary; they only take a few minutes.

- Do a set of Coffee Enemas in the morning and again in the afternoon, especially if the headache makes you feel nauseous.

- Do a Mustard & Cayenne Foot Soak for 45 minutes. This pulls toxins out through the feet, greatly increases circulation in the feet and legs, and helps eliminate headaches in general.

- Take the homeopathic remedy *Kali Bichromicum 200ck*, sometimes just called *Kali* or *Kali Bi*. Dissolve 3 tablets under your tongue once per hour for 3 hours. This is a total of 3 doses and 9 tablets. After the third dose, wait 3 hours then take 3 more tablets. Three hours after this, take 3 more tablets. This ends your first day's doses. The second day, take 3 tablets three times, with about 4 hours in between each dose. You should be feeling much better by the end of the second day, especially if you are drinking a sufficient amount of water. If the homeopathic remedy isn't working by the end of the second day, try a different remedy for two more days. *Kali Bichromicum* helps because it starts the drainage that brings relief.

- Note! If you have a lot of sinus headaches, it's a clear indication that you are eating something that doesn't agree with you. You're either unable to digest it because of lack of enzymes or a dysfunctional microbiome, and this leaves you with a lot of waste matter in your system that the liver must filter out, or you are allergic to something in your food, likely an additive of some sort, like sulfites or food coloring or "natural flavors" which are natural at all. Homeopathics, foot soaks, baths, and acupressure points may help, but if you want to be free of sinus problems, you simply must change your diet.

Herpes – Cold Sores and Genital

Cold sores and genital herpes are a huge nuisance to those who carry the virus. If you are plagued by either problem, you can control it or eliminate it.

- To control it, take L-Lysine regularly. A 500 mg capsule will keep it at bay as long as you drink enough water and don't get too stressed.

- If you have genital herpes, you might want to take Olive Leaf in order to ward off any possibility of having an outbreak. Start with one capsule a day for a week, then go to 2 capsules per day and maintain. If you're also taking L-Lysine, you should be protected. Be aware that the Olive Leaf must have 25% oleuropein in it in order to work, and the best place to get this kind of formula is from Olivus, https://www.olivus.com/OliveLeafMAX-Capsules--300-Count--Super-Strength_p_50.html.

- To eliminate cold sores and herpes of any kind, you can also invest in a frequency generator. This is a healing tool that uses frequency to destroy an organism. Frequency generators are expensive (up to $2500) but they can be used by anyone in the family, have no side effects like prescription medicines do, and can be used over and over for a wide range of problems. I would recommend a BCX Frequency Generator. A reputable dealer can be found at www.bioelectricsforhealth.com.

• If you should have an outbreak, heal it quickly using a docosonal cream, available over-the-counter. *Abreva* is a good formula. This is definitely a pharmaceutical drug, but sometimes you must compromise.

Infections – Bacterial or Viral

The rule of thumb in natural healing is, "When you don't feel well – *stop eating!* Doing so allows the body to focus 100% of its energy on healing and this is never more true than in the case of infection. Generally, if you eat anything cooked, you will notice that you feel worse, and healing will take longer. Once you have experienced the power of "not eating" to heal yourself, especially in the case of a cold or sore throat, you will not quibble over this fasting requirement.

That said, the next most important thing you need to know about healing an infection is, "What kind of infection is it?" Basically, there are two kinds of infection – bacterial and viral, and each needs a particular kind of environment to survive. A bacterial infection thrives in an acid environment, and a viral infection thrives in an alkaline environment.

If you have an infection that is bacterial, one of the most helpful things you can do to heal yourself is to quickly shift your body to the *opposite* environment needed by the infection.

We have already said that when you get an infection you should immediately stop eating, however, if you have a serious bacterial infection and need to quickly shift to an alkaline environment, doing the Purge will do exactly that but will require you to drink certain things. Although this appears to contradict the "no eating" rule, the Purge is a lifesaver.

Athlete's Foot or Other Yeast-based Infections

Athlete's Foot is a version of a yeast infection, which relies on sugar and an overly alkaline environment\.

• Change your diet to meat and vegetables and avoid sugars like the plague. Coffee, tea, and cream are okay, as are milk and eggs. For Athlete's Foot, put 2 TBSP of colloidal silver in a basin of warm water and soak your feet for 20-30 minutes, twice a day. When finished soaking, Rub with Tea Tree oil and wear cotton socks.

• All Yeast Infections: Take Caprylic Acid capsules, 4 capsules per day spread over the day. These are available from www.ProgressiveLabs. com.

Comments on healing Infections...

If you have taken antibiotics to help heal an infection, you will have to repair the damage done to the beneficial bacteria that live in your gastrointestinal system and make up your microbiome. Anytime you have taken an antibiotic, do a Colon Sweep to remove *all* bacteria from your gut and then immediately begin a program of ½ cup of Bravo Yogurt daily at bedtime for three months, followed by high quality probiotic capsules for another three months to help seed and then stabilize a broad range of healthy bacteria. A healthy microbiome creates a strong immune system, reduces allergies, sweetens breath and sweat, and promotes much better absorption of nutrients from the food you eat.

Infection in a Hand, Foot, or Leg

• If the infection is in a hand or foot, stop eating and start drinking 8-10 glasses of water per day.

• Soak the affected area for 30 minutes in a pan or bowl of hot water containing 1/2 cup of Epsom Salt or 1/2 cup of ordinary salt (sodium chloride) twice a day.

• If the infection is in an arm or leg and not able to fit into a bowl or pan, soak your entire self in a warm Salt and Soda Bath for 30 minutes. Salt is an amazing healer of infections!

• Use a heating pad a couple times a day to heat the area for two hours, as bacteria do not have much tolerance for temperatures over 106°. My husband spent a week in the hospital with a terrible, fast growing leg infection and was receiving three of the most powerful intravenous antibiotics known, but it was a heating pad that finally turned the tide toward healing. If you don't have a heating pad, use a hot saltwater compress on the infection. Keep changing the compress to keep it hot for at least 30 minutes. Heat 1 cup of Salt and 2 cups of water, or enough water to soak whatever size compresses needed to cover the site of the infection.

Strep Throat

- If you have strep throat, stop eating completely and drink 8 oz. of water every hour to equal 1 gallon of water daily. If you caught the infection early, you can probably end it by not eating for 3 or 4 days and only drinking water. If you didn't catch it early, do a 1-day Purge and then fast for 3-4 days. Take five doses of the homeopathic remedy *Mercurius Vivus 30x* or *200ck* as described above in the Colds and Sore Throat section, and gargle with salt water two or three times a day.

Peritonitis

- If you have a serious internal bacterial infection – let us use peritonitis as an example – stop eating and do the core part of the Purge which involves taking Epsom Salts and the citrus punch made from lemons, grapefruit, and oranges. Do not bother with the salads before or after the Purge and do not eat any solid food at all.

- Immediately after the Purge, go into a complete water fast for 4-10 days, drinking one 8 oz glass of water with a tiny pinch of salt in it every hour, consuming one gallon per day. You don't absolutely have to use the salt, but it helps increase the number of transactions going on in your body, it is a healing element in itself, and you will have a tad more energy while you're fasting. Don't use more than a pinch or you could trigger diarrhea. The infection will clear, usually within 3-5 days. Don't take iron supplements when you have a serious infection as it supports bacteria. Do not take antibiotics while you are drinking the citrus punch of the Purge. The grapefruit juice in the punch will cause you to absorb all of the antibiotic in a very short amount of time and this could overwhelm you. Never take prescription medicine with grapefruit juice!

Post-surgical Infections

If you have a post-surgical infection, there are several options.

- First, stop eating and do a 2-day Purge immediately, then begin drinking water at the rate of 1 gallon per day. Do not try to work; stay in bed and allow the body to rest and use its energy to heal.

- Second, make a salt compress of 1 cup of salt and 2 cups of water. Put the water and salt in a pan, warm slightly to help dissolve the salt, then soak several layers of cotton or a washcloth in the salt water, squeeze only enough to prevent major dripping, and place over the wound or site of infection. Put a piece of plastic over the compress and then put a heating pad over that. Leave in place for 2 hours. Repeat doing several rounds of salt compress + heat daily for several days until the infection is cleared.

- Once the infection has cleared, make a compress using a couple layers of cotton flannel or a sturdy woven fabric smeared thickly with honey. Raw honey is best, and Manuga honey is the very best, but not absolutely necessary. Use what you have, and put the honey compress on the place where the infection used to be. Leave on for up to 8 hours or overnight, then remove and discard. Use a honey compress for several days to nurture the new tissue forming at the site of the incision.

- if the infection is post-surgical and the surgical cut in the skin has mended itself to be sealed but now shows signs of infection, and go to step three below.

MRSA (methylin resistant staphylococcus aureus)

- Start with a honey compress using a couple layers of cotton flannel or a sturdy woven fabric smeared thickly with honey. Raw honey is best, and Manuga honey is the very best, but not absolutely necessary. Use what you have, and put the honey compress directly over the site of the MRSA infection. Leave on for up to 8 hours or overnight, then remove and discard.

- Replace with a new honey compress and leave it on for another 8 hours. Continue to apply a new honey compress at least every 8 hours until the infection has cleared. Honey is antibacterial, anti-viral, and anti-fungal. It also feeds the newly forming skin, greatly reducing scarring!

- Immediately begin taking an oxygen elixir like Oxy Life Force or OxyDHQ. 1 dropperful morning and evening the first day, diluted in juice, increasing to 2 droppersful, morning and evening on the second day. On the third day, increase to 3 droppersful twice a day, and maintain there for the next 4 days. One week will have passed. For the second week, increase to 4 dropperful twice a day and maintain there until the infection is gone. Take oxygen elixirs away from meals unless they upset your stomach, in which case a couple teaspoons of yogurt or a piece of toast will help. Be aware that oxygen is a powerful detoxifier. You may have headaches, loose stools, flu-like symptoms, and fatigue. To counter these detox reactions, do a set of Coffee Enemas at least once a day until the infection is healed.

- If the infection is MRSA and it's internal, start with a 2-day Purge if you can. Get someone to go to the grocery store to get the required amount of citrus.

If there is a danger of the infection becoming full-blown sepsis, add the following.

- Make and drink a trace mineral cocktail 1–3 times daily in addition to the oxygen elixir. If you don't have oxygen elixirs on hand, you can use the trace minerals to counter the infection until you get some oxygen elixir:

- Stop eating and start drinking water! This allows your body to focus on fighting the infection instead of digesting.

- ½ tsp of liquid trace minerals (ConcenTrace) stirred into ½ cup of orange juice made stronger by using slightly less water, which helps cover the taste of the trace minerals. Trace minerals will kill an infection, but they will also cause loose bowels and diarrhea because they create an alkaline environment, which does not support bacterial infections.

- To counter the loose bowels or diarrhea, take 1 TBSP of Bentonite clay in suspension (by Sonné) 1-3 times daily. The bowels may continue to be loose, and you may get cleaned out, but you don't want uncontrolled diarrhea.

- Drink 1-3 of these trace mineral cocktails per day over the first 48 hours. For the next five days, make and drink the trace mineral cocktail 2 or 3 times a day and keep the location of the MRSA infection covered with the honey compress until infection is gone. Do not make and drink the mineral cocktail if you are already taking an antibiotic. However, if the antibiotic is not making good headway in healing the MRSA infection, the honey and trace minerals will finish the job in a matter of days. If you don't have the trace minerals on hand, the honey will often do the job all by itself, even without the antibiotic!

Trace minerals are very powerful and so is honey. We have used these two substances to heal both nasty post-surgical infections and MRSA within 3-5 days.

Alternate plan for infection, in case you don't have the oxygen elixirs, or trace minerals, or Bentonite clay on hand and must order them, do this in the interim while you wait:

- 1 tsp of colloidal silver in a cup of water 2-3 x day along with the honey compress over the MRSA and salt compresses over any other infection. Silver is not as powerful as the trace minerals, but it does an excellent job. Be sure to stop taking the colloidal silver after 10 days because it is known to cause patches of gray, discolored skin that do not return to their natural color. If the gray patch were to appear on your face, you would be quite unhappy about it.

- 500 mg of garlic, 3 x day until the infection has cleared up, but only take garlic if the incision has closed. Garlic promotes a much more fluid blood and you may end up bleeding if the incision is still open. Yes, you will smell like garlic!

- When you do begin eating again, continue to avoid alcohol, sugar, caffeine, and iron supplements as much as possible! The alcohol, sugar, and caffeine make the body too acid, which is the perfect environment for *bacterial* infections. And bacteria *love* iron because it helps them be stronger. Sugar feeds infections, while alcohol and caffeine draw water out of your tissues, something you cannot afford during an infection. Instead, stick to fresh raw citrus fruits, fresh raw vegetable juices, and beef broth or chicken broth. An alkaline environment is preferred by viruses and fungi, therefore avoid citrus juice if you have a viral infection since citrus alkalinizes the body. Drink milk instead, which acidifies the body.

Sinus Infection

- If you have a sinus *infection*, stop eating immediately! Do not eat again until the symptoms are gone, usually 3 to 7 days, depending on how long you delayed before beginning the activities that allow the body to heal itself. Sinus trouble of any kind is a clear indication you are eating foods that do not agree with your body, and you are not paying attention to what it needs. Constant sinus problems also indicate that you either have, or are developing, allergies.

- Drink 64 oz of water every day that you have the problem. Drink 8 oz at a time, putting a tiny pinch of salt in each glass. In addition, drink another 24 oz of water with the juice of 2 lemons squeezed into it. Drink this total of 88 oz of water each day until your sinuses clear.

- If the infection does not clear after a couple of days, do the Purge for 1-2 days.

- Take *Mercurius Vivus 200ck* and *Kali bichromicum 200ck* using three doses (either 3 tablets or 5 pellets per dose) over three hours, followed by a fourth dose 3 hours later, and a fifth dose three hours after that. Over the next 2 days, take 3 doses spread out over the course of the day.

- Use a Neti pot with ¼ tsp of salt in warm water morning and evening.

Prostate Troubles & Urinary Difficulties (Men and Women)

Start with the Basic Healing Program, especially the exercise, detox procedures and the Bravo Yogurt. In addition to the supplements in the Basic program, I would do the following:

Water and Additional Supplements

- Being sure to drink 6-8 glasses of water every day.

- For a time, *limit* alcohol, stress, and coffee until the symptoms recede and healing has a good start.

- Make and drink 1 pint of carrot juice, 3 x week.

- Zinc, in picolinate form, 60 mg/day for 3 months, then reduce to 45 mg/day for 3 months, then reduce to 30 mg/day for maintenance.

- Vitamin C, 1,000 mg, 4 x day, unless you have a history of kidney stones, in which case do not take any extra Vitamin C. Instead, take Glutathione, 500 mg, 4 x day.

- Extra Vitamin A, 15,000 i.u. daily.

- Copper, 1-2 mg, daily.

- FOR MEN: Saw palmetto berry capsules, 160 mg, 2 x day. Limit commercial chicken for 3-4 months because it is often loaded with estrogens, which play a role in the swelling of the prostate. Do not avoid lovemaking altogether, but don't engage in prolonged lovemaking. If you do not have a spouse or lover, yet still have a functioning sex drive, masturbate through to ejaculation routinely to keep things moving in the genital area. Saw palmetto berry tends to accentuate your sexuality, so don't fight your own healing or wonder what has gotten into you lately that you're suddenly in need of more sexual activity.

- Alternate daily: ½ cup of pumpkin seeds on Day 1; ½ cup of sunflower seeds on Day 2; 10 almonds on Day 3, then begin again.

- FOR WOMEN: Get a formula with D-Mannose in it and follow the directions on the package.

- Drink 1 cup of unsweetened cranberry juice twice a day.

- Take 1-2 droppersful of CBD oil twice a day.

- For MEN and WOMEN - probiotics are critical. It is time to begin rebuilding your microbiome.

Exercises

- Walk briskly for 30-60 minutes every day. Walking not only increases circulation to the affected areas, it raises your level of energy, which is important for the male ego.

- Several times a week, lie down on the floor next to a wall, with your body perpendicular to the wall. Raise your legs straight up and rest them against the wall. Lie there with your legs up the wall for at least 10 minutes, less in the beginning if necessary, and more if you can, working up to 25 minutes as you build yourself toward good health.

- Do a set of 25 Kegle exercises every morning and every night. These are simple. Just stand in place and tighten up all of the muscles you would normally use to stop urination, count to 3, then relax. This tightens the lower abdomen, upper legs, hips, and works all of the organs in the lower part of the body.

- Do a Salt and Soda Bath each week for 6 weeks.

Comments on healing Prostate and UT troubles

You should notice significant improvement for a urinary tract infection in a few days, and a great deal of relief in 4-6 weeks for prostate problems on this healing program, but should stay on it for at least 3 months and go a full 6 months if you can.

Once your prostate and urinary tract have returned to normal, you can go off the saw palmetto or the D-Mannose and embark on a full detox program and a regular supplement program, with careful attention to diet and ongoing stretching and walking. If the difficulties return, which is unlikely if you're still taking the full spectrum of vitamin and mineral supplements, keeping up with your exercise, and including the flaxseed oil and probiotics, then start the program again for another 3-6 months while continuing to reduce stress and improve your lifestyle.

These are only a few of the possible healing programs that can be created using natural healing approaches. Remember, the body will do the healing and it is your job to support its efforts.

When you first read through some of the natural healing programs, you may immediately feel overwhelmed by the number of things that are listed and the perceived complexity of the healing processes. However, start with what appeals to you and keep adding things as you go along. You will develop an appreciation for old-fashioned nursing skills as you nurse yourself back to good health. You will probably be surprised at how much you will learn regarding how to use everyday foods and techniques to such wonderful effects. You will also come to enjoy the patience that comes from working with the body, as well as the deep pleasure that is experienced in nurturing yourself back to health, vitality and high levels of calm energy.

I love some of the new, modern medicines and technologies, although they are very expensive and sometimes out of reach for many. Yet even though I celebrate the new, I think it is critical to hang onto the old knowledge, partly because modern medicines are so expensive, partly because they have awful side-effects, and partly because we have no guarantees that we will continue to move forward with modern medicines without interruption or backsliding, and partly because natural healing is so effective. If we should suddenly hit a serious global event that sets us back a few centuries, knowing how to use the foods and the processes that will restore us is critical. It could mean the difference between survival and extinction.

I am also acutely aware that taking all of the supplements that may be necessary is neither cheap nor is the availability of supplements guaranteed should a market or global catastrophe occur. My goals have been to learn as much as I can about food and how to grow it and what it does in the body, all while I am taking advantage of the supplements that are at hand.

Although healing yourself may seem daunting, my experience has been that when you do your first Liver Flush, Coffee Enema, or Castor Oil/Olive Oil Sweat bath, you will quickly see that the reality of these procedures is not nearly as overwhelming as it first appears. It is more difficult to read the list of steps that describe the process than to actually do them! It is even more challenging to be patient with the body that is doing the work. Just try to keep in mind that what you are doing is rebuilding yourself, almost from scratch!

By far, the biggest challenge you may have will be finding, trying, and getting used to new foods and new routines in the kitchen. However, once you discover the taste of real food and experience the power of natural healing, I think you will embrace the new lifestyle with gratitude and grace. To make things easier in the supplement department, many of the vitamins and minerals can be purchased as a vitamin powder or a liquid, making them much easier to take. And the exercises often turn out to be something you enjoy doing because the results are so powerful.

One day, you will look out at the world through new eyes fully aware that the body is an intelligent, self-healing system. Give it what it requires and there are few illnesses and diseases that cannot be healed, or conditions that cannot be greatly improved. ❖

Appendix A
Personal Healing Checklist

Name _____

Condition _____

Date _____

  The Personal Healing Checklist is one of the things I keep on hand as well as hand out in my classes on getting well because I found that when I was ill, my thinking was cloudy and uncertain about what to do. I would forget the huge range of options at my fingertips or be foggy about what supplement might be best to increase or even start. The checklist is also a good tool for sparking intuitions about what to do, and you can make a photocopy of it to keep a record of what you did to heal yourself for a given condition. As mentioned earlier, if a condition shows up and you figure out how to reverse it, and then it shows up again in the distant future, you might not be able to remember all the details of what you did to heal the condition originally. Think like a doctor and keep at least a few notes of what you've suffered with, how old you were, and what you did to restore good health. If you are a parent, keep notes of your children's health and conditions as well. The notes don't have to be fancy, and they might be a godsend later if something challenging occurs.

  The checklist presented here lists the basic tools that can be used to heal yourself and serves as a reminder of the information discussed in this book so you don't have to go digging through a ton of writing at a moment when you're in a crisis. Note that the Supplements show only the Recommended Daily Allowance (RDA), which is the minimum you must take to stay alive! And remember, everyone's response to supplements is unique, so approach them as the powerful tools they are.

  In any program of healing, take into account what you put *into* the body and what you want to *clean out*. To heal permanently, you must make permanent changes in your life. Regardless of the disease or illness, recognize that *your body already knows how to heal itself*. Your job is to provide support in that effort. Remember, you are the best doctor you will ever have.

Procedure	Detoxification Accomplishes	How often	Used?
Parasite Removal Program	Removes parasites from tissues and G.I. tract	Annual	Yes No *See Ch. 17*
Liver Flush	Flushes toxins, plaque, and waste materials from the liver, gall bladder, kidneys, and cardiovascular system.	Quarterly	Yes No *See Ch. 19*
Colon Sweep	Removes goop, yeast overgrowth, toxins, and unfriendly bacteria from colon	Quarterly	Yes No *See Ch. 20*
The Purge	Removes toxins, mucous, dead tumor tissue, dead cellular material, pus, inflammation, and cell wastes from the entire body, esp. lungs and joints	Quarterly	Yes No *See Ch. 21*
Chelation - Intravenous EDTA	Removes plaque from the arteries	As needed	Yes No *See Ch. 18*
Chelation - Subcutaneous DMPS	Removes heavy metals from tissues of the body	As needed	Yes No *See Ch 18*
Castor Oil/ Olive Oil Sweats	Forces toxins out of the skin	Annual	Yes No *See Ch. 22*
Coffee enemas	Causes the liver to dump toxins, which then allows it to continue filtering poisons/ wasts from the blood	Daily, during detox, or as needed	Yes No *See Ch. 23*
Fasting, water or juice fast	Gives body a rest from digestion, gets rid of poorly built cells, relieves pain, allows rebuilding. For water fast, read *Fasting Can Save Your Life.* For juice fast, read *How to Get Well.*	3-day, 5-day, 7-day, 10-day, 21-day, 35-day, or intermittent.	Yes No *See Ch. 17*

Minerals	*Supplements*	*RDA*	*Overdose*
Amino Acids	Provide the body with the basic materials needed to continuously rebuild its structures and tissues, fluids, enzymes, and hormones.	See label	Yes No
Calcium	Supports bones and teeth; maintains regular heartbeat and transmission of nerve impulses; lowers cholesterol & risk of colon cancer; prevents muscle cramps.	800 – 1500 mg / day	Risk of kidney stones, estrogen-like effects, acidosis
Magnesium	Allows the body to utilize calcium and potassium; essential for enzyme activity; helps prevent depression and fatigue; supports lungs and heart; eases dozens of conditions from asthma to insomnia to IBS	400 – 750 mg / day	Loss of appetite, renal difficulty, diarrhea, severe edema
Sodium	Maintains proper pH, good water & fluid balance; helps prevent cramps, depression, fatigue, gas, poor memory, recurring infections, loss of taste, headache, heart palpitations, nausea, and anorexia	1100 – 3300 mg / day	Edema, high blood pressure, potassium deficiency, liver & kidney disease
Potassium	Maintains nervous system and regular heart beat; prevents stroke; lowers cholesterol; assists in transfer of nutrients through cell membranes; prevents constipation, nervousness, thirst, fatigue, headache, respiratory difficulties, and salt retention	1800 – 5600 mg / day	G.I. upset, nausea vomiting, severe fatigue, diarrhea, general weakness

Iron	Produces hemoglobin; oxygenates red blood cells; essential for enzyme activity; prevents anemia, hair loss, ridged nails, obesity, dizziness, difficulty swallowing, and slow mental reactions	18 mg / day	Constipation & digestive trouble, headaches, light sensitive; kills under age 4
Zinc	Maintains protein/enzyme synthesis; heals wounds; restores taste and smell; protects liver & prostate; assists bone formation; increases utilization of Vit. A; prevents infertility, poor memory; fights infection; speeds healing	15 mg / day	Anemia, copper deficiency, stomach upset, lethargy, impaired muscle control, lowers HDL
Iodine	Produces thryoid hormones; prevents cancers and cysts; promotes healthy hair and nails; guards against dry skin; helps with weight loss and regular sleep; prevents goiter and fatigue	125 mcg/ day,	Heart palpitations
Vitamins	*Needed For*	*RDA Dose*	*Overdose*
Vitamin A (oil soluble)	Healing!! Maintains healthy eyes, lungs, tissues, digestive organs, bones, genitourinary tract, and cell membranes. Can be toxic in large doses over 50,000 iu/day for sustained period. Need goes up *sharply* when ill.	RDA Dose: 4000-5000 iu/ day	Anemia, enlarged spleen & liver, hair dry or falls out, clubbed fingers/toes, dbl. vision
Beta Carotene (oil soluble)	Same as Vit. A, however, carotene may *not* be converted to Vit. A when diabetes, hypothyroidism, or liver malfunction is present	RDA Dose: 5000 iu / day Toxic: None	None

Vitamin B-1 Thiamine (water soluble)	Digests carbohydrates; maintains healthy appetite, digestive tract, & nervous system; protects from effects of smoking, alcohol, aging; prevents fatigue, forgetfulness, irritability	RDA Dose: 2 mg / day Toxic: 10,000 mg / day for many months	Headache, rapid pulse, trembling, weakness
Vitamin B-2 Riboflavin (water soluble)	Digests proteins, carbohydrates, and fats; healthy eyes; burns calories; cracks in corners of mouth or between fingers/toes signals deficiency. Note: Riboflavin *deficiency inhibits some cancers.*	RDA Dose: 1.7 mg / day Toxic: None, or very rare	Antibiotics destroy B-2
Vitamin B-3 Niacin (water soluble)	Lowers cholesterol; turns carbohydrates into energy, assists in metabolism of proteins and fats; maintains circulation and healthy skin; needed for bile and stomach fluids; reduces dementia, insomnia, low blood sugar	RDA Dose: 20 mg / day Toxic: 750 mg / day for over 3 months	Dry itchy skin, liver damage, skin pigmenting, low blood pressure, too much worsens diabetes
Vitamin B-5 Pantothenic Acid (water soluble)	Lowers stress; increases stamina; required by every cell in body; assists production of adrenal hormones, antibodies; aids metabolism; produces neurotransmitters	RDA Dose: 7 mg / day Toxic: none	None
Vitamin B-6 Pyridoxine (water soluble)	Involved in more bodily functions than any other nutrient! Maintains physical & mental health; produces enzymes & HCL; needed for DNA, RNA, & hemoglobin; metabolizes proteins, carbohydrates & fats; produces serotonin and other neurotransmitters	RDA Dose: 2 mg / day Toxic: 2000-6000 mg / day for some months	Sensory neuropathy, difficulty walking, makes allergies worse, L-dopa conflict

Vitamin B-12 Cyanocobalamin (water soluble)	Prevents anemia, helps with cell formation; required for digestion and absorption; maintains fertility; assists memory & learning; protects nerve sheaths.	RDA Dose: 3-6 Mcg./ day	None, but conflicts with anti-convulsants, TB, cancer, and cholesterol drugs
Biotin (water soluble) Part of the complex of B-vitamins	Aids in cell growth & development, metabolism, & use of other B-vitamins; helps relieve muscle pain, prevent hair loss (Under good conditions, our body manufactures some biotin.)	Dose: 100-300 mcg / day (No RDA)	None known
Choline (water soluble) Part of the complex of B-vitamins.	Maintains proper nerve transmissions, brain function & memory, liver function, gall bladder, and hormone production (Under good conditions, our body manufactures some choline.)	Dose: 400-900 mg / day (No RDA)	"Fishy" odor to body, diarrhea, depression
Folic Acid (water soluble) Part of the complex of B-vitamins	Maintains healthy blood; prevents birth defects; protects DNA/RNA; strengthens immunity; feeds the brain; eases breathing and memory problems Oral contraceptives increase need for folic acid. Our body manufactures some folic acid.	Dose: 400 mcg / day Toxic: 3000-15,000 mcg /day (No RDA)	Nausea, disturbed sleep, irritability; conflicts with epilepsy & schizo-phrenia drugs.
Inositol (water soluble) Part of the complex of B-vitamins	Reduces cholesterol; prevents hardening of arteries; needed for hair growth; metabolizes fats and cholesterol; has calming effects; prevents irritability and mood swings. (Under good conditions our body manufactures some inositol.)	Dose: Unknown Toxic: Unknown	

Vitamin C Ascorbic Acid (water soluble)	Fights infection; necessary for metabolism and collagen formation; speeds healing, helps absorb iron, lower cholesterol and blood pressure, lessens bruising	RDA Dose: 60-80 mg / day Toxic: 30,000 mg / day by mouth	Diarrhea; increases pain perception; masks copper deficiency; kidney stones
Vitamin D Ergocalciferol and Cholecalciferol Cholecalciferol (oil soluble)	Regulates calcium and phosphorus use; needed for bones and teeth; promotes regular heartbeat; enhances immunity; necessary for thyroid function, good eyes, weight loss & healthy appetite	RDA Dose: 200-400 iu / day Toxic: can be as low as 1000 iu/ day in some, and 1,000,000 iu / day in others.	Nausea, thirst, vomiting, headache, confusion, delirium, coma, shock & death, kidney failure, osteoporosis, calcification of organs & blood vessels
Vitamin E Tocopherol (oil soluble)	An antioxidant that improves circulation, tissue repair; needed for fat metabolism; lowers cholesterol & blood pressure; works as skin/hair conditioner; keeps nerves healthy; helps prevent cancer and heart disease	RDA Dose: 30 iu / day Toxic: 600iu/day in a few, and 2000 iu/day in most others.	Severe weakness and fatigue; gas, diarrhea, hives, chapped lips
Vitamin K (oil soluble)	Needed for bone repair and formation; production of prothrombin, healthy liver, resistance to infection, and longevity; protects against cancers that form inside organs	RDA Dose: unknown Toxic: unknown	Flushing; toxic to fetus in utero

	Glandulars		
Raw Adrenal	Supports adrenals, helps the body manage stress, is useful in diabetes		
Raw Brain	Supports brain function, memory		
Raw Heart	Supports the heart and the heart-lung relationship		
Raw Kidney	Supports the kidney		
Raw Liver	Supports the liver, helps make liver enzymes		
Raw Lung	Supports the lungs and lung function in asthma, allergies, cancers, etc.		
Raw Mammary Gland	Supports the breast in cases of breast cancer		
Raw Ovary	Supports the ovaries in cases of PMS, hysterectomy, cysts, etc.		
Raw Pancreas	Supports the pancreas, helps the body produce digestive and other enzymes		
Raw Parathyroid	Supports the parathyroid glands, manages calcium metabolism, helps prevent loss of hair, gruff voice, etc.		
Raw Pituitary	Supports the pituitary function, keeps the body fluidified		
Raw Spleen	Supports the spleen and making of new red blood cells		
Raw Thymus	Supports the thymus and the entire immune system		

Raw Thyroid	Supports the thyroid and the dozens of functions it has, inc. diet, weight, osteoporosis, etc.		
Raw Orchic	Supports the testicles and helps maintain normal function in males		
Enzymes	**Function**	**Source**	
Amylase	Works with other enzymes to digest sugars and starches, improves the absorption of nutrients from food.	Aspergillus	
Lipase	Works with pancreatin to digest fats, improve the function of the pancreas, and improve digestion overall	Aspergillus	
Protease	Works with other enzymes to digest proteins and improve digestion overall	Several sources	
Chymotrypsin	Helps the immune system identify tumors and can dissolve the fibrin covering of cancers; reduces the blood stickiness that helps tumors/ growths spread	Animal organs	
Trypsin	Accelerates healing of injuries, assists your immune system, reduces blood stickiness from phlebitis, emboli, and thromboses. Also dissolves the fibrin covering on cancer cells.	Ox pancreas	
Bromelain	Helps reduce swelling and inflammation of joints, injuries; aids in amelioration of burns, thrombosis, cellulitis, and skin infections; accelerates the healing of bruises, abrasions, and contusions	Pineapple stem	

Pancreatin	An important family of enzymes in the digestion process. Improves digestion in older people	Animal organs	
Papain	Reduces inflammation and stimulates Tumor Necrosis Factor (TNF) which destroys growths. Destroys bacteria associated with stomach disorders like gastritis and ulcers.	Papaya	
Rutin	A free-radical scavenger that also destroys viruses and numerous bacteria. Rutin is a repairman of varicose veins and capillaries.	Several plants	
	Exercise		
The Five Rites of the Fountain of Youth by Peter Kelder	Ancient yoga-like exercises out of Tibet that stimulate the endocrine system, reverse aging, and create an amazing amount of physical, mental, and emotional energy that lasts for approximately 2 ½ days each time you do them	Do the entire set at least 3-4 times a week. Do up to 21 of each rite.	
Yoga	Any good yoga tape or instructor can provide you with guidance in performing the stretches this system offers.	20-30 minutes each day is ideal	
Walking	Go outside and walk – not fast – but at a good pace, with arms swinging naturally.	Walk at least twice a week for 30 min.	
Free weights	Use to maintain upper body strength	15-20 min. 3 times/wk	

Affirmations, Imagery, and Dreams

It is very important to maintain a positive attitude and engage in practical thinking. Don't panic!! If you take a turn for the worse, stop and assess what is happening. Think back over the past four to seven days and ask yourself what you might have done to trigger the situation as it is, or what the body is trying to accomplish. It could be a useful healing crisis manufactured by the body to accomplish its own goals. Trust your body. It knows what it is doing. Listen to the signals and pay attention to the messages it sends you.

Affirmations are also important. Come up with at least one statement or thought that affirms your self, your healing, your body, your courage, or some other aspect of the healing journey you are on. Write it down and post it where you can see it every day. When a specific fear comes up, face the fear until you get to the bottom of it to unearth its core belief about yourself or life. Usually the belief is simply not true. Then create an affirmation that specifically counters the belief and soothes the fear.

Examples of this might be your abject fear of dying…or of worsening pain…of serious scars…of being disabled…of your resistance to what you are experiencing…of embarrassment over your situation… or the belief that an infection (or perhaps a cancer) cannot be healed. Affirmations that counter these might be something like "I am alive, living in the light, and loving it" or "I am able to put my attention anywhere I want it to be" or "My body knows how to heal itself perfectly and I am listening to it and doing what it needs me to do" or "I am excited about the healing journey I'm on and ready to do whatever is needed for good health" or "My body and I can figure out how to heal anything, and we have the patience and persistence to do so."

If you are seriously ill, spend time at least once a day doing some healing imagery. This can be anything from seeing yourself going into the problem area, cleaning it out, and removing the difficulty to imagining you are constructing an entirely new body, to visualizing yourself doing something you have always wanted to do in a setting in which you're perfectly healthy.

In your mind, pick out several symbols of your own healing. For instance, give yourself the instruction that every time you notice a particular item, hear a certain song, or notice a certain color, it will be a reminder of your whole, healed Self. Then ask your body/mind system to bring the symbols to your attention as often as possible so that you are constantly reminded and reassured of the healing processes taking place inside you. When one of your healing symbols comes to your attention, be sure to thank yourself for noticing it, then spend a moment or two picturing yourself as completely healed and functioning normally.

Pay attention to your dreams, especially healing dreams or dreams that bring deeply buried issues or a reassuring awareness into consciousness. Write them down and study them until you have grasped the subtleties of their message to you. If they point to an action or a direction, take that action or go in that direction. Use the awareness to deepen your healing abilities.

Repetitive thoughts that keep coming to you:

Affirmations spontaneously created right now:

Recent Dreams that had an impact on you:

Daydreams that recur and seem to have significance:

Intuition

Pay attention to the miscellaneous thoughts and intuitions that cross your mind. When a thought comes to you more than once or twice, there is often some valuable reason for it. Pay special attention to those thoughts that take the form, "Maybe I should…" or "This doesn't feel right… I should stop doing (or eating) this…"

Above all, live as if you are going to live. Each day is a decision point in life!

Support

In your efforts to change your life and embark on a healing journey, who will nurture and support you? It's really important to have at least one person who will encourage and push you to keep going with your healing program. Ideally, that would be a spouse or family member. A true friend is also a good choice. Name at least two people who might be willing to support your healing program.

Support Person #1:

Support Person #2:

Obstacles

Are you willing to take the time needed for healing? If so – Why? What is in the way? Nothing is more important than your health. Note here your biggest obstacles, whether physical, mental, emotional, or spiritual, and evaluate what you would have to face to get past the obstacle.

Physical: (e.g. money, relationships)

Mental: (e.g. uncertainty, not enough information)

Emotional: (e.g. self-worth, fear of what you might have to do)

Spiritual: (e.g. what will this mean about you or your life?)

Other obstacles I would have to deal with:

Your Space

Is your physical space set up to promote a healing lifestyle? Take a look around your kitchen. You may need new, updated, or additional small appliances in your kitchen. Jot down the most obvious things you would have to move, install, change, rearrange, or purchase and set up to make your kitchen work as one of the major support centers of a healing home.

Then take a look around your entire house, especially the bathroom, bedroom, even the yard. You might need space for exercise, a healing bathroom, a meditation space, an herb garden or small vegetable garden for fresh organic foods at least several months out of the year, different colors in your bedroom or living room, or some other arrangement. What would you do first? Second? Third? Jot down the changes needed in your space arrangements.

Kitchen:

Bathroom:

Bedroom:

Living Room:

Yard:

Other rooms:

Sleep and Rest

I need _____ hours of sleep each day/night in order to get the rest needed for healing.

Normal sleep habits can suffer when you are ill, but it is very important to get extra sleep *and* rest. Sleep is sleep. Rest is rest. Sleep can be rest, but rest is not necessarily sleep. Therefore, if you aren't sleeping well, it becomes all the more important to rest.

During a recent period of extreme stress and overwork, I found myself waking up in the night. At first, I was waking at 4:30 am, soon it was 3:30 am. Before long I was going to bed at midnight and waking at 1:30 am after only an hour or so of sleep. I'm not a napper and couldn't sleep during the day, so it was clear to me I was running on adrenaline. Since I couldn't see any way out of the situation, I ignored the sleeplessness until I crashed and burned. Of course, then I needed almost a year to repair and rebuild.

If you aren't getting enough sleep, it becomes doubly important to just rest. To rest is to relax, and while it can mean lying down for a while, it can also mean doing something that brings you great pleasure and doesn't require interaction with others. This can be going to the beach to watch a sunrise or a sunset, perhaps a walk in the woods, time to daydream, read, paint, fish, cross-stitch, putter in your shop, listen to music, or enjoy any light activity that brings a sense of renewal, peace, and satisfaction.

If you aren't sleeping, try a cup of melatonin tea about an hour before bedtime. If you're already in bed tossing and turning, do some very deep breathing as follows.

1. Using your diaphragm to pull upwards on the bottom of your lungs, exhaust as much air from your lungs as you can, hold for a moment until you feel the need to breathe in.

2. Breathe in through your nose, if you can, letting air flow in effortlessly, slowly, and as deeply as possible, allowing yourself to feel the expansion of your belly, your back, your sides, your neck, your feet, and your entire body as you completely fill your lungs. See the breath entering golden-pink light that goes directly to the place in you that needs healing. When you can't breathe in any longer, release and exhale through slightly pursed lips, envisioning that you are exhaling the illness and all of its symptoms.

3. When all the air is exhausted, pull up on your diaphragm at the very end of the exhale to exhaust the last drop of air and empty yourself completely. Hold for a moment.

4. Breathe in again, relaxing the diaphragm, and filling your lungs and your entire body as in Step 2. When filled with golden-pink light, count to 8 slowly, and then release the air through pursed lips.

5. Repeat until you have done somewhere between 10 and 20 deep breaths. Then go to sleep. You will probably sleep deeply and well. Oxygen is a great relaxer!

Intuitive Checklist

At this point, after reading through the entire book, you should have at least some idea of the foods, detox procedures, minerals, vitamins, glandulars, enzymes, and exercises that make up a healing program. If you have also read the first part of this appendix, you have considered affirmations, support issues, personal obstacles, and the physical changes that might be needed in your living space.

Now, without reviewing the book, and working solely on the basis of intuition, check off those procedures, supplements, foods, exercises, and changes that the all-knowing part of you feels would be important for you to include in your personal healing program.

Fasting:

    Water Fast   _____

    Juice Fast   _____

    Herbal Tea Fast   _____

Exercise:

    Fountain of Youth   _____

Yoga _____
Walking _____
Physical labor _____
Daily Detox:
    Coffee enema _____
    Mustard Foot Soak _____
    Castor Oil Pack _____
    Clay for Parasites _____
    Salt and Soda Bath _____
Water:
    64 oz/day _____
    128 oz/day _____
Weekly Detox:
    Chelation – EDTA _____
    1-day Juice Fast _____
    3-day Juice Fast _____
    5-day Juice Fast _____
    3-day Water Fast _____
    5-day Water Fast _____
    8-day Water Fast _____
    Castor/Olive Oil Sweat _____
Monthly or Annual Detox:
    Liver Flush _____
    Colon Sweep _____
    The Purge _____
    Chelation – DMPS _____
    Full Parasite Program _____
Supplements:
    Amino Acids _____
    The Basic 6 Minerals _____
    Vitamin A _____
    Vitamin B-Complex _____
    Vitamin C _____
    Vitamin D _____
    Vitamin E _____
    Specific, extra
      vitamins/supplements _____
      that you know about _____
      or have used with _____
      success & which _____
      might be useful _____

_____
    Digestive Enzymes _____
    Pancreas Enzymes _____

Additional Useful Supplements:

        Liquid Trace Minerals   _____

        Sulfur/MSM   _____

        Copper   _____

        Boron   _____

        Silica   _____

        Silver   _____

        Gold   _____

        Selenium   _____

        Germanium   _____

        Manganese   _____

        Iodine   _____

        Glucosamine   _____

        Gingko Biloba   _____

        Saw Palmetto   _____

        Hawthorne Berry   _____

        DHEA   _____

        Bilberry   _____

        Milk Thistle   _____

        Nettle   _____

        RNA/DNA   _____

        Bentonite clay   _____

        Primrose Oil   _____

        Borage Oil   _____

        Black Currant Seed Oil   _____

Glandulars:

        Raw Adrenal   _____

        Raw Brain   _____

        Raw Heart   _____

        Raw Kidney   _____

        Raw Liver   _____

        Raw Lung   _____

        Raw Mammary   _____

        Raw Ovary   _____

        Raw Parathryoid   _____

        Raw Pancreas   _____

        Raw Pituitary   _____

        Raw Spleen   _____

        Raw Thymus   _____

        Raw Thyroid   _____

        Glandular Complex   _____

Organic Foods:

        Beef   _____

        Chicken   _____

Lamb _____

Pork _____

Fish _____

Milk _____

Buttermilk _____

Butter _____

Yogurt _____

Cheese _____

Eggs _____

Flaxseed Oil _____

Hempseed Oil _____

Raw Vegetables _____

Raw carrot juice _____

Raw fruits _____

Raw fruit juice _____

Raw almonds _____

Freshly ground whole
  wheat breads _____

14-Grain Cereal _____

Breads made from spelt,
  oats, rye, etc. _____

Organic wine (red) _____

Green tea _____

Black tea _____

Herb teas _____

Homeopathic remedies to keep on hand:

Oscillococcinum _____

Pulsatilla _____

Mercurius vivus _____

Kali bichromicum _____

Belladonna _____

Apis mellifica _____

Aconite _____

Staphysagria _____

Arnica montana _____

Hepar sulfuris _____

Spongia tosta _____

Hypericum perf. _____

Arsenicum album _____

Ipecac _____

Allium cepa _____

Bryonia _____

Cantharis _____

Rhus toxicodendrum _____

Foods to reduce, temporarily avoid, or compensate for:

      Coffee (more than 1-2 c/day)   _____

      Cigarettes (consider growing
        your own tobacco)   _____

      Alcohol   _____

Foods to avoid forever:

      White flour products   _____

      White sugar products   _____

      Soy   _____

      Margarine   _____

      Polyunsaturated fats   _____

      Foods in bottles, boxes,
        and cans   _____

Once you have used your intuition to check off the things you think would be helpful in your healing program, combine it with your common sense and logic to decide what you will actually do, where you will begin, what you can afford, etc. When your healing program is under way, refer back to the checklist from time to time, as there will be things you forgot to implement, as well as new intuitions to guide you.

In closing, it should be obvious that you will have to make some lifestyle changes during the time you are healing. A friend of mine with cancer did not want to bother with the detox routines that are so critical for liver and tissue support. He said he didn't have time for that sort of thing and turned his nose up at the coffee enemas. He only wanted to change what he ate. I argued to no avail. He turned out to be right about not having time because his time on the planet ended and he is no longer with us.

Educate yourself to do the majority of your own healing. Take time to reconnect with Mother Nature and the soil. Take time to find good sources of high-nutrition food and do the detox routines. Develop the strength to change your life. As I have pointed out before, it is not your job to heal your body. Your body will heal itself. Your job is to figure out how to support and nurture the healing process going on within you.

Act! Even if you have some doubts. You will learn as you go along. I can't count the number of people who thought it was hopeless in the beginning when it wasn't. They waited until it was too late, then frantically tried to take action. Don't stand around waiting for a magic button or a magic pill.

On the other hand, I have seen miracles and sometimes I think it is never too late. Just remember this…you are a body/mind system with individualized needs. Begin filling them wisely and well in accord with how Mother Nature intended, and you will heal. Whether the miracle takes 20 minutes or 20 months is not important. What is important is that you take action at all levels – physically, mentally, emotionally, and spiritually.

May your efforts be blessed with success, everlasting good health, and wisdom. ❖

Appendix B

Suggested Reading and Reference Books for Your Healing Library

THE FOLLOWING IS A VERY PARTIAL listing of books that would be good to have in your library. Everyone who intends to heal either the self or anyone else in the family should maintain a small library of books containing a combination of accurate knowledge, hands-on techniques, reference material, and old and new wisdom. Hopefully these references will also impart a level of sensitivity and awareness to people, plants, animals, and the Earth. I have put an asterisk next to those I consider to be basic, necessary references that should be on every family bookshelf. The rest are all important in one way or another and are critical to a full understanding of the issues currently facing us today if we want to live and be well.

A Promise Made, A Promise Kept: One Son's Quest for the Cause and Cure of Diabetes by Dr. James Chappell, DC, ND, PhD, MH; BL Publications, Detroit Lakes, MN, 2005. ISBN 1-890766-3152995.

Biomimicry by Janine M. Benyus; Wm. Morrow and Co. Inc., New York, 1997. ISBN 0-688-13691-5.

Dead Doctors Don't Lie by Dr. Joel Wallach, DVM, and Dr. Ma Lin, MD; Wellness Publications, 2nd Edition, March 2004; ISBN 978-0974858104.

* *Dr. Wright's Guide to Healing With Nutrition* by Jonathan V. Wright, MD; Keats Publishing Inc., 1989. ISBN 0-87983-530-3.

Empty Harvest by Dr. Bernard Jensen and Mark Anderson; Avery Publishing Group, Inc., Garden City Park, NY, 1990. ISBN 0-89529-558-X.

* *Encyclopedia of Natural Medicine* by Michael Murray, ND and Joseph Pizzorno, ND; Prima Publishing, Rocklin, CA, 1998. ISBN 0-7615-1157-1.

* *Enzyme Nutrition: The Food Enzyme Concept* by Dr. Edward Howell; Avery Publishing Group, Inc. 1985. ISBN 0-89529-300-5.

* *Fasting Can Save Your Life* by Herbert M. Shelton; American Natural Hygiene Society, 1991. ISBN 0-914532-23-5.

Fats That Heal, Fats That Kill by Udo Erasmus; Alive Books, Burnaby, BC, Canada, 1997. ISBN 0-920470-38-6.

Fit For Life by Harvey & Marilyn Diamond; Warner Books Inc. 1985. ISBN 0-446-30015-2.

From Fatigued to Fantastic by Jacob Teitelbaum, MD; Avery Books, New York, NY, 2001. ISBN 1-58333-097-6.

* *Gut and Psychology Syndrome: Natural Treatment for Autism, Dyspraxia, ADD, Dyslexia, ADHD, Depression, Schizophrenia* by Dr. Natasha McBride-Campbell; Medinform Publishing, 2010. ISBN 978-0-954852023.

Gut and Psychology Syndrome: Natural Treatment for Allergies, Autoimmune Illness, Arthritis, Gut Problems, Fatigue, Hormonal Problems, Neurological Disease and More by Dr. Natasha McBride-Campbell; Medinform Publishing, 2020. ISBN 978-0-95485207.

How To Get Well by Paavo Airola, PhD; Health Plus Publishers, 1974. ISBN 0-932090-03-6.

In The Absence of The Sacred by Jerry Mander; Sierra Club Books, San Francisco, CA, 1992. ISBN 0-87156-509-9.

* *It's All In Your Head* by Hal S. Huggins, DDS; MS, Avery Publishing, NY, 1993. ISBN 0-89529-550-4.

Living Water by Olof Alexandersson; Gateway Books, Bath, United Kingdom, 1996. ISBN 0-946551-57-X.

Living Cuisine by Rene Loux Underkoffler; Avery Publishing, New York, NY, 2003. ISBN 1-58333-171-9.

Minerals and the Genetic Code by Charles Walters; Acres USA Publishing, 2013; ISBN 978-0911311853

* *Plague: One Scientist's Intrepid Search for the Truth about Human Retroviruses and Chronic Fatigue Syndrome (ME/CFS), Autism, and*

Other Diseases by Kent Heckenlively, JD and Judy Mikovits, PhD; Skyhorse Publishing, February 2017. ISBN 978-1510713949.

* *Nourishing Traditions Cookbook* by Sally Fallon; ProMotion Publishing, San Diego, CA, 1995. ISBN 1-887314-15-6.

Nutrition and Mental Illness: An Orthomolecular Approach to Balancing Body Chemistry by Carl C. Pfeiffer, PhD, MD; Healing Arts Press, Rochester, VT, 1987. ISBN 0-89281-226-5.

* *Nutrition and Physical Degeneration* by Weston A. Price, DDS.; Keats Publishing, 1989. ISBN 0-87983-502-8.

Nutrition and The Mind by Gary Null, PhD; Four Walls Eight Windows Press, New York, NY, 1995. ISBN 1-56858-021-5.

* *Our Earth, Our Cure* by Raymond Dextreit, translated and edited by Michel Abehsera; Citadel Press Book, Carols Publishing Group Edition, New York, 1993. ISBN 0-8065-1013-7.

Permaculture by Bill Mollison; Tagari Press; Tyalgum, NSW, Australia, 1996. ISBN 0-908228-01-5.

* *Prescription for Nutritional Healing, 5th Edition* by James F. Balch, MD & Phyllis A. Balch, CNC; Avery Publishing Group, October 2010. ISBN 978-1583334003.

* *Prescription for Herbal Healing 2nd Edition* by Phyllis A. Balch, CNC; Avery Publishing Group, April 2022. ISBN 978-1583334522.

Robes – A Book of Coming Changes by Penny Kelly; Lily Hill Publishing, Lawton, MI. ISBN 0-9632934-2-7.

Solved: The Riddle of Illness by Stephen E. Langer, MD and James F. Scheer; Keats Publishing, CA. ISBN 0-658-00293-7.

* *Stolen Harvest* by Vandana Shiva; South End Press, Cambridge, MA, 1999. ISBN 0-89608-607-0.

* *Sugar Blues* by William Dufty; Warner Books Inc., NY, 1993. ISBN 0-556-34312-9.

* *The Ancient Secret of The Fountain of Youth* by Peter Kelder; Doubleday, NY, 1998. ISBN 0-385-49162-X.

The China Study by T. Colin Campbell, PhD and Thomas M. Campbell II; BenBella Books; Dallas, TX, 2006. ISBN 978-1932100-66-2.

* *The Healing Power of Herbs* by Michael T. Murray, ND; Prima Publishing, Rocklin, CA, 1995. ISBN 1-55958-700-8.

The Right Dose: How to Take Vitamins & Minerals Safely by Patricia Hausman, MS; Ballantine Book, NY, 1992. ISBN 0-345-335877-5.

The Rodale Book of Composting, ed. Deborah L. Martin & Grace Gershuny; Rodale Press, 1992. ISBN 0-87857-991-5.

The Secret Life of Plants by Christopher Bird and Peter Tompkins; Harper Collins Publishers, New York, NY, 2002. ISBN 0600915870.

The Secrets of The Soil by Christopher Bird and Peter Tompkins; Harper & Row Publishers, New York, NY, 1989. ISBN 0-06-091968-X.

Tissue Cleansing Through Bowel Management by Bernard Jensen, DC; Bernard Jenzen Enterprises, Escondido, CA, 1981. No ISBN. www. bernardjensen.com.

Vitality Foods for Health & Fitness by Pierre Jean Cousin & Kirsten Hartvig, Duncan Baird Publishers, London, UK, 2002. ISBN 1903296889.

Water: For Health, for Healing, for Life by F. Batmanghelidg, MD; Warner Books, New York, NY, 2003. ISBN 0-446-69074-0.

What Your Doctor May Not Tell You About Menopause: The Breakthrough Book on Natural Progesterone by John R. Lee, MD; Warner Books, New York, NY, 1996; ISBN 0-446-67144-4.

* *Your Body's Many Cries for Water* by F. Batmanghelidj, MD; Global Health Solutions, Inc, Falls Church, VA, 1995; ISBN 0-9629942-3-5.

Your Third Brain: The Revolutionary New Discovery to Achieve Optimum Health by Peter Greenlaw, Dr. Marco Ruggiero, and Drew Greenlaw; Greenlaw Group, May 2015; 978-0-988277144

Reading these books will give you a broad, fairly deep, and well-integrated idea of health, what it should be, and what must be corrected in our thinking, our choices, and our lifestyles. We do not need to be sick, dysfunctional, disabled, or diseased! Begin to educate yourself and you will be stunned at how much we weren't taught about our bodies or the world we live in. Correcting situations in ourselves or in the world around us is not that difficult once you have the bigger picture. ❖

Index

Penny Kelly is a writer, teacher, author, publisher, consultant, Naturopathic physician, and researcher of consciousness. Early in her career she was an engineer for Chrysler Corporation, but left there in 1979 after a full, spontaneous awakening of kundalini to study the brain, consciousness, intelligence, intuition, and cognition. This was followed by 18 years of work as an educational consultant specializing in Accelerated and Brain-Compatible Teaching and Learning, working with both schools and corporations.

After purchasing acreage in 1987, she raised grapes for Welch Foods for a dozen years while also building Lily Hill Farm. For 15 years, she worked with Dr. Wm. Levengood, biophysicist at Pinelandia Lab near Ann Arbor, MI, studying materials from crop circles and animal mutilations, and researching plasma, energy, and consciousness.

Penny started Community Gardening in Kalamazoo and Battle Creek, MI through grants from the Kellogg Foundation, and she was a member of the Tipping Point Network whose focus is sustainability in all sectors of life. She maintains a worldwide counseling and coaching practice, teaches a half-dozen courses in *Developing Intuition*, as well as courses in *Organic Gardening*, and *Getting Well Again Naturally*. She produces regular videos for Patreon, YouTube, BitChute, and other platforms. She also travels widely to speak and teach.

Penny holds a degree in Humanistic Studies from Wayne State University and a degree in Naturopathic Medicine from Clayton College of Natural Health. She is the mother of four children has co-written or edited 23 books with others, and has written nine books of her own.

Lightning Source UK Ltd.
Milton Keynes UK
UKHW012007030921
389864UK00001B/56